The
Ordinary.

Clinical Formulations
with Integrity.

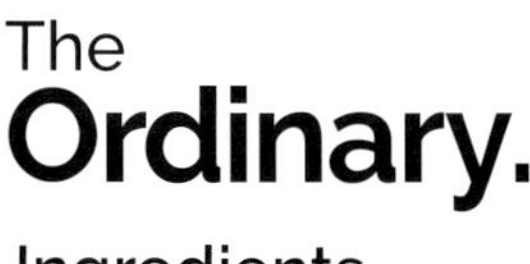

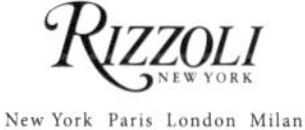

Table of contents.

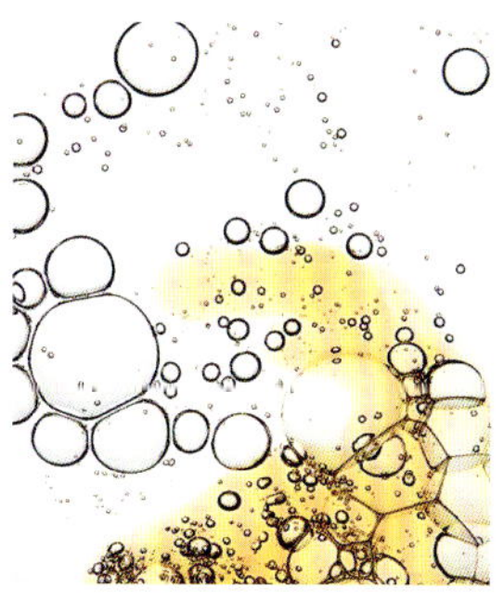

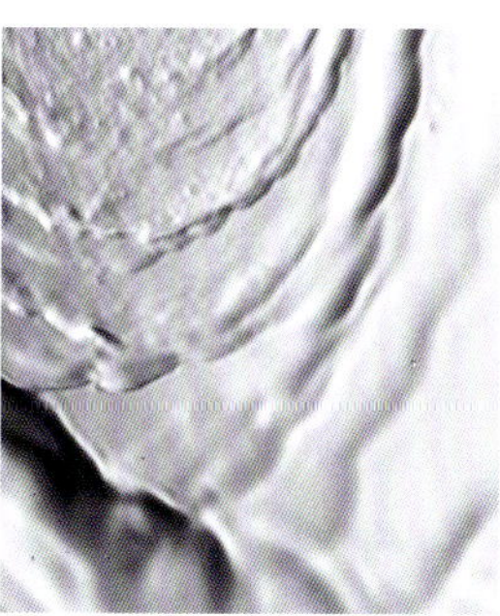

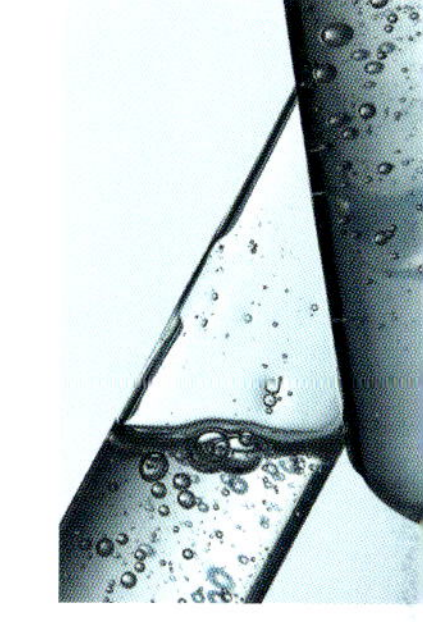

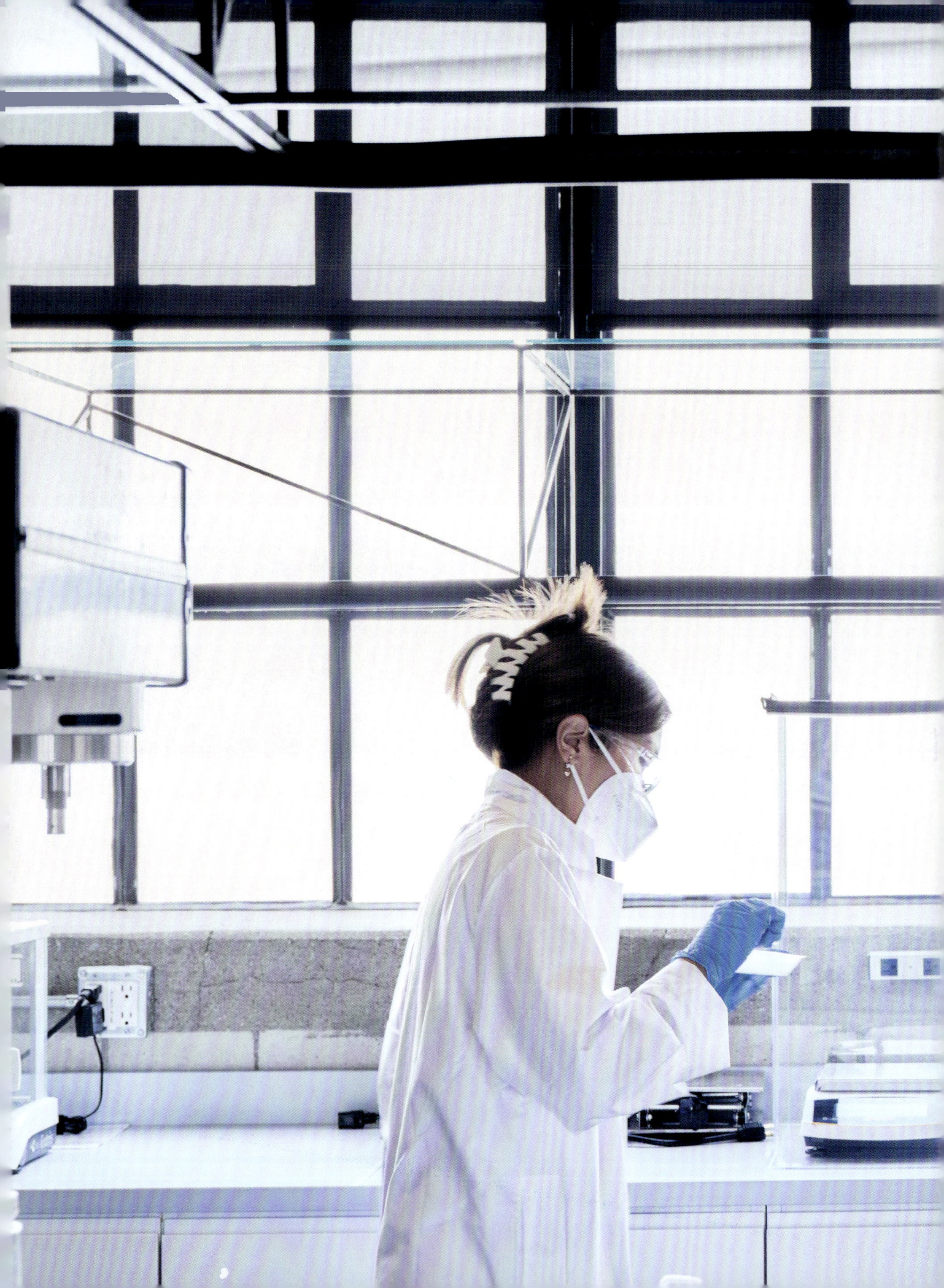

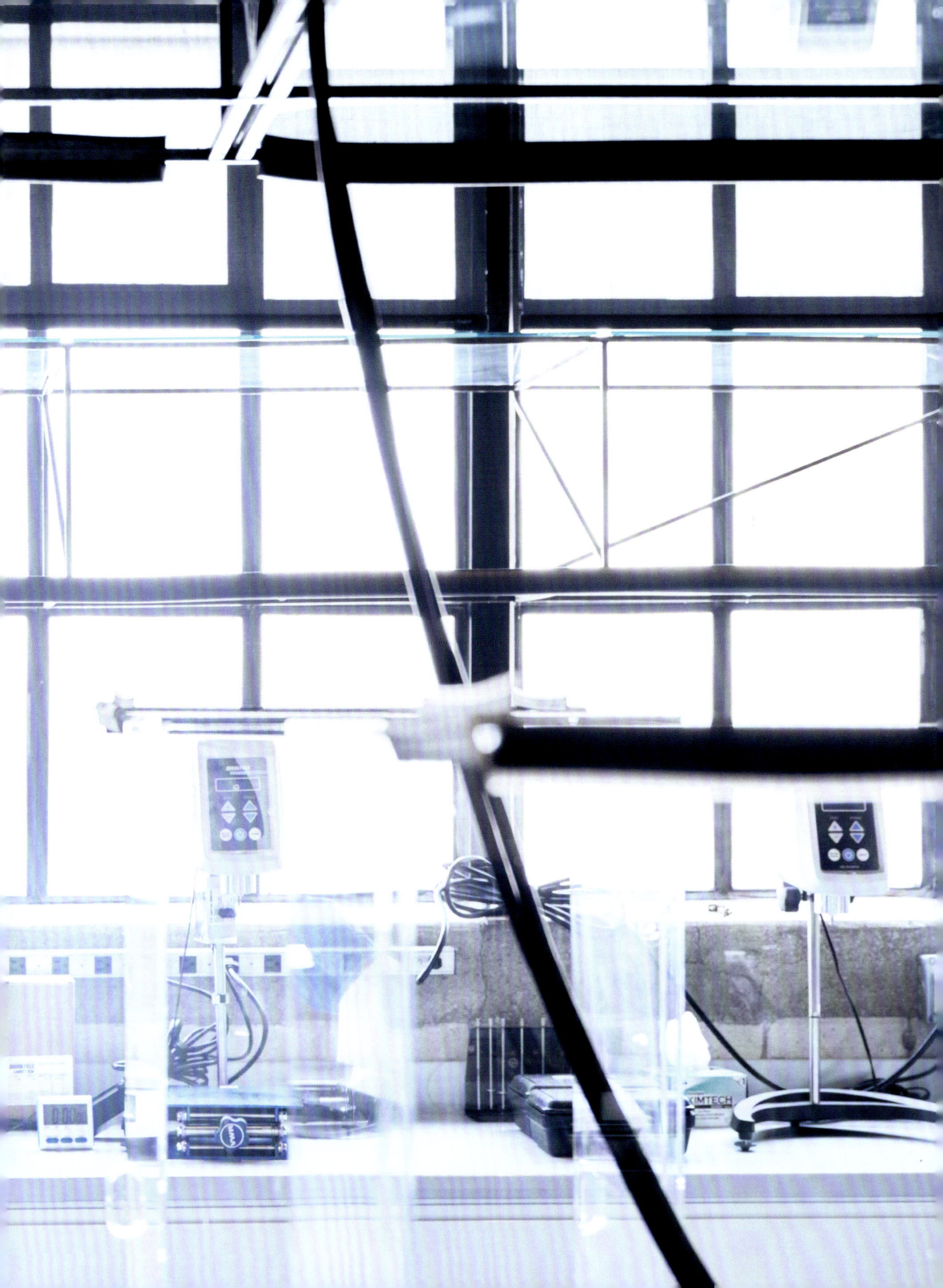

Dear Reader,

Welcome to a book of science. A book of transparency. A book of ingredients. A book of The Ordinary.

When I walk through the 20,000 square feet of labs in our Toronto HQ, I am always blown away by the level of thinking of our scientists. Not only the clear high level of academia, but the limitless good they have, the warmth in their eyes, and their desire to follow science as the guiding truth in serving our community.

This dedication comes from the roots instilled by our late founder, Brandon Truaxe. Brandon designed an incubator called DECIEM to be our own micro-world of beauty that operates with love, integrity, humility, passion, and a deep desire for innovation.

DECIEM is the proud creator of The Ordinary.

The Ordinary is clinical formulations with integrity. But this book isn't about our products, it's about the ingredients that make them.

Because we don't believe that marketing should lead over science, or that celebrities should be lauded ahead of researchers. We believe, above all, in transparency. In an industry that often complicates what should be simple, we are always honest, and stand by our commitment to create skincare that is effective and accessible to everyone.

That's why The Ordinary exists—to champion integrity in the industry.

Skincare isn't magic. It's science. And that's what makes it powerful.

To Brandon, we continue your vision for transparency and integrity.

My love always,
Nicola <3

Nicola x

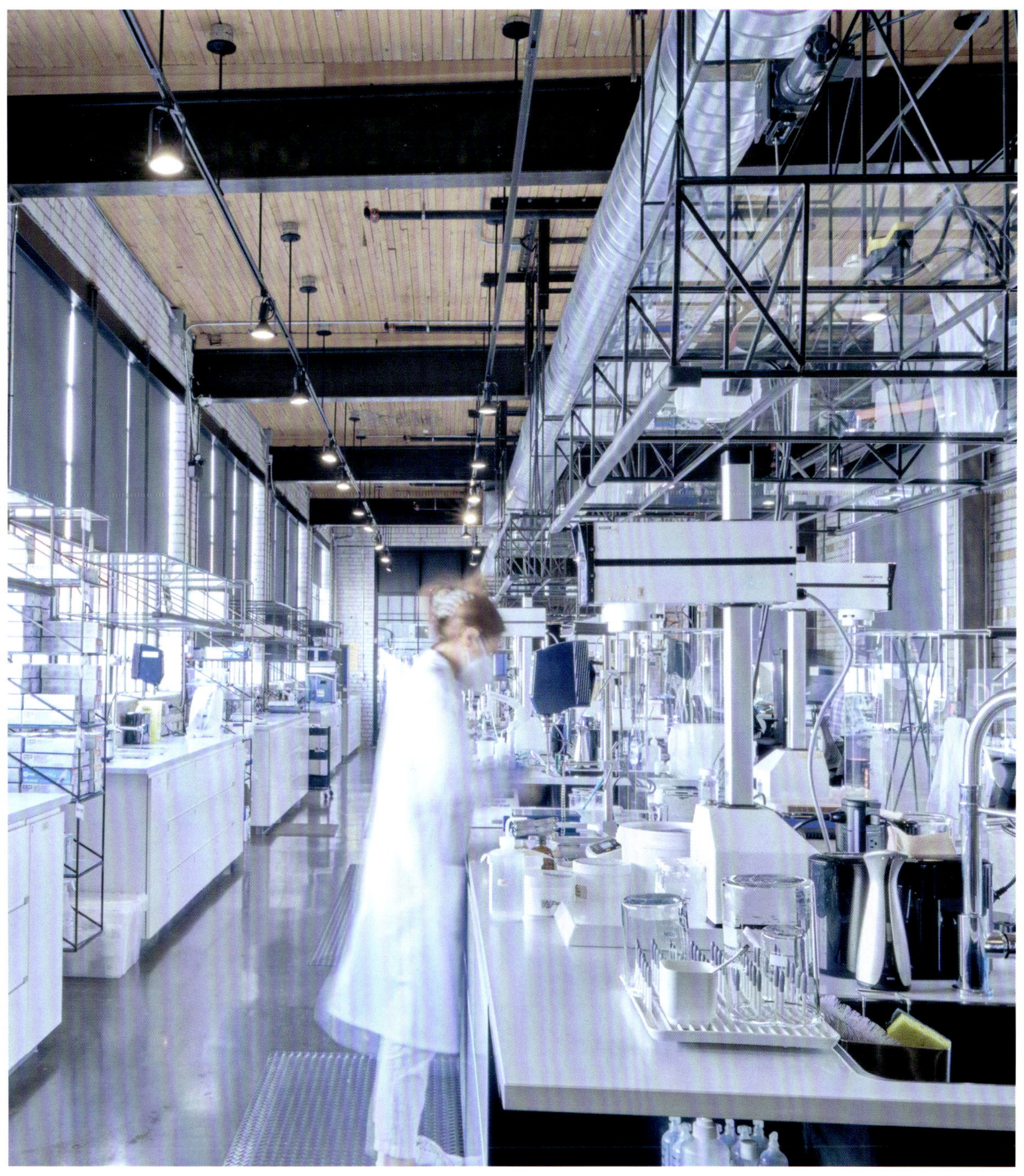

Our Story

When The Ordinary launched in 2016, it was the eleventh brand that Brandon and Nicola created at DECIEM, and had, at its heart, a very simple proposition. It was about skincare in its purest form. About shining a light on the science and ingredients of skincare that, up until that point, were all too often hidden behind marketing. The Ordinary was a riposte to the smoke and mirrors, jargon-filled, celebrity-endorsed, three-figure price tag lotions and potions that seemed to dominate the beauty industry.

In this context, it was revolutionary. Rather than using buzzwords and glossy advertising, the idea was to strip everything back; to educate the consumer about ingredients with a proven track record when it came to helping skin—and to sell them these relatively inexpensive ingredients with the minimum of fuss and fanfare.

Interviewed by Vox in 2020, Nicola said, "The idea was, let's start to communicate these trusted ingredients because they're so affordable." So, rather than hiding active ingredients on the back of a bottle, The Ordinary made them the stars of the show, complete with their concentrations. No fancy product names, no magic claims, just formulations that told you exactly what they were, such as Lactic Acid 5% + HA and Vitamin C Suspension 23% + HA Spheres 2%.

The north stars were transparency, science, and minimalism, and everything about the brand spoke to this. The name itself, The Ordinary, reflected it—no pretense, just honesty and simplicity. As did the packaging and labeling. From the stark and clean typography of the logo to the distinctive white aesthetic, every aspect of The Ordinary's design was meant to reinforce the brand's core message of clarity and honesty. The design was not just about being visually striking; it was about reflecting the brand's commitment to transparency in every possible way.

Packaging was another area where The Ordinary set itself apart. In an industry where flashy packaging was often the norm, a clean, simple, and functional approach was chosen instead. Transparent bottles allowed consumers to see the product inside, reinforcing the sense of honesty that underpinned the entire brand. The easy-to-use droppers were designed with practicality in mind, ensuring that the focus remained on the formulations themselves rather than unnecessary packaging details.

And at its heart were those formulations that—to this day—although straightforward are backed by years of meticulous scientific research, rigorously tested, and contain proven ingredients at concentrations shown to be effective. No inflated claims, no overblown promises. Just products that work at accessible prices.

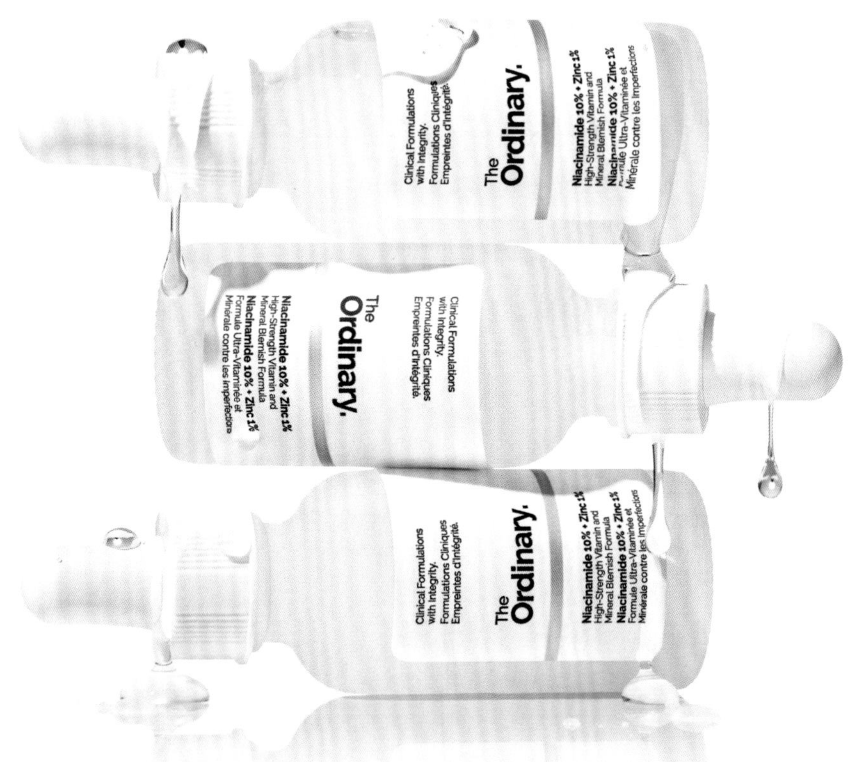
The Ordinary.
Clinical Formulations with Integrity.
Formulations Cliniques Empreintes d'Intégrité.
Niacinamide 10% + Zinc 1%
High-Strength Vitamin and Mineral Blemish Formula
Niacinamide 10% + Zinc 1%
Formule Ultra-Vitaminée et Minérale contre les imperfections

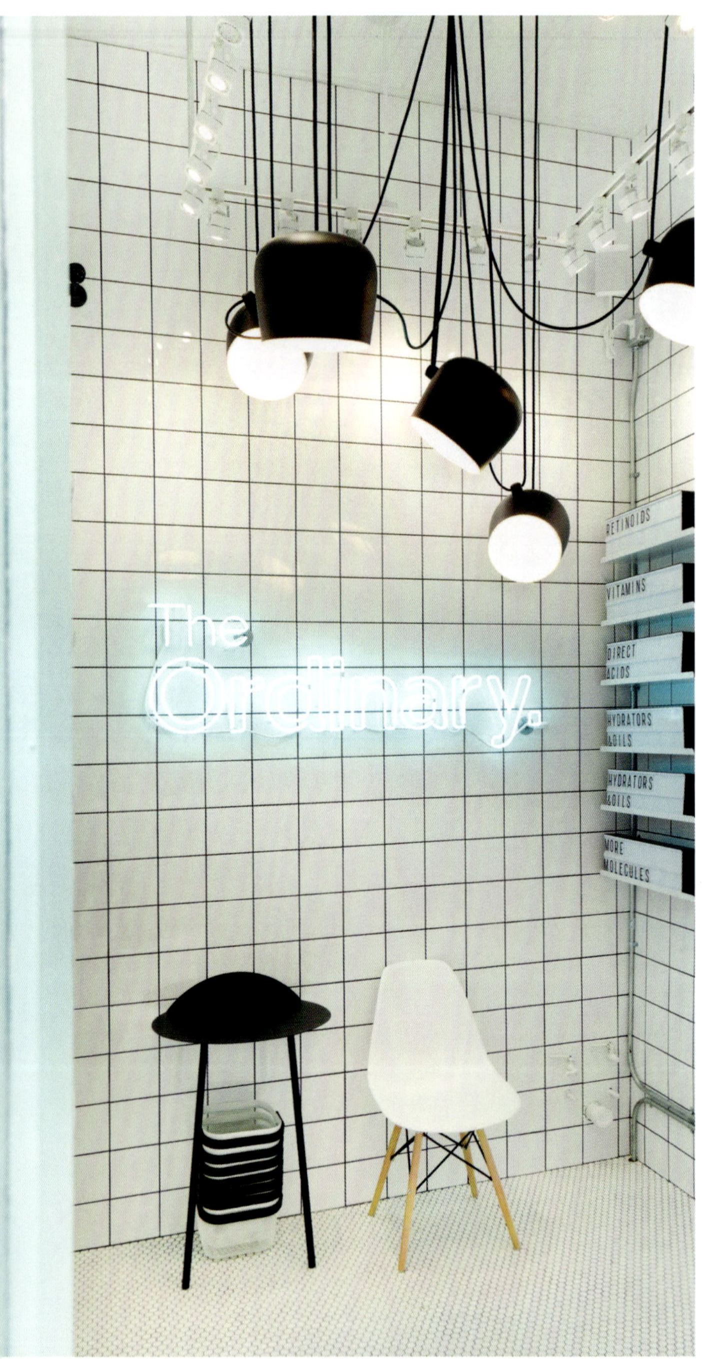

With the benefit of hindsight, it was a no-brainer, what consumers had been waiting for. But the industry didn't immediately get it.

When we pitched The Ordinary to some of the biggest retailers in the world, we were met with rejection after rejection. The feedback was often harsh: "It's too complicated," "It's too cheap," "It's too white."

In fairness to them, it represented such a departure from the norm that it was hard to comprehend who would want to buy it. From a price perspective, it looked like a mass market brand, but it didn't seem to be targeting the mass market. The very nature of the product meant that it demanded a very educated audience who understood ingredients and were prepared to choose efficacy and science over appearance and marketing.

And that audience was growing. The Ordinary was born at a time when what's been dubbed "skintellectualism" was on the rise. A growing number of consumers were eager to know more about the products they were using, and the ingredients they contained. Online, they found like-minded communities where they shared their discoveries, and—initially—it was consumers like this who instinctively understood, and valued, what the brand stood for.

When we set out to launch The Ordinary, we were fully aware of the challenges we faced. We were not just competing with other skincare brands; we were confronting an entire industry and what had become commonplace. But we knew we had something real. We knew we had something consumers desired, even if they didn't fully realize it yet. We were offering a skincare brand that prioritized their education over their consumption, that respected their intelligence and empowered them with the knowledge they needed to make the best choices for their skin.

The original 50 sq. ft store at 410 West Broadway, New York

And so we stayed true to the vision and the ethos and—eventually—it paid dividends. Despite the initial rejections, despite the skepticism, The Ordinary began to make a name for itself. Slowly but surely, we built a community of people who appreciated what we were doing—people who didn't just want to buy products, but wanted to understand the science behind them. We weren't just selling skincare; we were offering a new way of thinking about skincare. It was revolutionary, not because we were selling new, never-before-seen formulations that broke the mold, but because we were selling a new, never-before-seen way of approaching skincare.

The success of The Ordinary has been about more than just the products themselves. It has been about education, transparency, and unwavering belief in the importance of science. It has been about rejecting the status quo in favor of authenticity and integrity.

Today, as we reflect on The Ordinary's journey, we are proud of the impact we've made and how far we've come. As of the start of 2025 we have a dedicated—and growing—team of more than 150 scientific experts in toxicology, biology, chemistry, and cosmetic science. But we're not finished. Nowhere near. We remain committed to our mission of making skincare transparent, accessible, and science-driven.

This book is an extension of that mission, a way for us to continue educating and empowering our community—and beyond. It's not about our products; it's about some of the most important and functional ingredients used in skincare—the ones that can make a real difference. And it's our hope that through this book, more people will have access to the knowledge they need to make informed decisions about their skin and their skincare.

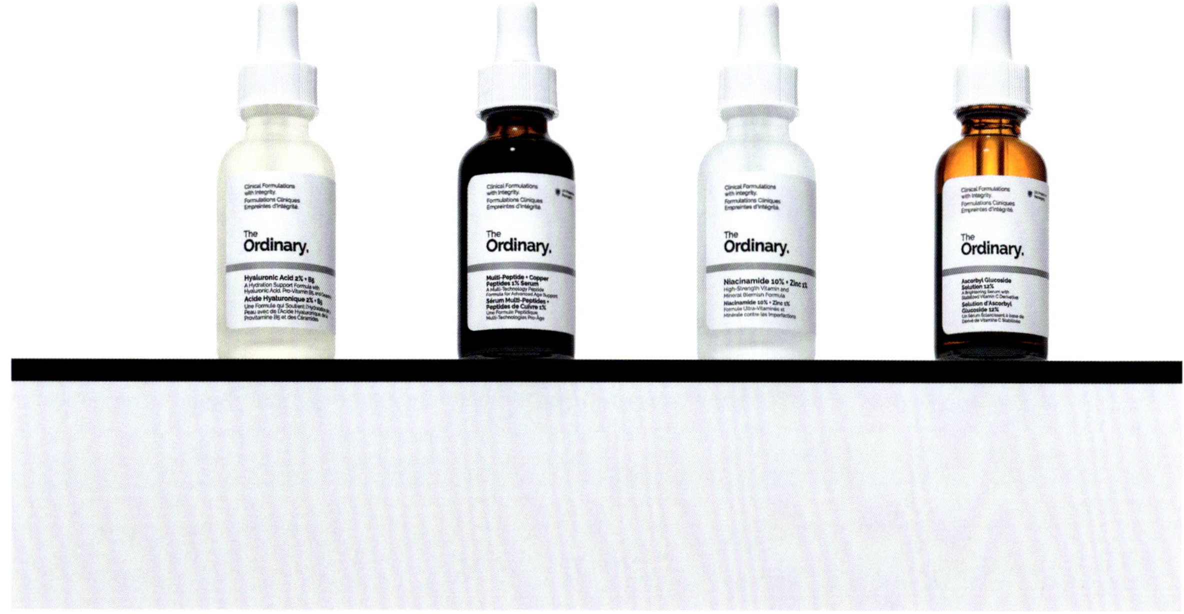

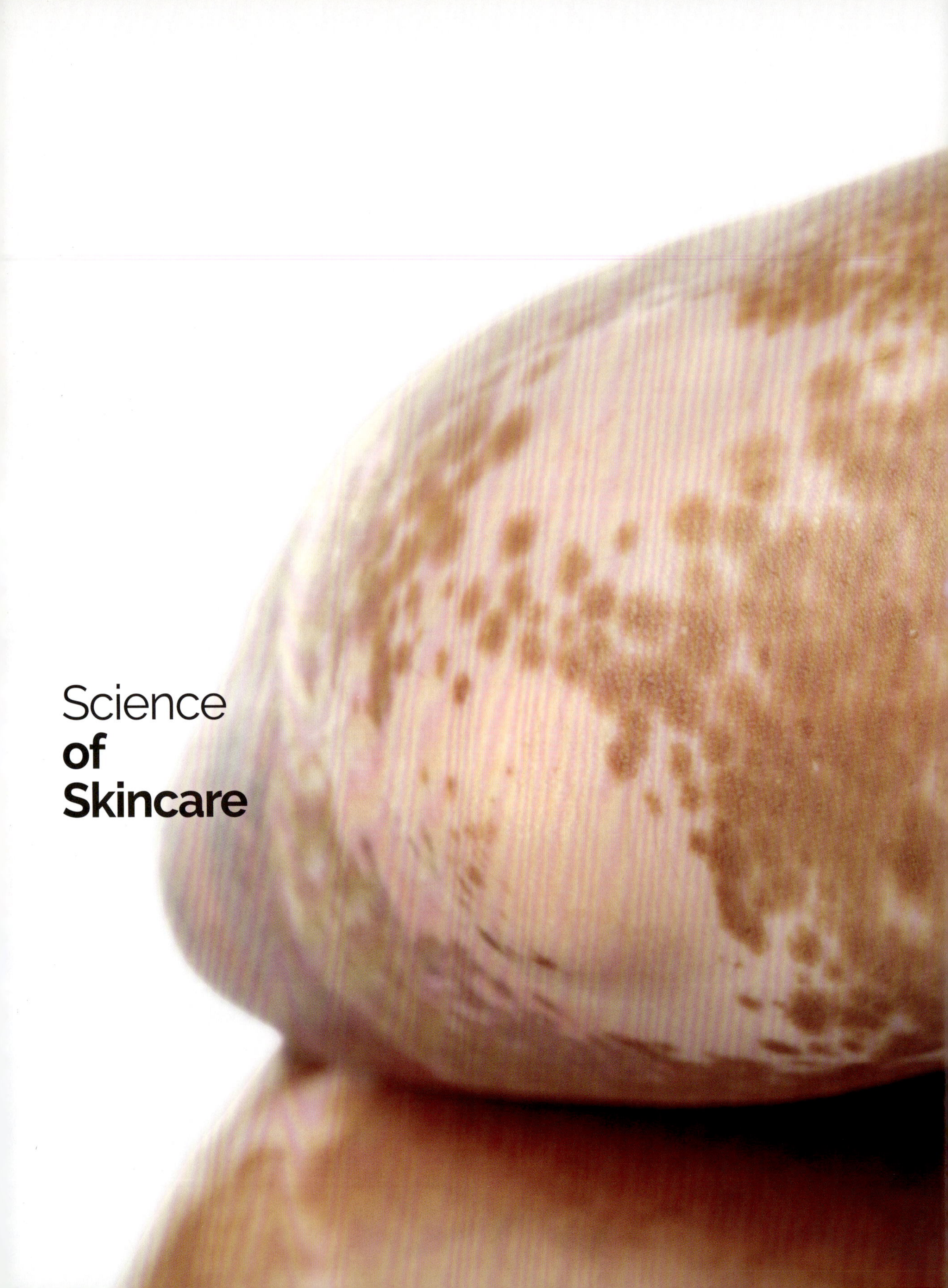
Science
of
Skincare

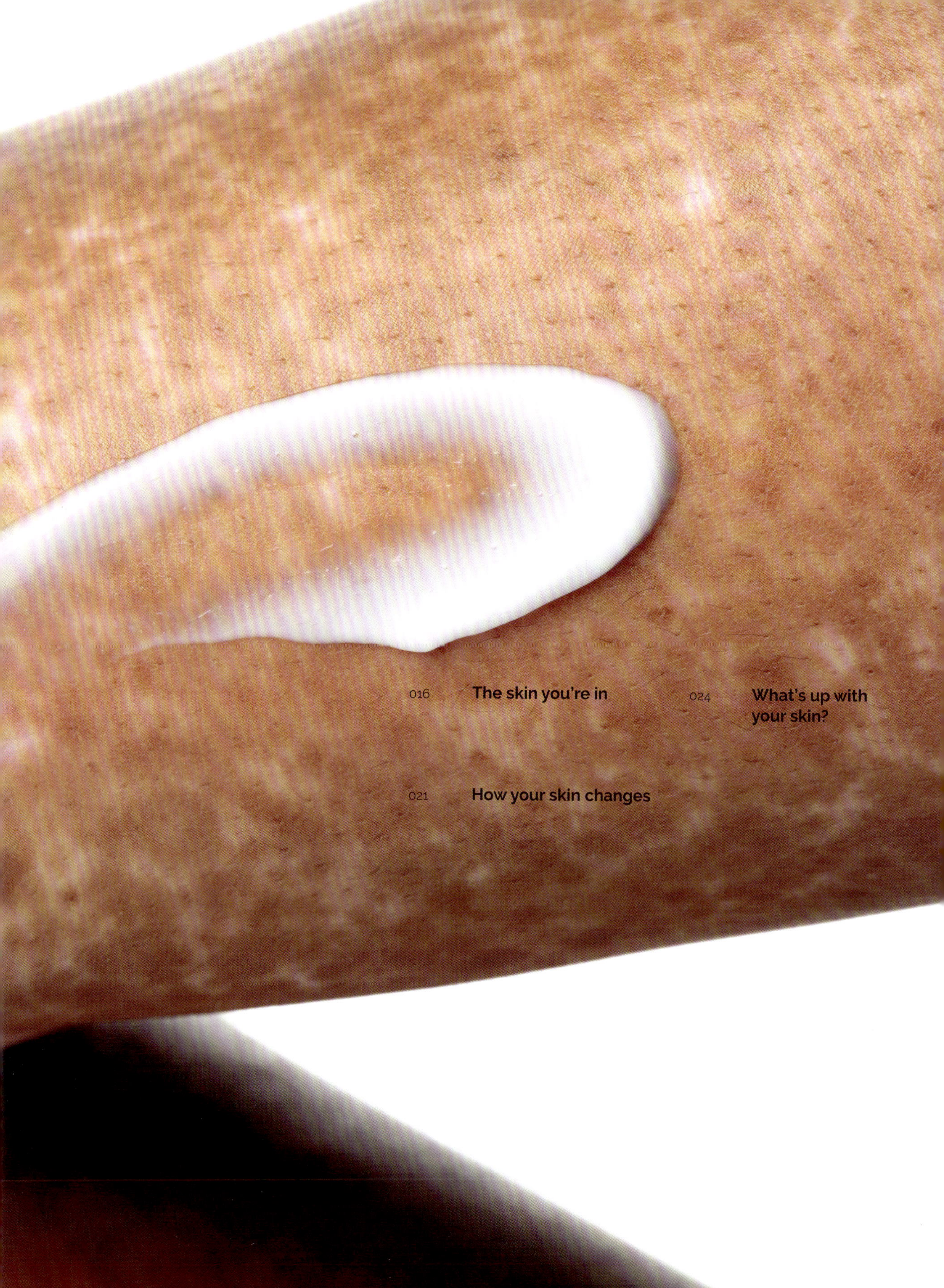

Science of Skincare

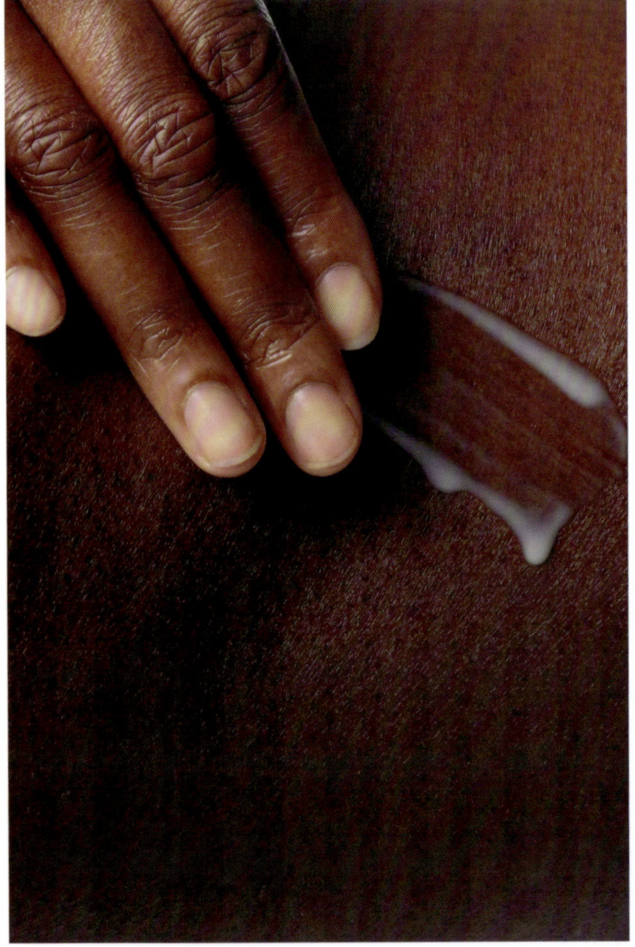

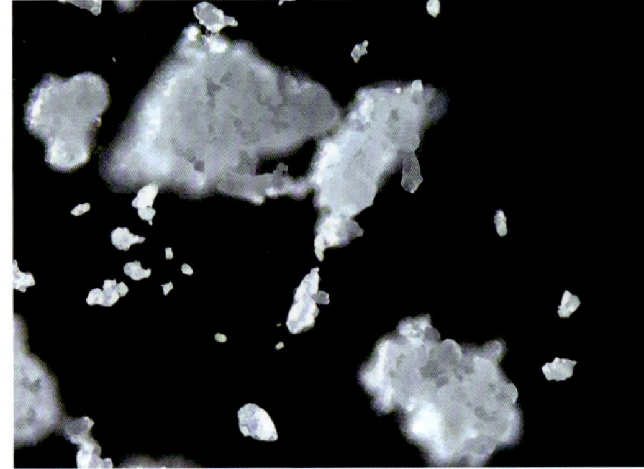

The skin you're in

The skin is the body's largest—and most visible—organ. Most human adults have an incredible 16,000 to 18,000 square centimeters of skin on their bodies. It is our interface with the outside world, and one of its key functions is to protect us from that world—from dirt, bacteria, pollution, sunlight, water, changes in temperature, and much more. As well as keeping things out, it also has a role to play in keeping things—such as blood and water—in. Additionally, it acts as a store room for minerals and vitamins that the body needs, and as a factory, helping to produce hormones and other essential compounds.

This amazing and complex organ is made up of several components, some of which include...

The dermis

The dermis is the deepest layer of the skin and is composed of a number of molecules, including collagen and elastin—the proteins that give skin its firmness, bounce, strength, and elasticity—and glycosaminoglycans (GAGs)—which attract water. They work with collagen and elastin to help support the skin and give it structure. One of the most well-known, and abundant, is hyaluronic acid.

Down in the dermis, you'll also find structures such as hair follicles, sebaceous (or oil) glands, and sweat glands—all of which originate here and run to the surface. Some areas of the body have more of these structures than others. For example, the scalp has more hair follicles than anywhere else on the body, and the face and scalp have the highest density of sebaceous glands—as many as 900 in a single square centimeter. In fact, the only parts of the body that have no hairs or sebaceous glands at all are the palms of your hands and the soles of your feet.

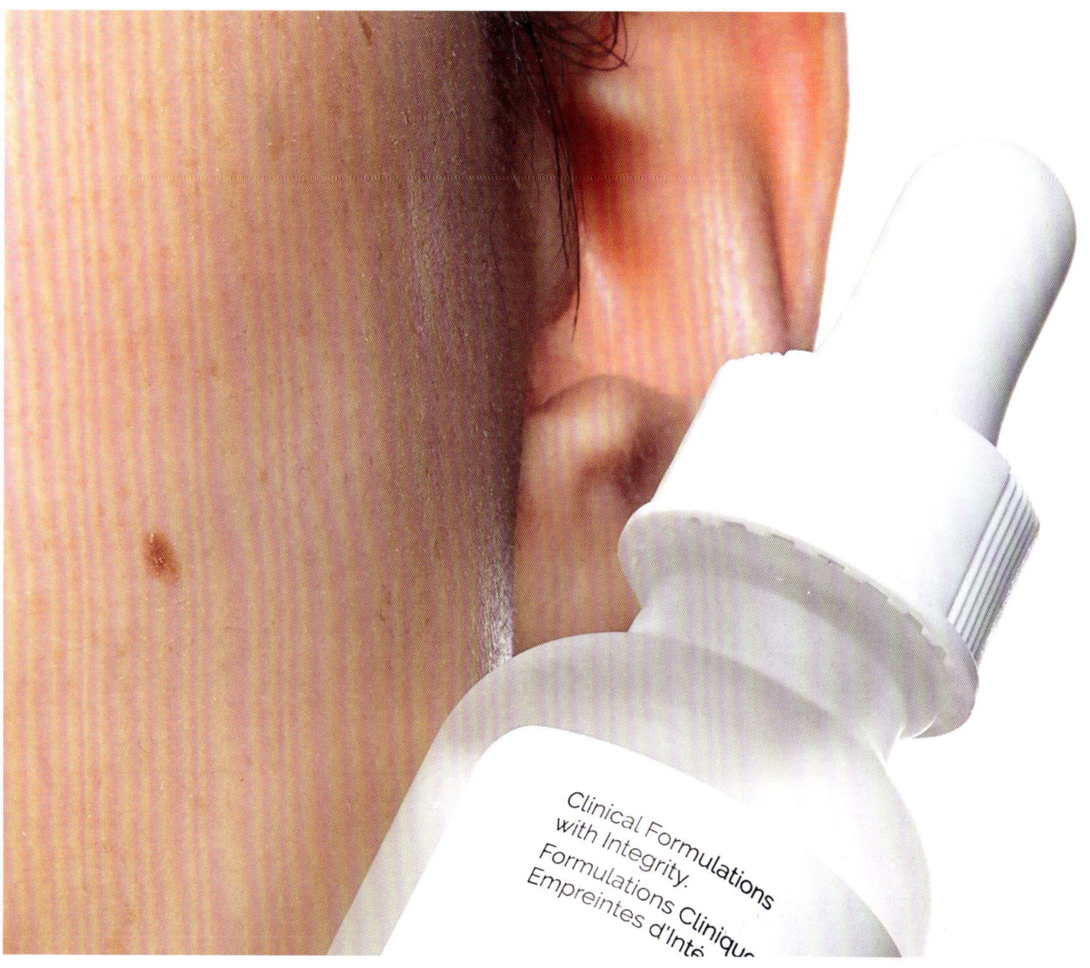

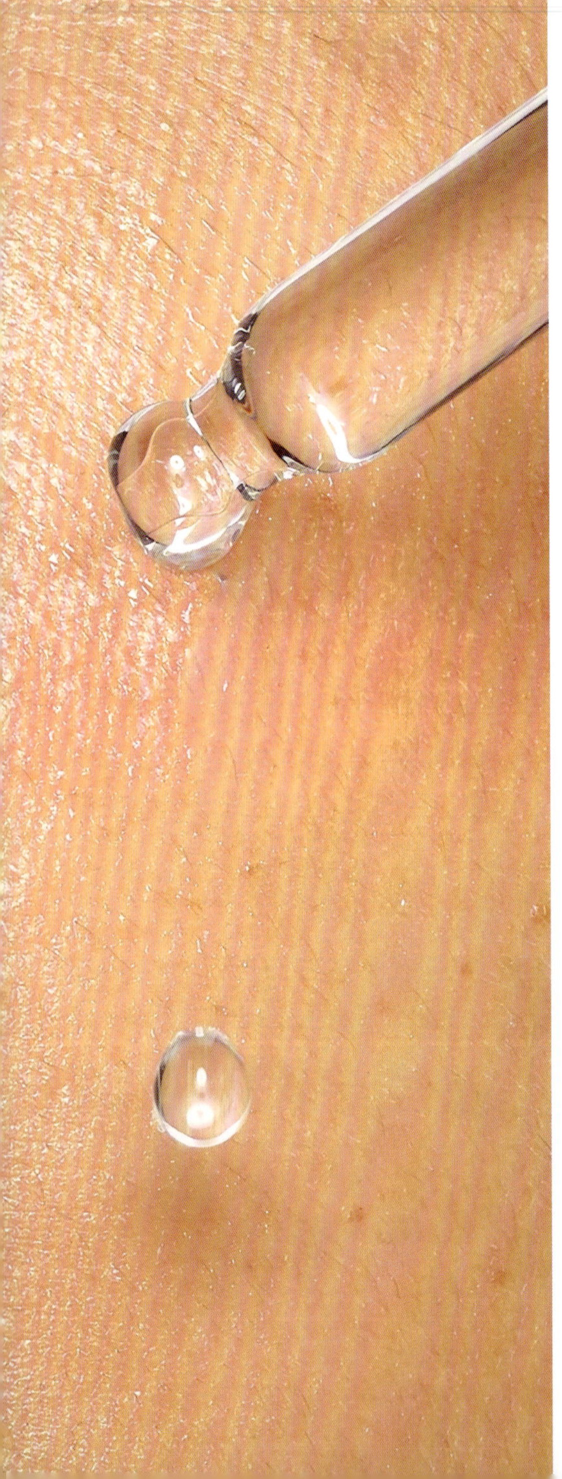

The epidermis

Sitting on top of the dermis is the epidermis, the top layer of the skin. The uppermost part of the epidermis is known as the stratum corneum, and this is the primary physical barrier between your body and the outside world. The stratum corneum is made up of skin cells in what is often described as a bricks-and-mortar structure. The skin cells are the bricks, while a mix of lipids (fats and oils, such as ceramides, cholesterol, and fatty acids) are the mortar in between, holding them together.

The skin cells and lipids work with Natural Moisturizing Factors (NMFs)—compounds found inside the skin cells that attract and hold water—to help the skin fulfill its function as a barrier. The skin cells provide a physical barrier; the lipids stop water being lost from the skin; and the NMFs maintain water balance within the cells, helping the skin to stay supple so the surface is less likely to be damaged.

While the stratum corneum is the part that we see, the epidermis is also home to a number of other layers—including the stratum granulosum and stratum spinosum. These layers are vital to the function of skin, containing structures that help to keep foreign bodies out and water in.

The deepest part of the epidermis, known as the stratum basale, contains cells called melanocytes. These cells produce the melanin pigment that gives skin its color. All humans have roughly the same number of melanocytes, but the quantity of melanin produced within these cells varies widely, resulting in our diverse skin tones.

The stratum basale also contains special cells called stem cells. They give skin its ability to regenerate. Because the epidermis is exposed to the outside world and consequently experiences a lot of wear and tear, it constantly undergoes a shedding process, known as desquamation. This means it needs to be renewed continuously, and stem cells are the key to this process.

Over a period of around 28 days, stem cells become skin cells and make their way up through the layers of the epidermis, displacing the cells above them, until they reach the surface and become part of the bricks-and-mortar structure of the stratum corneum mentioned above.

This is known as a complete skin cycle and it's the reason why, if you're trying a new skincare product, you should give it at least a month before you can expect to see noticeable changes. That way you'll know that all the skin cells on the surface of the skin have had a chance to respond to the product.

The microbiome

Traditionally, models of the skin haven't included the microbiome, the collection of more than 10,000 species of bacteria, fungi, and viruses that live on the surface of the skin. But research has started to show what an important role these organisms play in how our skin behaves. After all, before anything even gets to our skin, it has to interact with the microbiome that sits on top of it.

Your microbiome is as unique to you as your fingerprint, and the exact combination of organisms it contains is dictated by both your genes and the environment. That means that the microbiome varies across your body—areas where there's more moisture (such as in the armpit, where there are more sweat glands) or more oil (such as on your scalp, where there are more oil glands) will have a different microbiome from drier areas, such as the shin.

Almost anything that you put on your skin—soap, chlorine, hand sanitizer—can temporarily have an impact on the balance of organisms that make up the microbiome. But, after a relatively short period of time, it will return to its usual state. That's not to say that at the age of 60 you'll have the same microbiome as you did when you were born, though.

There is evidence that the composition of the microbiome can change gradually over time. Broadly speaking, the microbiome of older skin looks different from the microbiome of younger skin, and the microbiome of healthy skin generally looks different from the microbiome of skin that suffers from a condition such as eczema or acne.

Science has shown that certain skincare ingredients can temporarily have an impact on the microbiome, but it's not yet possible to make permanent changes so that a diseased, or older, microbiome can be transformed into a healthy, or younger, one.

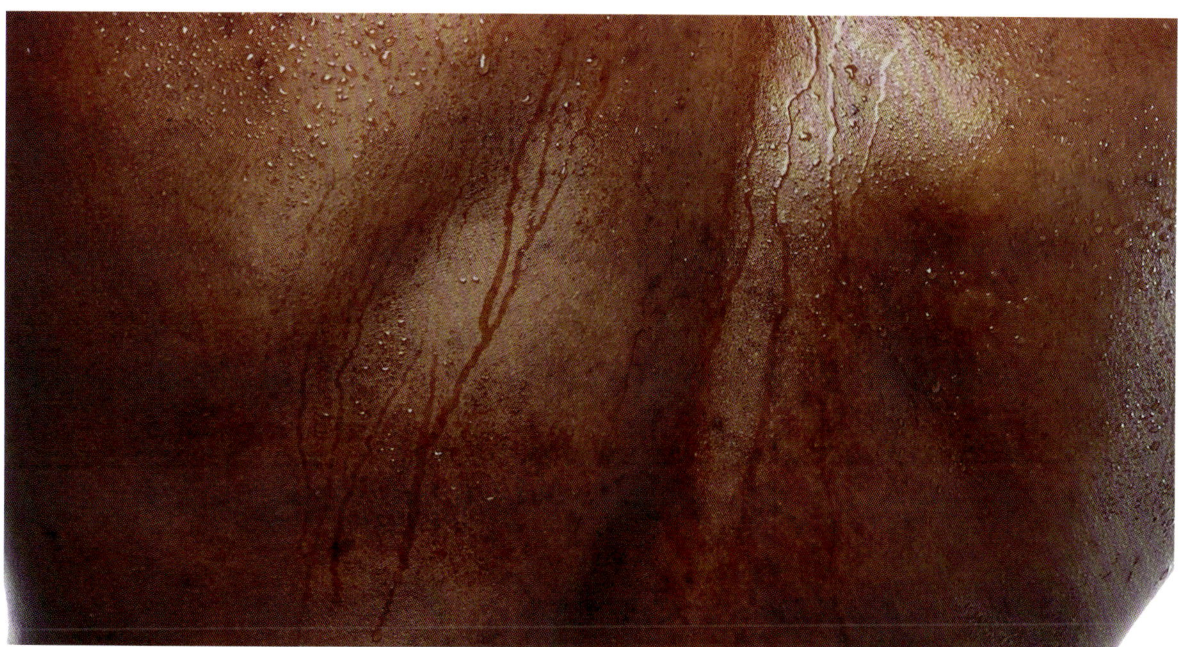

Probiotics, prebiotics, and postbiotics

The buzz around the skin microbiome means that increasingly you'll see skincare products claiming to be "microbiome friendly," or including ingredients called prebiotics, probiotics, or postbiotics, so here's a quick rundown of what it all means:

+ Prebiotics are ingredients, such as inulin, that act as food for your microbiome.

+ Probiotics are live bacteria and yeasts that theoretically promote healthy skin. But you're unlikely to find live bacteria in a skincare product as it would be very difficult to formulate in such a way that also prevents the growth of unwanted microorganisms.

+ Postbiotics are any ingredients that are byproducts derived from bacteria. These may be fermented ingredients or fractions of bacteria. The theory is that these types of ingredients can offer similar benefits to probiotics but, as they aren't live organisms, can be more stable.

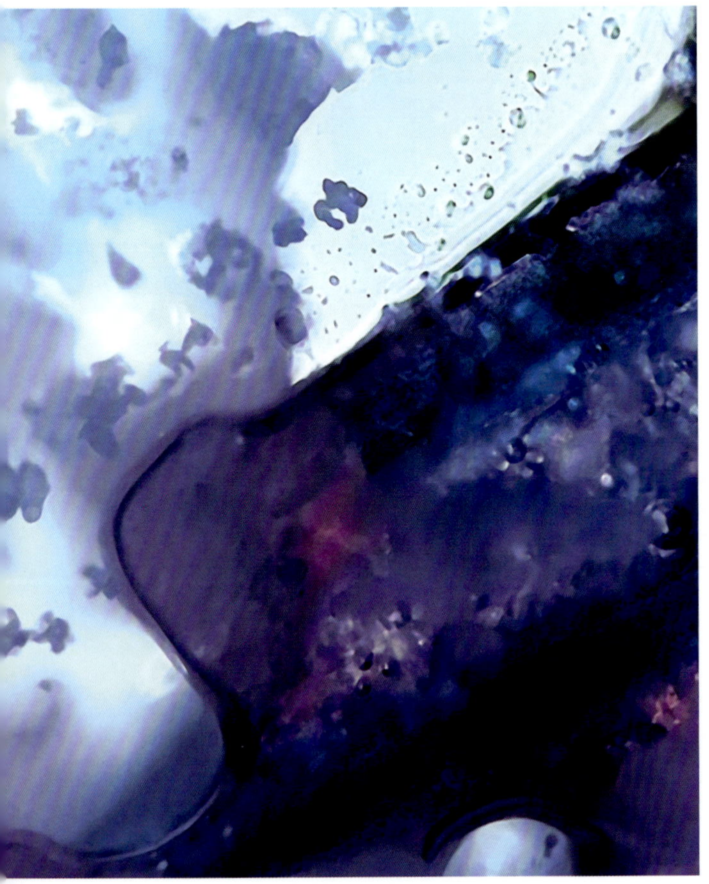

Some formulations aim to ensure microbiome compatibility by removing ingredients that might have a negative impact on the microbiome. Although there are tests that allow brands to make certain claims about how products impact the microbiome, the term "microbiome friendly" isn't yet legally regulated. It's also worth keeping in mind that, while external factors—such as cosmetic ingredients—can temporarily influence the microbiome, there remains little evidence that they have a lasting disruptive effect on the microorganisms that reside on our skin over the longer term.

How your skin changes

While the skin's basic structure largely stays the same throughout our lives, there are a number of factors that affect the way skin changes as we age, and the way skin looks and behaves at various stages.

For example, while all the structures of the skin are present in babies and young children, they're not necessarily working optimally. That means that babies and children can be more likely to suffer from skin conditions such as eczema, where skin is dry, itchy, red, or sore, because their skin barrier function hasn't fully developed.

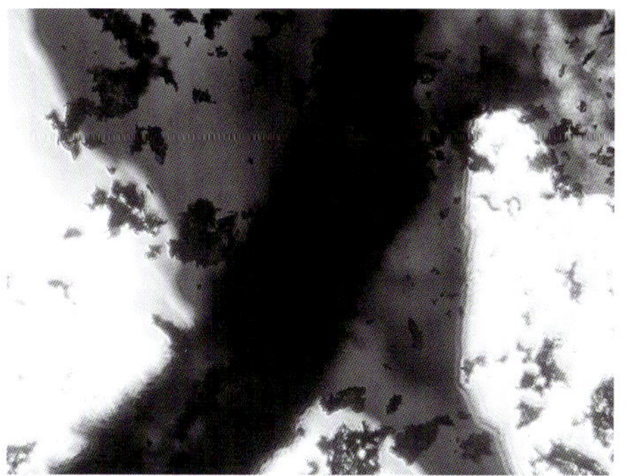

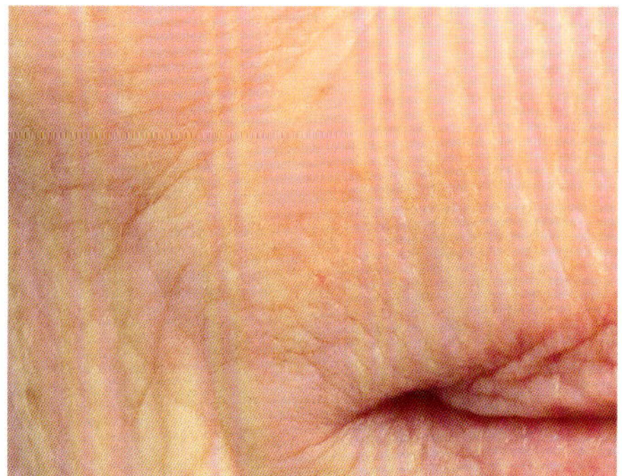

Puberty is the next big milestone for skin. Hormonal changes in the body can lead to increased levels of sebum—or oil—and, in turn, cause the skin to become more prone to blemishes.

Then, for many people—although not for everyone—once the hormonal storms of teenage life are over, there's, biologically speaking, a sweet spot when things should settle down and the skin should be functioning optimally, with balanced levels of sebum, efficient production of collagen and elastin, and swift turnover of skin cells.

This lasts until anywhere from the mid-20s to the mid-30s, depending on the individual. At this point, certain processes in the skin start to slow down or become less efficient. This doesn't happen overnight, and it may take decades before you can see the visible results of these changes, but this is when it begins. The changes are:

Less collagen and elastin is produced by the skin, and the way in which these proteins are laid down within the skin changes. So not only do you have less of them, but what you do have is more disorganized, resulting in skin losing its elasticity and firmness.

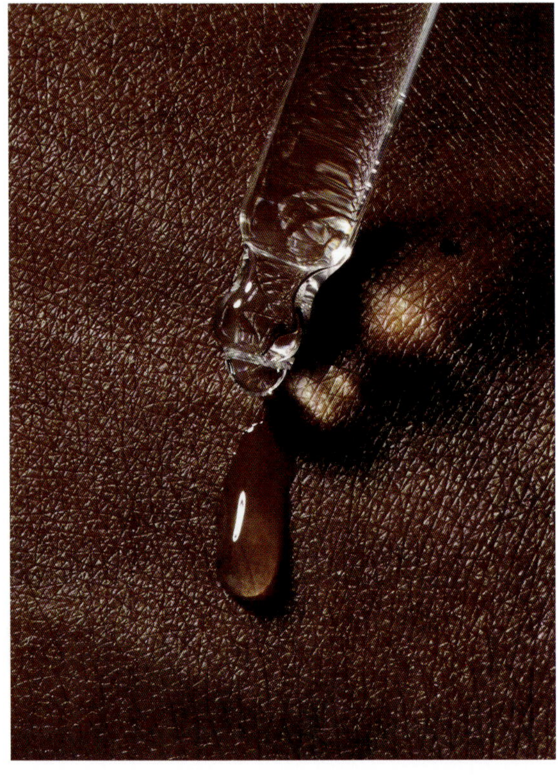

The process of making new skin cells slows down, so the skin cycle becomes longer and, as a result, the skin texture can become uneven and dull.

Layers of fat that sit beneath the skin start to become thinner, contributing to wrinkling and sagging.

The number of melanocytes in the skin decreases, meaning skin can become paler.

Sweat glands and sebaceous glands become less active, so skin can feel drier.

The epidermis becomes thinner, making the skin feel more fragile.

While everyone is subjected to these changes as they age, people who go through menopause may find that these issues are exacerbated due to the drastic drop in levels of the hormone estrogen, which plays an important role in several skin processes, including the production of oil and collagen.

These changes are entirely unavoidable; they're a part of the way that we evolve and grow from helpless babies through to fully formed adults. While they may differ slightly from individual to individual based on our genetics, they are changes that happen internally as we age and not something we have any control over. This is known as intrinsic aging.

But there are other reasons why skin changes as we get older. External factors—such as exposure to UV light, cigarette smoke, pollution, and weather—can accelerate the rate at which we see these changes in the skin, and this is known as extrinsic aging.

One of the reasons external factors like this are so damaging to the appearance of the skin is because they generate unstable compounds called free radicals. Free radicals can be neutralized by antioxidants, such as vitamin C and resveratrol, which may be found naturally in the body but can also be applied via topical creams. But if free radicals aren't neutralized by antioxidants, they can cause damage to many of the important structures within skin, including proteins and lipids, resulting in the same sorts of visible changes that intrinsic aging can cause.

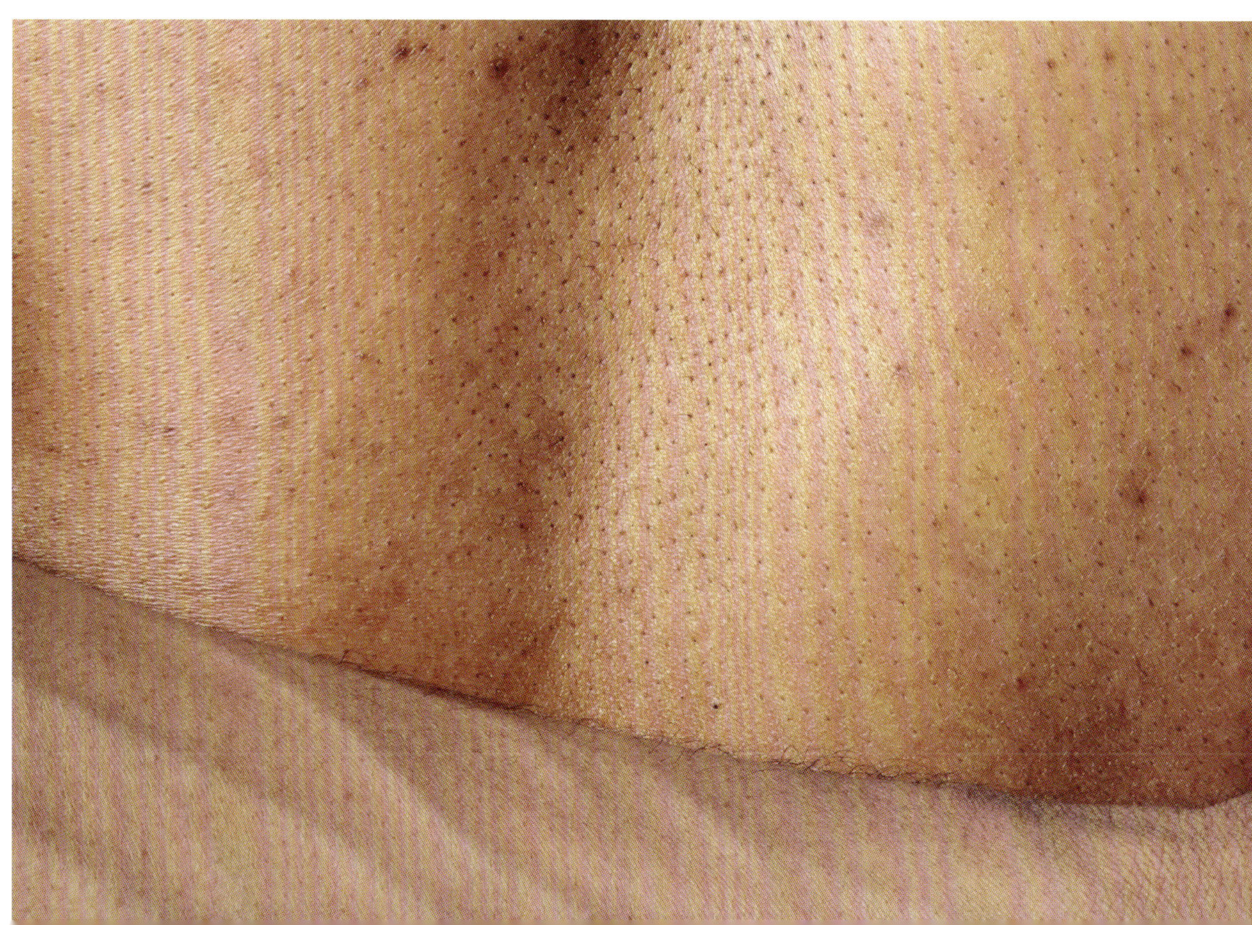

What's up with your skin?

As we have seen, our skin changes throughout our lives and, at various points, may present concerns that skincare products might be able to help address. These can include:

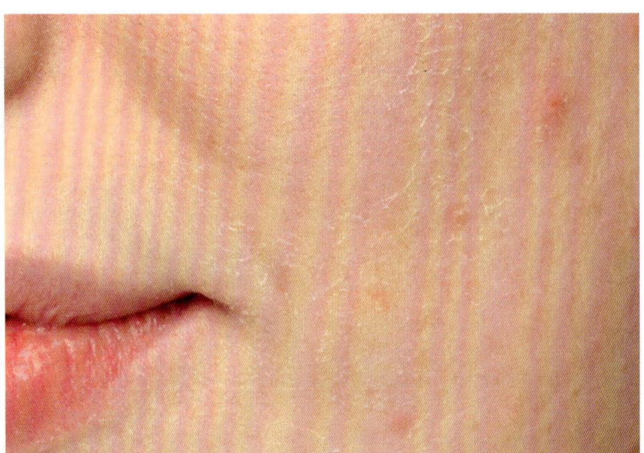

+ Dryness

When skin is dry, it may feel tight or sore, and can appear rough, flaky, red, or scaly.

Dry skin lacks moisture. Low levels of both NMFs and lipids such as ceramides, cholesterol, and fatty acids mean moisture leaves the skin faster than it can be replenished, and the skin barrier isn't working efficiently.

Skincare products that can help dry skin include those that help to strengthen the skin barrier by supplementing skin with NMFs and lipids. Other ingredients that can help are those that draw water to the skin, known as humectants, and ones that lock moisture in, known as emollients.

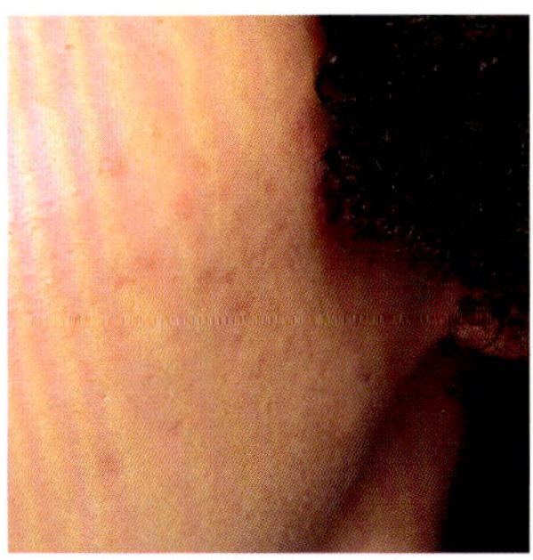

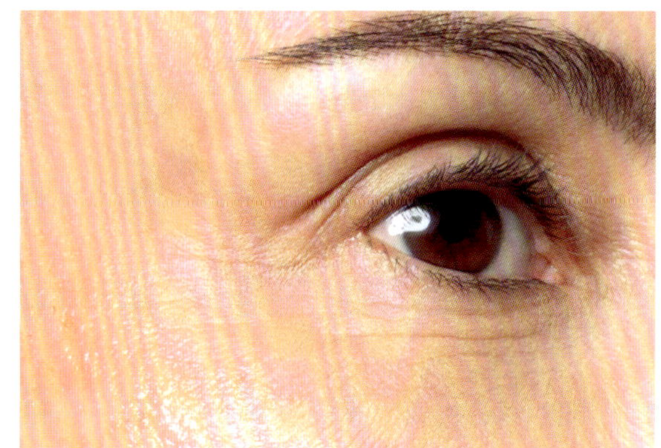

+ **Breakouts**

Breakouts can take the form of red or white spots and blackheads. Breakouts can occur when sebum and dead skin build up in the pores, blocking them. These bumpy blockages are known as comedones. Everyone has sebum and dead skin but not everyone has breakouts. Genetic and hormonal factors may play a role, but research has suggested that stress, pollution, diet, and hygiene may also have an impact.

When looking to skincare to tackle breakouts, regular cleansing is important. But there are also active ingredients that can help address the levels of sebum in the skin, and help clean out the pores.

+ **Fine lines and wrinkles**

When skin is dehydrated, temporary fine lines can appear. Deeper wrinkles tend to happen with age and are the result of a decrease in the amount of collagen and elastin in the skin, and the fact that these proteins aren't as tightly woven. This can also lead to skin looking less firm.

Keeping skin well moisturized is the first step in addressing fine lines and wrinkles. Other ingredients that can help include those that support the skin's natural collagen and elastin, and those that can help protect the skin from further damage from external factors, which will help reduce the rate at which collagen and elastin are broken down.

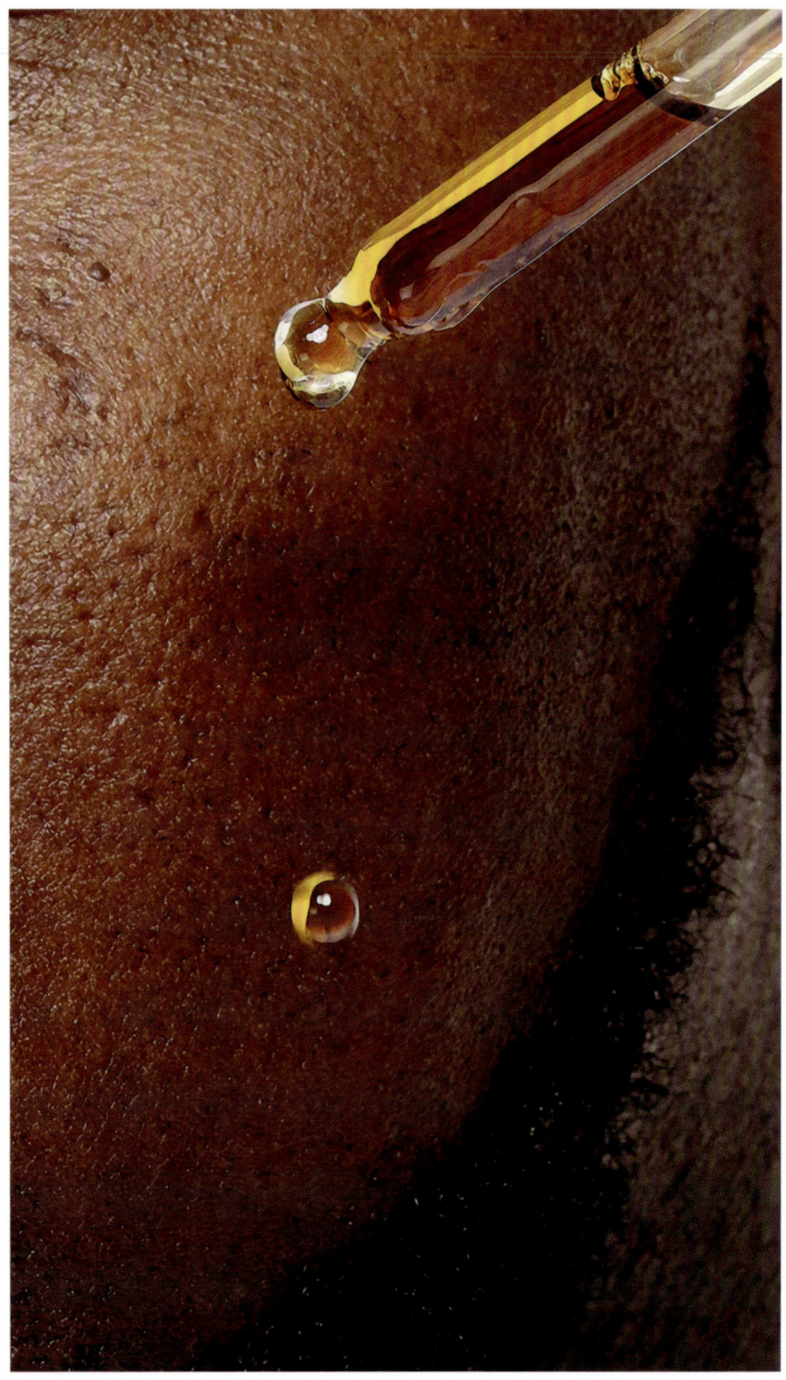

+ Dark spots and discoloration

In even-toned skin, the melanocytes, the skin's pigment-producing cells, work evenly to ensure that the surface of the skin is a uniform color. If these cells start to work inefficiently, or start to over- or under-produce melanin, you can end up with lighter or darker patches on the skin.

UV exposure, genetics, hormones, and injuries can cause the melanocytes to function in an unusual fashion.

Discoloration can be tricky to address because there are a number of contributing factors. Skincare ingredients that help tend to be those that can target several of these factors. It's important to combine ingredients that help disrupt the creation of new discoloration with ingredients that help fade existing discoloration and dark spots.

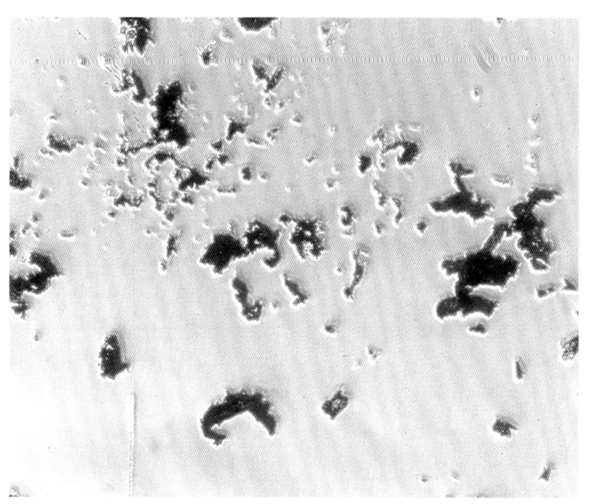

+ Uneven texture and/or dullness

We often talk about healthy-looking skin having a glow to it. This is because healthy skin tends to be very smooth, and smooth surfaces reflect more light. Skin that is uneven doesn't reflect light as well and so can look rough, flat, or dull.

A build-up of dead skin cells on the surface of the skin can make it look dull. But other skin issues, such as dryness and breakouts, can also cause the skin's surface to be uneven.

Ingredients that help slough off dead skin cells and speed up the rate at which new skin cells are produced will help to improve the appearance of flat, dull skin, increasing its ability to reflect light and appear more radiant.

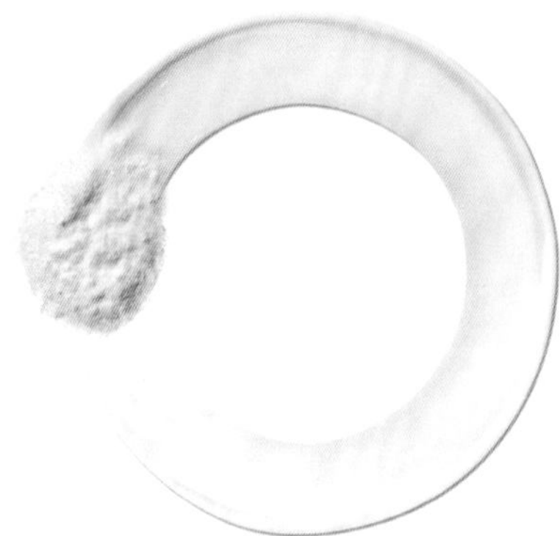

While some of these issues might relate to age or be triggered by intrinsic factors, they can also be precipitated by changes in our external environment. That might be anything from a change of season or a change of location to a new skincare product or stress. This means that, even if "normally" your skin tends to be dry, you could still get breakouts. And it also means that a 25-year-old who lives in the country and works outdoors may have very different skincare needs from a 25-year-old who lives in an urban environment and works in an air-conditioned office.

That's why a more effective way to think about skincare is to look at solutions for specific concerns. This means that rather than over-simplifying skin into dry, combination, or oily, or marketing products based mainly on age, it's about selecting products based on what your skin needs at that particular moment in time, which might be very different from what it needs in a few months' time, when the climate is different, or you're getting over a cold, or you've got a big work project.

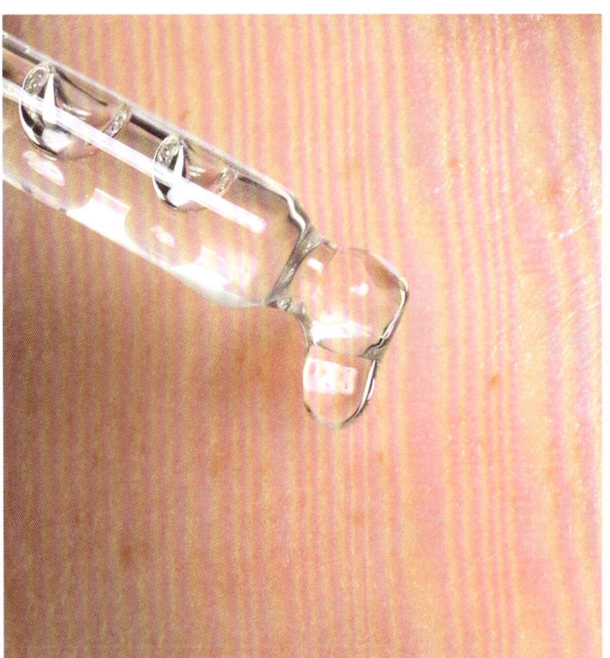

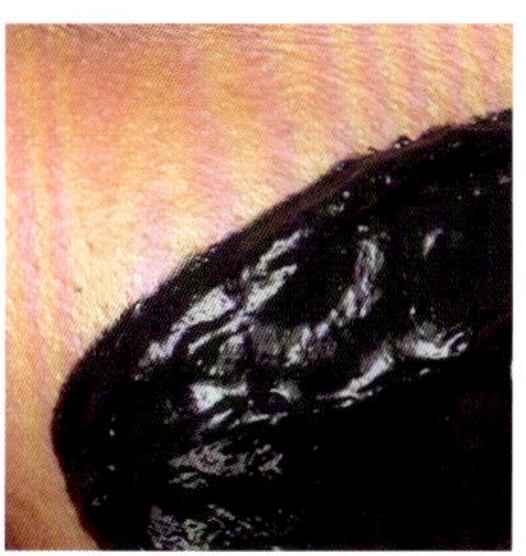

As you can see, there is so much more to your skin than meets the eye. It's a unique and constantly changing entity that fulfills so many essential functions. When you know how to interpret what it's telling you, you can help it to perform to the best of its ability—and keep it looking and feeling its best.

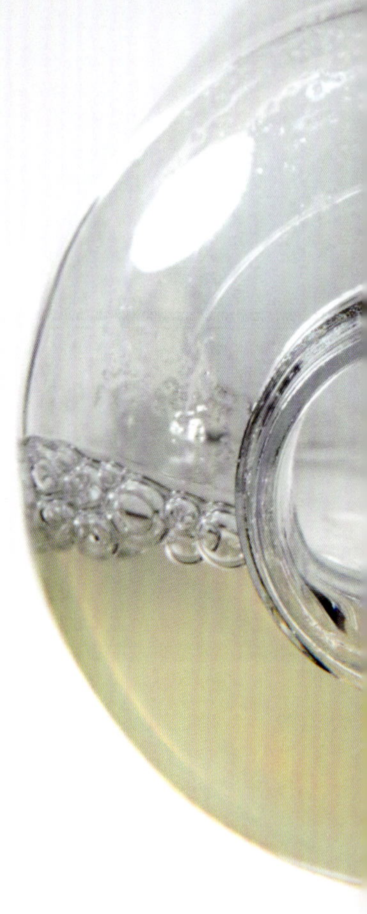

Beyond **the Label**

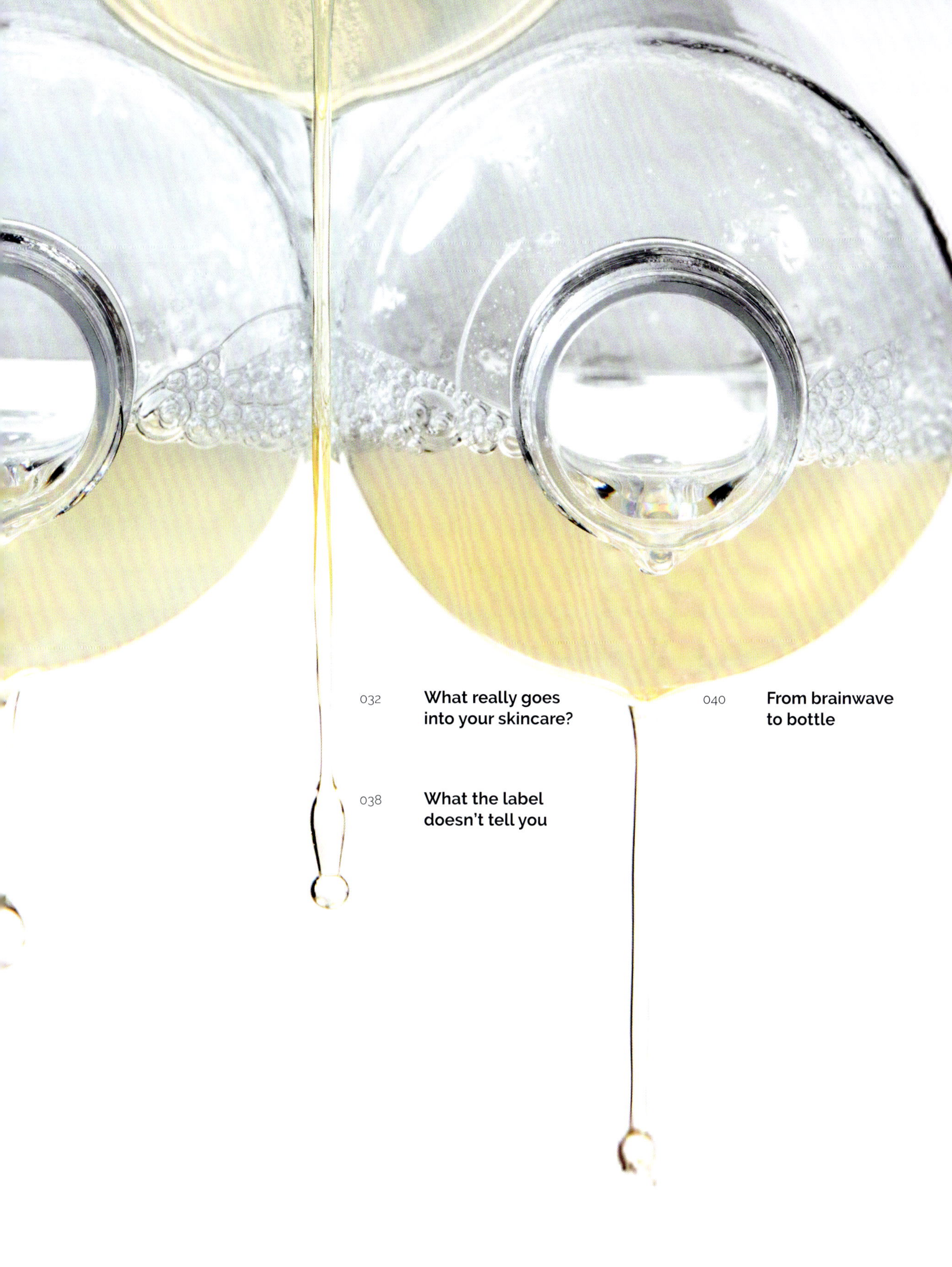

Beyond the Label

What really goes into your skincare?

So now you know all about the skin you're in, but what about what's in your skincare?

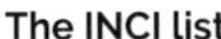

The INCI list

From one perspective, it's very easy to find out what's in a skincare product. Every cosmetic product must, by law, feature a label that lists the ingredients it contains. This list of ingredients is known as the International Nomenclature of Cosmetic Ingredients list—or, more commonly, the INCI (pronounced inky) list.

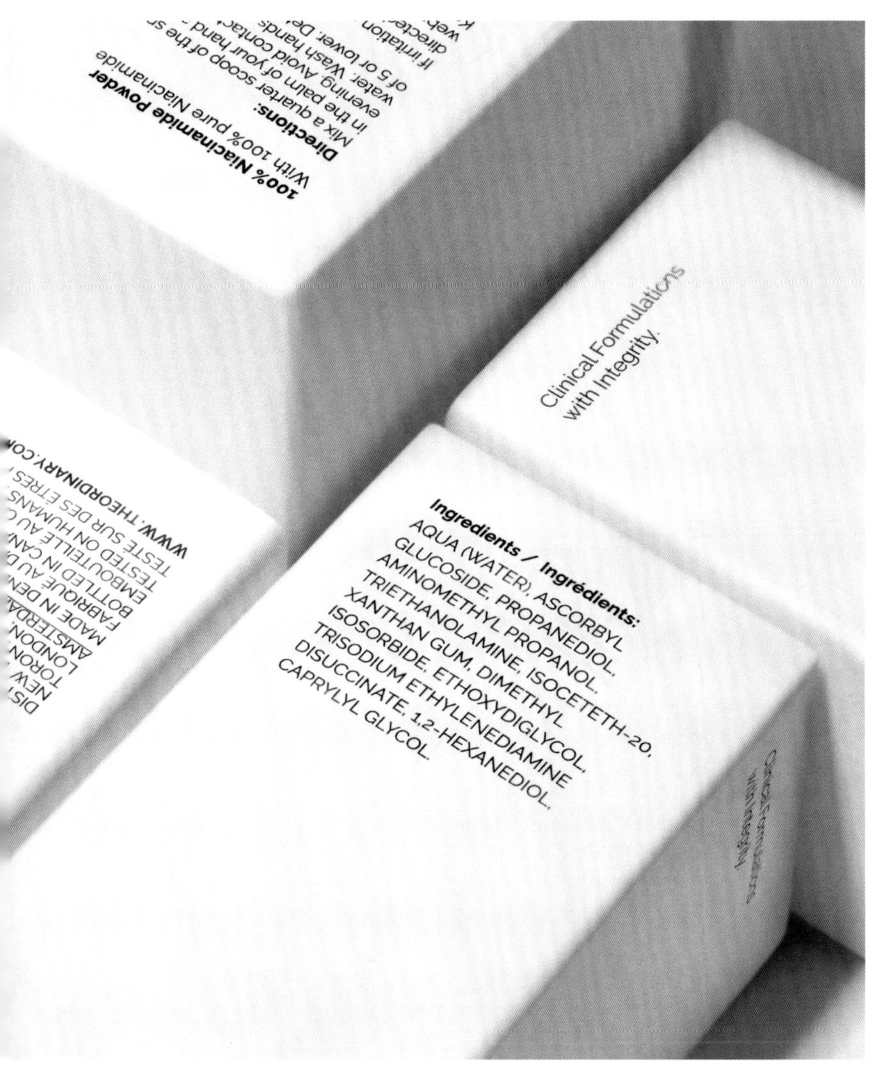

The INCI list sets out, in descending order of weight, the ingredients that make up more than 1% of the product. So, as with the ingredients list on food packaging, the ingredients at the top of the list form a higher percentage of the product than the ones at the bottom. Ingredients that form less than 1% of the product still have to appear in the list, but they can be listed in any order, after those with a concentration of more than 1%.

Because of different regulations in different parts of the world, the way that the INCI list is presented may differ slightly depending on where you are. For example, different names may be used. In the U.S. you might see the words "water" and "fragrance" used, whereas in the E.U. it would be "aqua" and "parfum." More often than not, you'll see both together—"water (aqua)" or "fragrance (parfum)"—so that a product can be sold in multiple territories without needing to be repackaged.

There are some other differences too. For instance, the European Union has a list of over 80 ingredients that can potentially cause reactions in people who are allergic to them, and these must be listed separately if they are present at concentrations that could cause a reaction.

Active ingredients vs inactive ingredients

When you see a long list of ingredients, you might be wondering what they all do and whether they're really necessary.

There is so much more to a product than just its active ingredients. Although those are the stars, the compounds that address specific skin concerns, there are other ingredients that contribute to the formulation, how it functions, and the consumer's experience of it. A single ingredient on its own doesn't usually make a skincare product.

It's a bit like how, if you wanted to make a chocolate cake, you wouldn't just use chocolate. You'd need flour to make a batter,

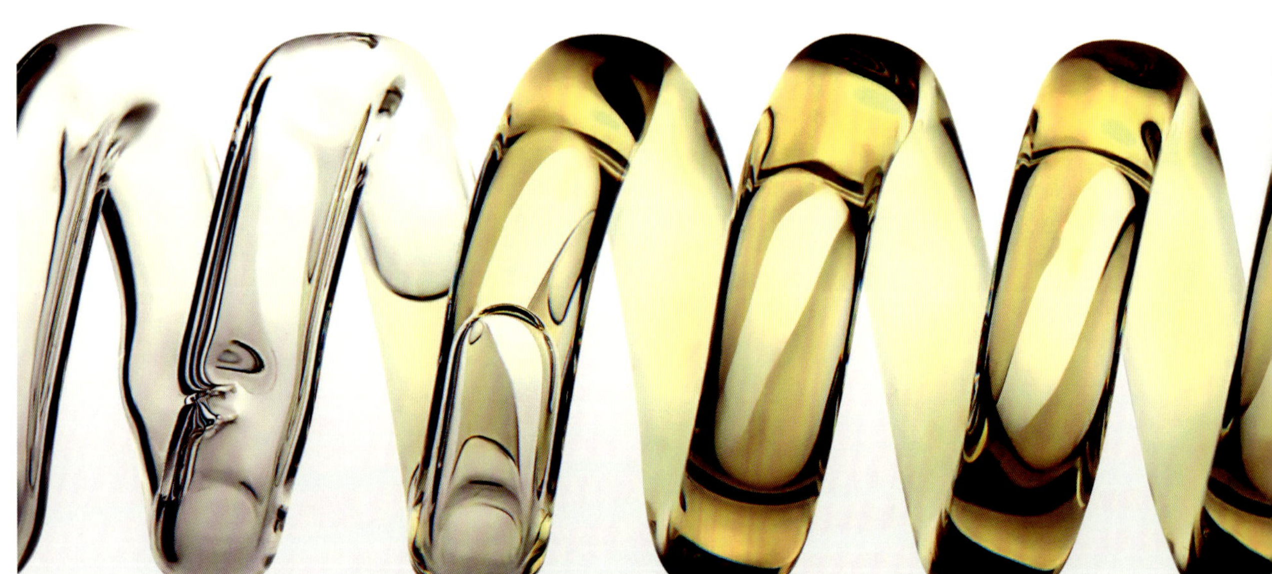

sugar to make it taste sweeter, vanilla essence to enhance the flavor of the chocolate, milk and butter so it isn't dry, and eggs and baking powder to make it rise.

Similarly, a skincare product typically needs to be made from more than just one—or more—active ingredients. It needs a delivery system to ensure that the ingredients get to where they need to be in the skin. That might mean encapsulating, or wrapping, one ingredient in another. It needs ingredients that will make sure that the active ingredient—and the product itself—remains stable throughout its shelf life and doesn't, for example, separate. It needs a preservative system so the product won't be contaminated once it's exposed to the air or people dipping their fingers into it. And depending on the product, and the customer it's being designed for, it might also include color or fragrance to make the experience of using it more pleasurable.

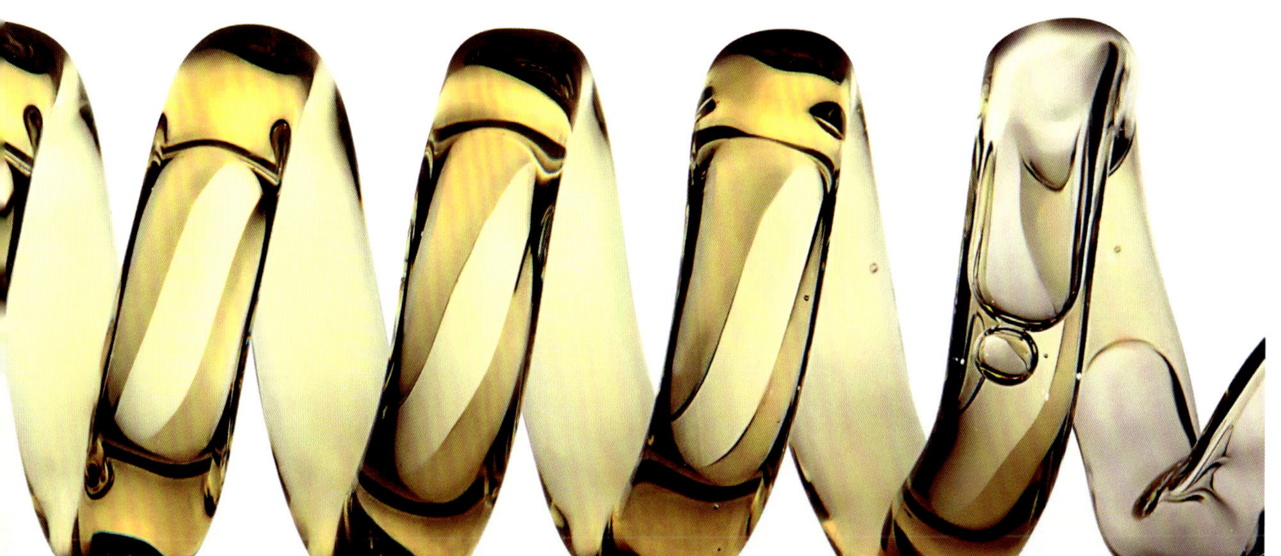

Other examples of inactive—but essential—ingredients include:

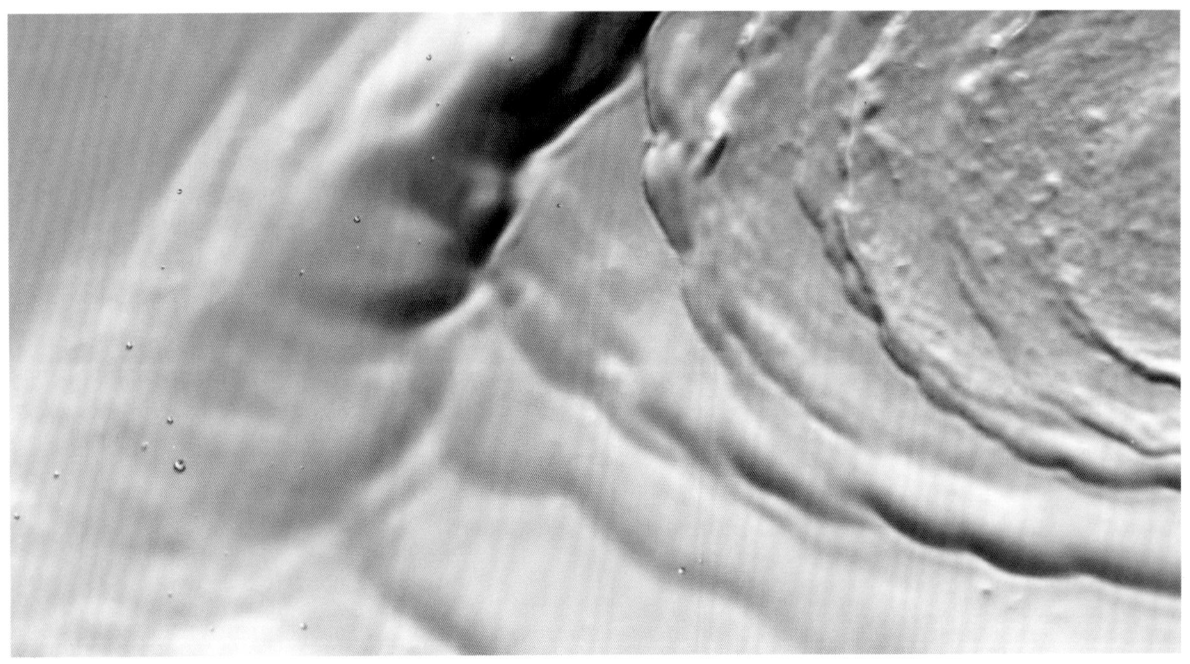

+ **Solvents:** used to dissolve something so that it can be appropriately included in a formulation and applied to the skin. Much like coffee without water would be undrinkable, most cosmetic products without solvents would be unusable.

+ **Viscosity enhancers:** the best product in the world is no use if you can't pump it out of the bottle or spread it over the skin. These ingredients can help improve these qualities by changing the texture of the formulation.

+ **Surfactants or emulsifiers:** used to help water and oil bind together, in the same way that mustard helps oil and vinegar mix together when you're making a salad dressing.

+ **pH adjusters:** some ingredients work better, or interact better with the skin, at a certain pH, or acidity level, so you might need pH adjusters to get the formulation to the right level.

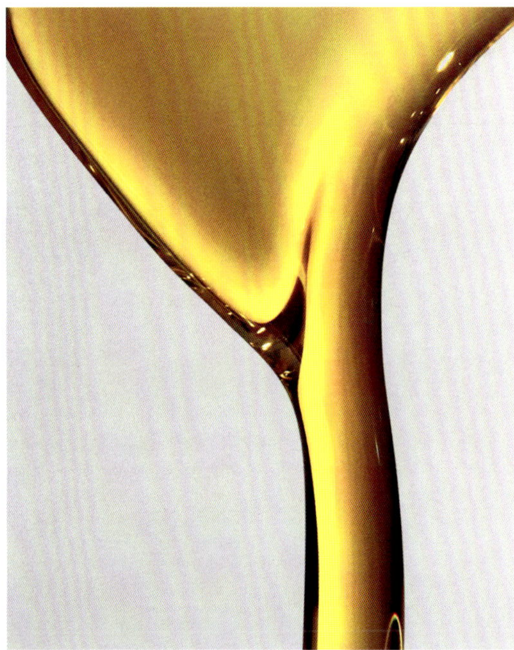

What the label doesn't tell you

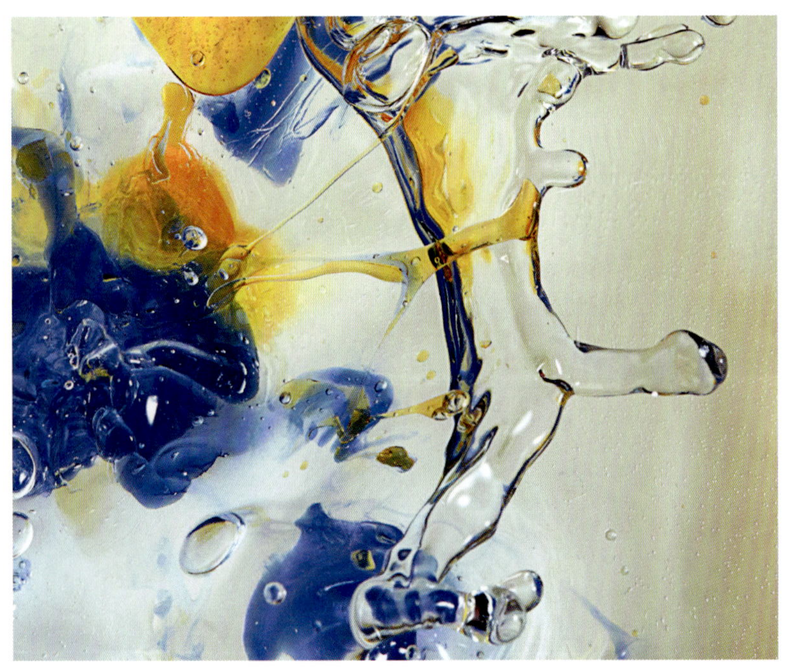

The INCI list can tell you a lot about what's in a product, but it doesn't tell you everything. For example, the efficacy of an ingredient depends on various factors, including the strength of that ingredient. The fact that the ingredient is listed doesn't tell you how much of it is there, or what delivery system is being used. Similarly, the name of a plant extract doesn't tell you anything about how it was grown, or how it was processed—both of which can have an impact on how it will interact with the skin. Then there's the sensory aspect—changing the concentration of an emulsifier by just 0.1% can make the difference between the product being a gel or a cream.

That's why even cosmetic scientists who've studied for years can't look at an INCI list and know how the product will look, feel, smell, or perform. These subtle yet important aspects of a formulation, as well as others such as the pH, are all a part of the product development process and will affect how a consumer responds to a product, but don't always show up on the label.

Ultimately the INCI list allows consumers to avoid a product that contains an ingredient they know they have an allergy or sensitivity to, and to select a product that contains ingredients that they think will help their skin. It's down to the formulators and developers to ensure that those ingredients are there at the right concentration for efficacy, in the right base for stability, and that the product has been tested to ensure it's stable, safe, and effective.

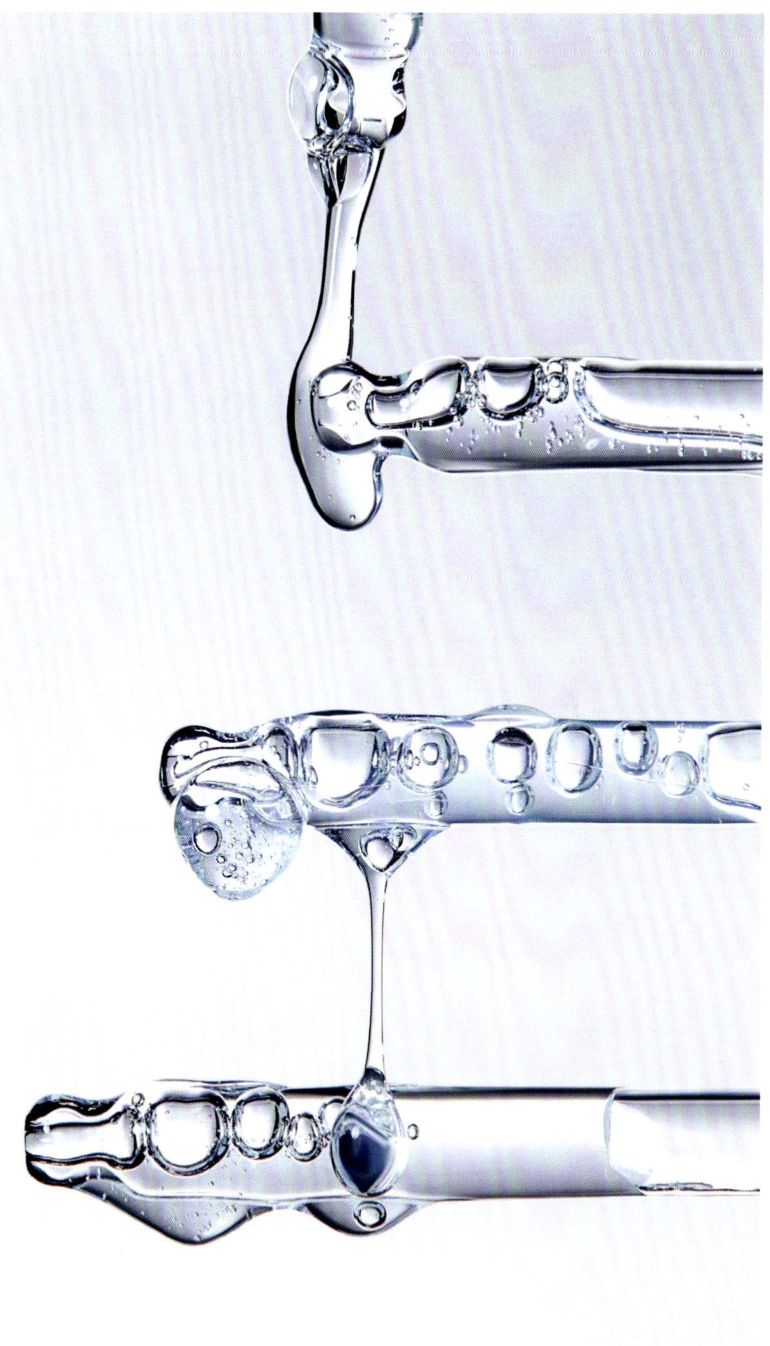

From brainwave to bottle

The journey from product concept to an actual cream you can buy may differ between cosmetic companies but the overall approach is similar—and can take years...

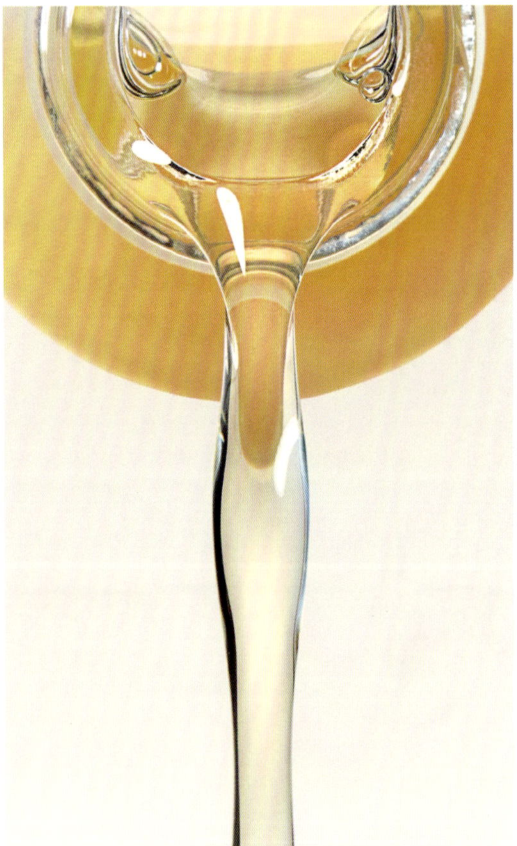

+ The idea

It starts with an idea. With some brands that might come from the marketing department, but at The Ordinary it starts in the lab. The Applied Research team investigates new technologies and scientific innovations presented in journals or at conferences. They listen to customer feedback—in store, on social media, or through customers making direct contact with the brand—and look at market insights and trend reports.

+ The brief

The idea then needs to be translated into a brief. The brief is essentially a written sketch that gives as many details of the end product as possible. It will detail its intended function and performance, as well as what it should look, smell, and feel like. Other details, such as the planned size and packaging, may also be included in the brief.

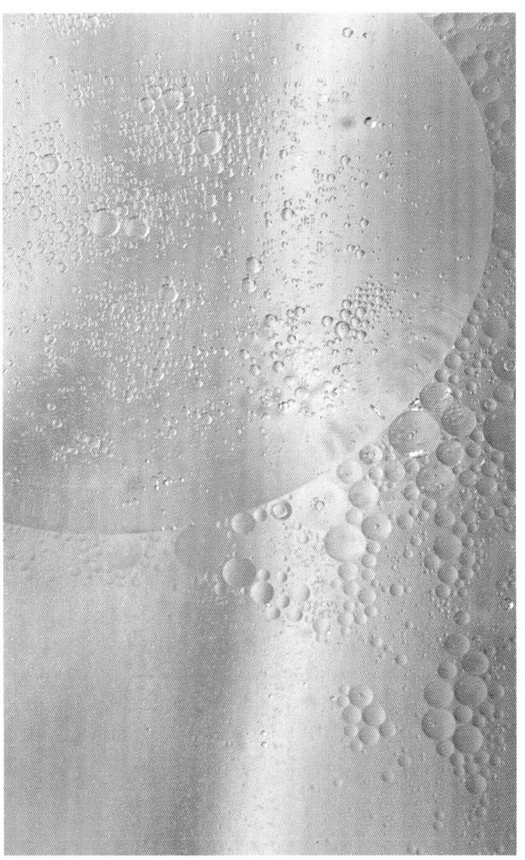

+ The research

Once the Research & Development (R&D) team has the brief, they will go through the scientific literature relating to technology and ingredients, as well as looking at data and research from ingredients suppliers. The aim is to ensure they have a full understanding of the ingredients, how they relate to the intended product, and how best to formulate and manufacture that product.

+ The formula

When a selection of ingredients has been agreed upon, the R&D team will come up with a formula, or recipe, that they think might work. They will then develop samples of this, tweaking the formula as necessary. This might mean adjusting the level of certain ingredients, or trying the same ingredient from various suppliers because it has a different texture or smell. There may be multiple iterations of a sample formula before it is finalized.

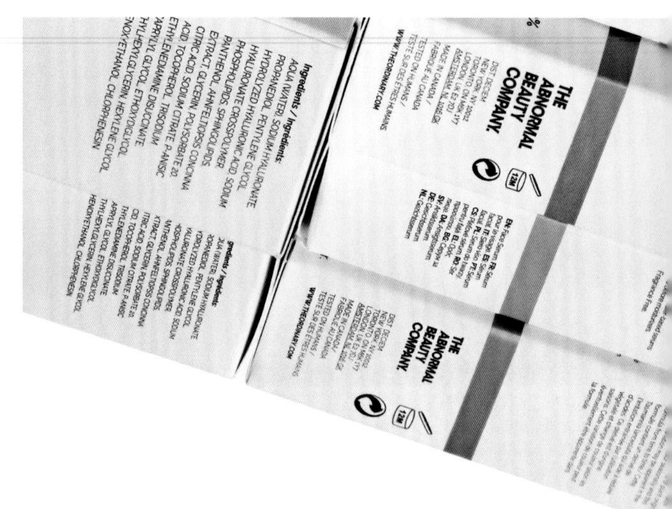

+ The testing

The team may think they've created a product that looks, smells, feels, and performs exactly how they want it to, but it needs to go through a number of tests before it can be sold to the public. The safety and efficacy of a product are assessed through regulatory and literature evaluations and tests on cell cultures (in vitro), on skin samples (ex vivo), and eventually on human volunteers (in vivo).

Before it can be tested on humans, the safety and regulatory teams must assess the ingredients and the product overall to ensure it complies with global regulatory requirements and is safe for its intended use.

At the same time, the product is tested to ensure that it will remain stable for its expected shelf life. This is typically done by placing it in a scientific oven at a temperature higher than room temperature, around 113°F (45°C), for an extended period. This process helps simulate how the product might behave at room temperature over a longer duration. Other tests will check that it will be able to withstand the extremes of temperature it might be subjected to during transport and storage.

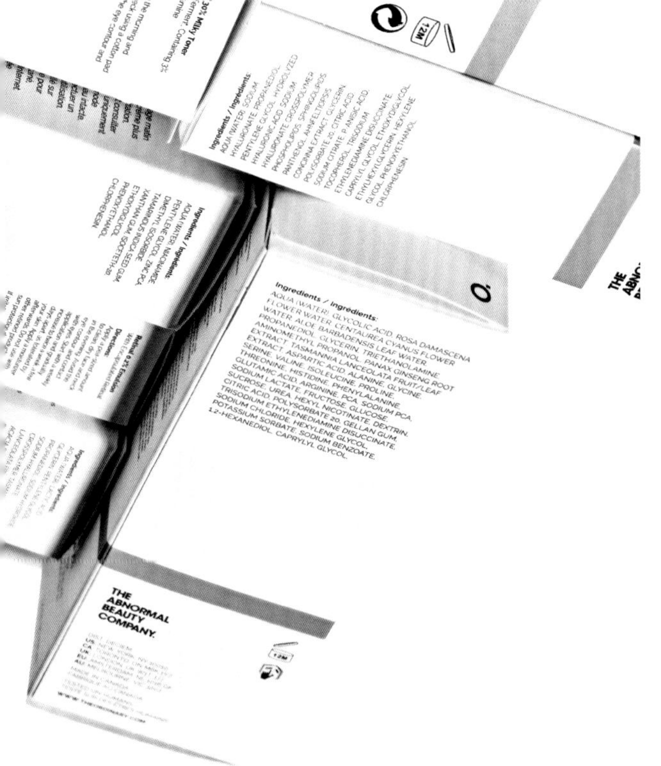

Other tests might include checking that the product can be easily dispensed from the intended packaging, and artificially contaminating it with microorganisms to check that the preservative system is working. If the formula doesn't pass all these tests, it has to be reworked and tested again until a version is found that does.

+ The communication

Throughout the process, numerous teams—including the clinical research team, the scientific communications team, the brand team, the legal team, and the regulatory team—work together to create the messages about the product that will reach consumers. This might include everything from drafting the wording that's printed on the packaging and educating retail staff in how to talk to customers about the new product to social media posts about the product and how it works.

+ The regulation

Before the new product can be sent out into the world, the regulatory team will ensure that all aspects, including the packaging, comply with all the regulations in the countries where it will be sold. Finally, the quality control team will assess the color, density, viscosity, and stability of each batch of finished product that comes off the production line to ensure it is within its set parameters.

Hopefully you now have a better understanding of the people, the processes, and the ingredients involved in creating a skincare product, as well as a clearer picture of what that ingredients list does—and doesn't—tell you.

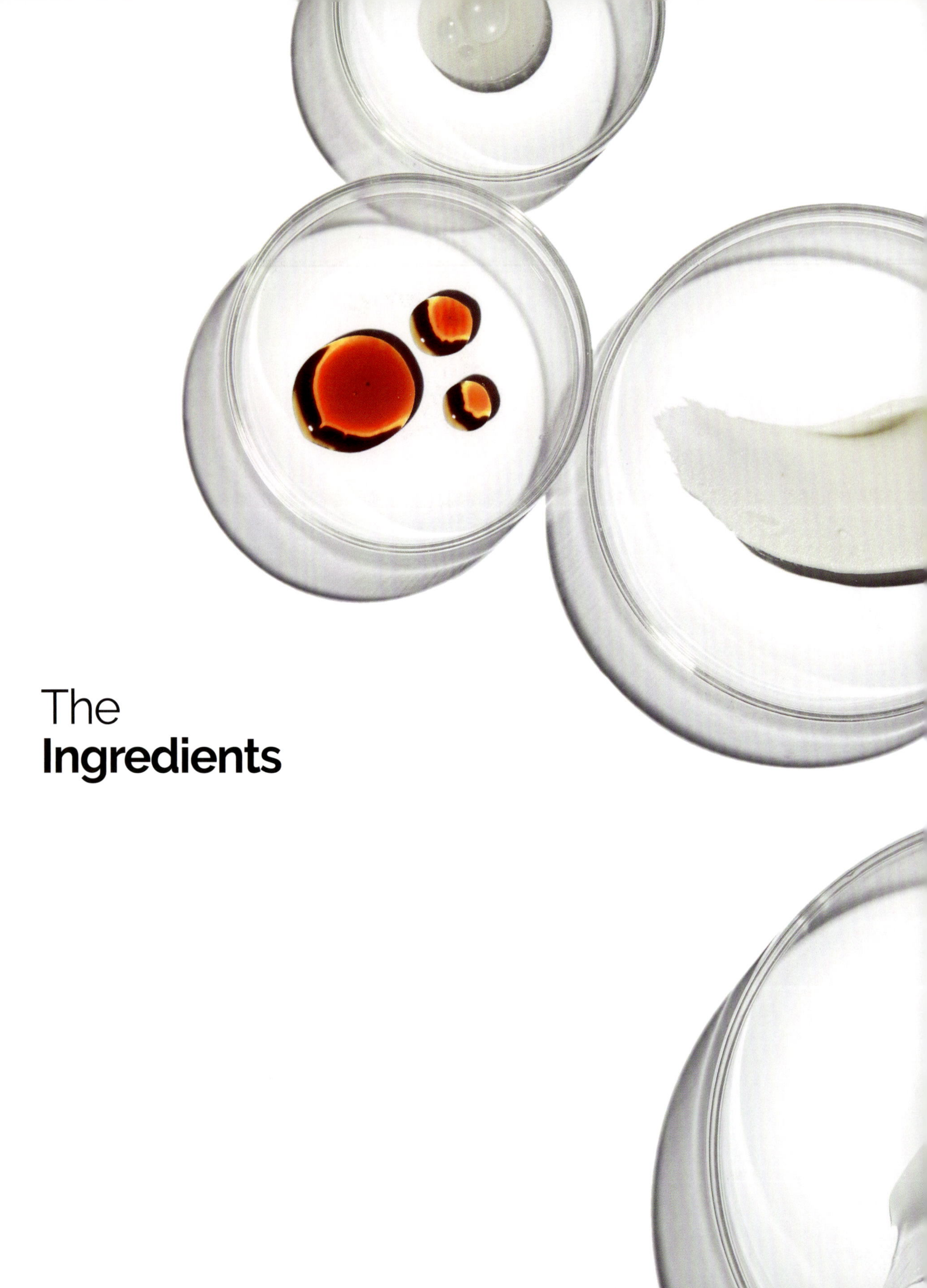

The **Ingredients**

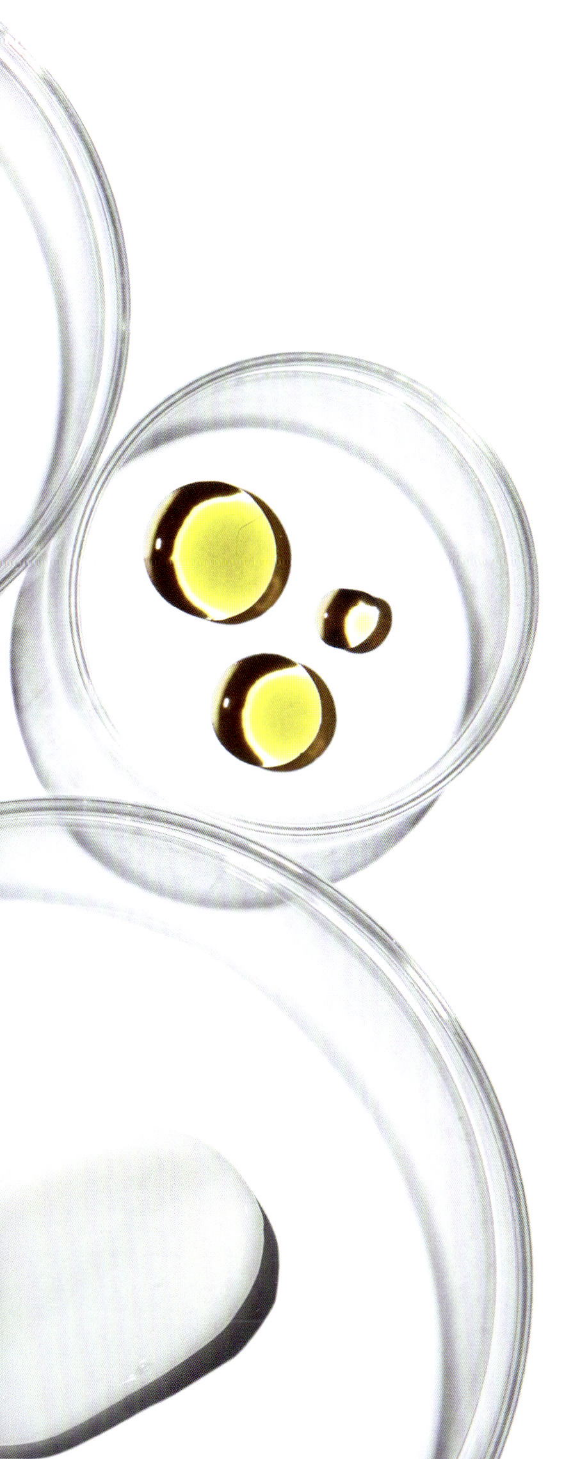

Aloe

001	**INCI Names:**	Aloe barbadensis
002	**Common/ Other Names**	Aloe, aloe vera
003	**Classification**	Humectant
004	**Primary Function**	Hydrating, soothing
005	**Phonetic Spelling**	AL-oh VEH-rah
006	**First Discovered**	Used for centuries in various cultures, with early records dating back to ancient Egypt (around 1500 BCE)
007	**Clinical Concentration(s)**	Can be used up to concentrations of 100% in formulations, depending on the product type

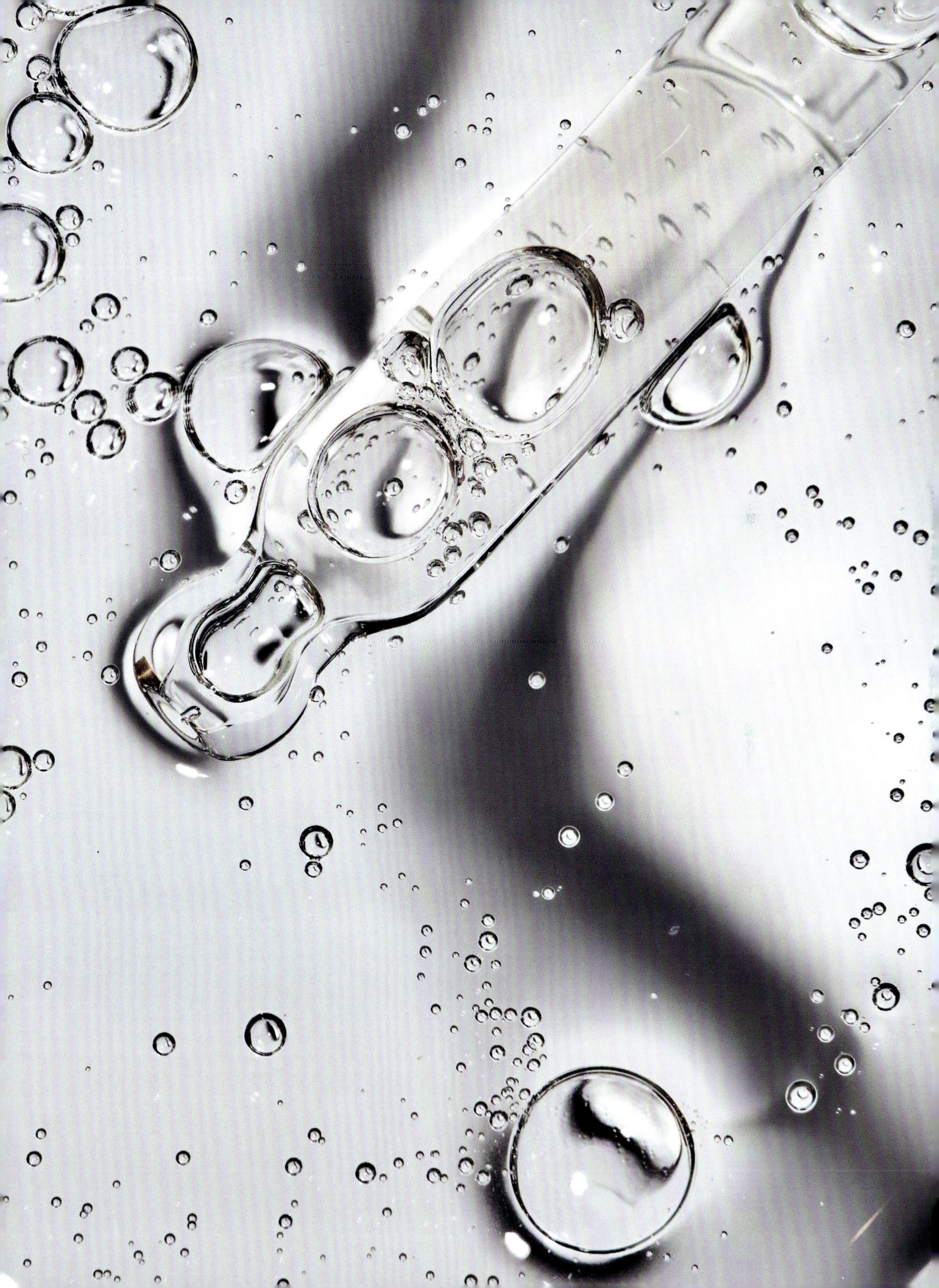

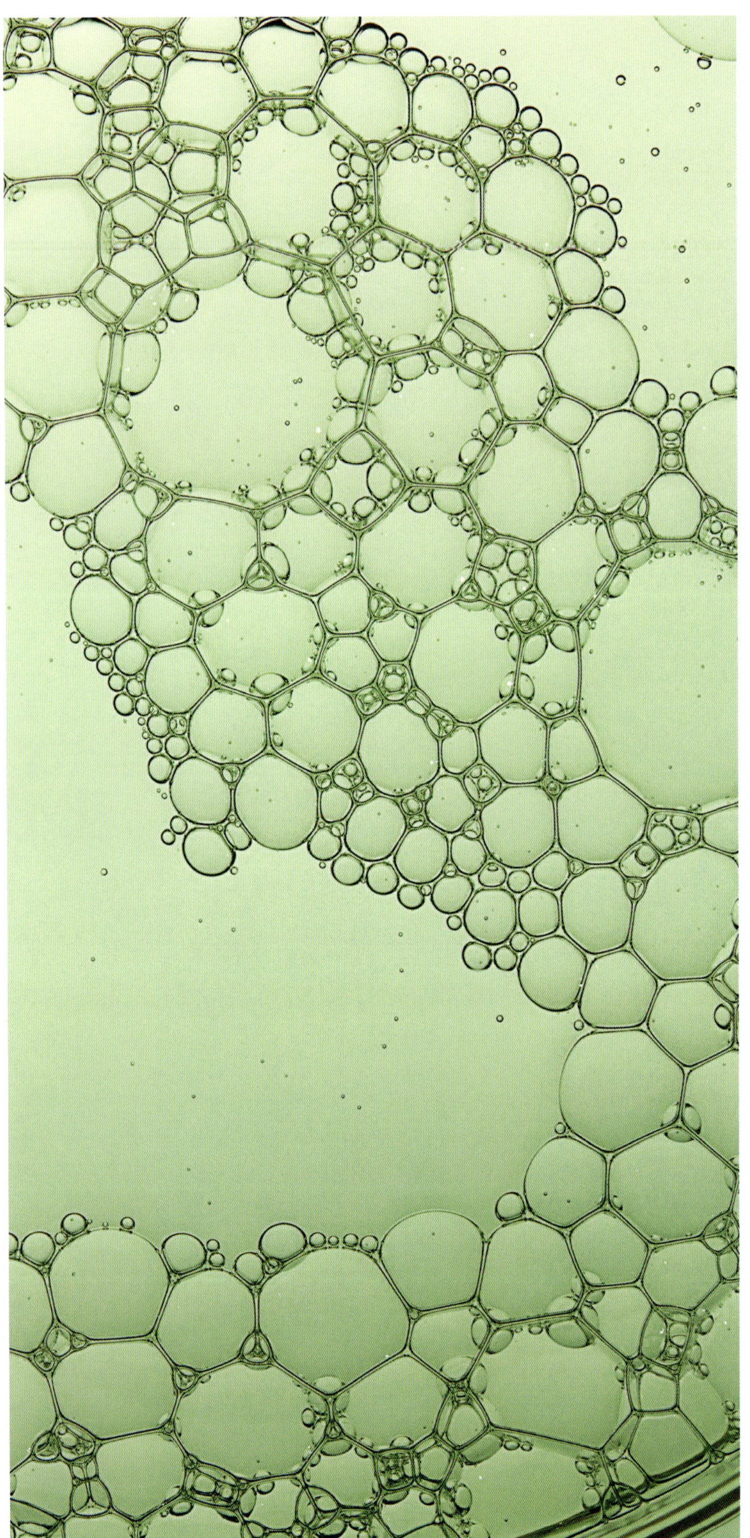

What it is

Aloe is a genus of flowering succulent plants that contains over 600 species. Often referred to as "true aloe," aloe vera is the most widely known aloe species. It grows in dry, hot climates and is recognized by its thick, fleshy leaves. The leaves store water and nutrients, which allow it to survive dry conditions. The plant is easy to grow indoors, making it a popular houseplant as well.

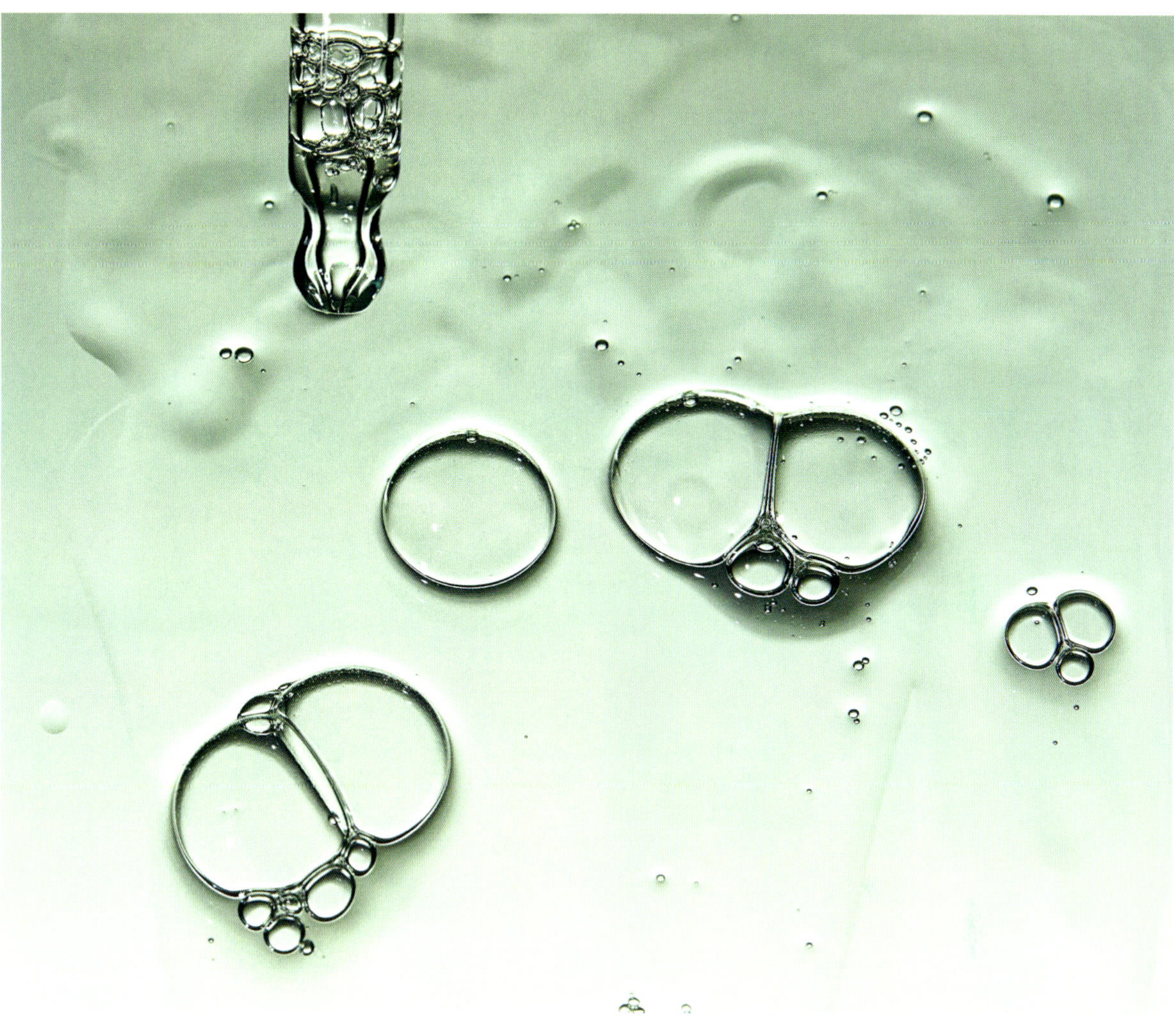

What it's used for

At present, aloe vera gel is popular in cosmetics, haircare, and health products. Aloe is a widely used ingredient in cosmetics, particularly known for its soothing and hydrating properties. The gel extracted from the leaves of the aloe vera plant is packed with water and essential nutrients, making it a go-to moisturizer for both dry and oily skin types. It helps to replenish the skin's moisture balance without leaving a greasy residue, making it suitable for a variety of formulations, from lightweight lotions to more hydrating masks and serums. Aloe is often included in products aimed at soothing irritated skin, thanks to its calming effect, which is why it is frequently found in after-sun treatments and products designed for sensitive skin.

In addition to its moisturizing and calming benefits, aloe vera is rich in antioxidants, such as vitamins C and E, which can help protect the skin from environmental stressors like pollution and UV exposure. These antioxidants support the skin's natural defense mechanisms, promoting a healthier-looking complexion. Aloe also contains enzymes that can gently exfoliate the skin, helping to improve skin texture and promote a more even tone.

Mechanism of action

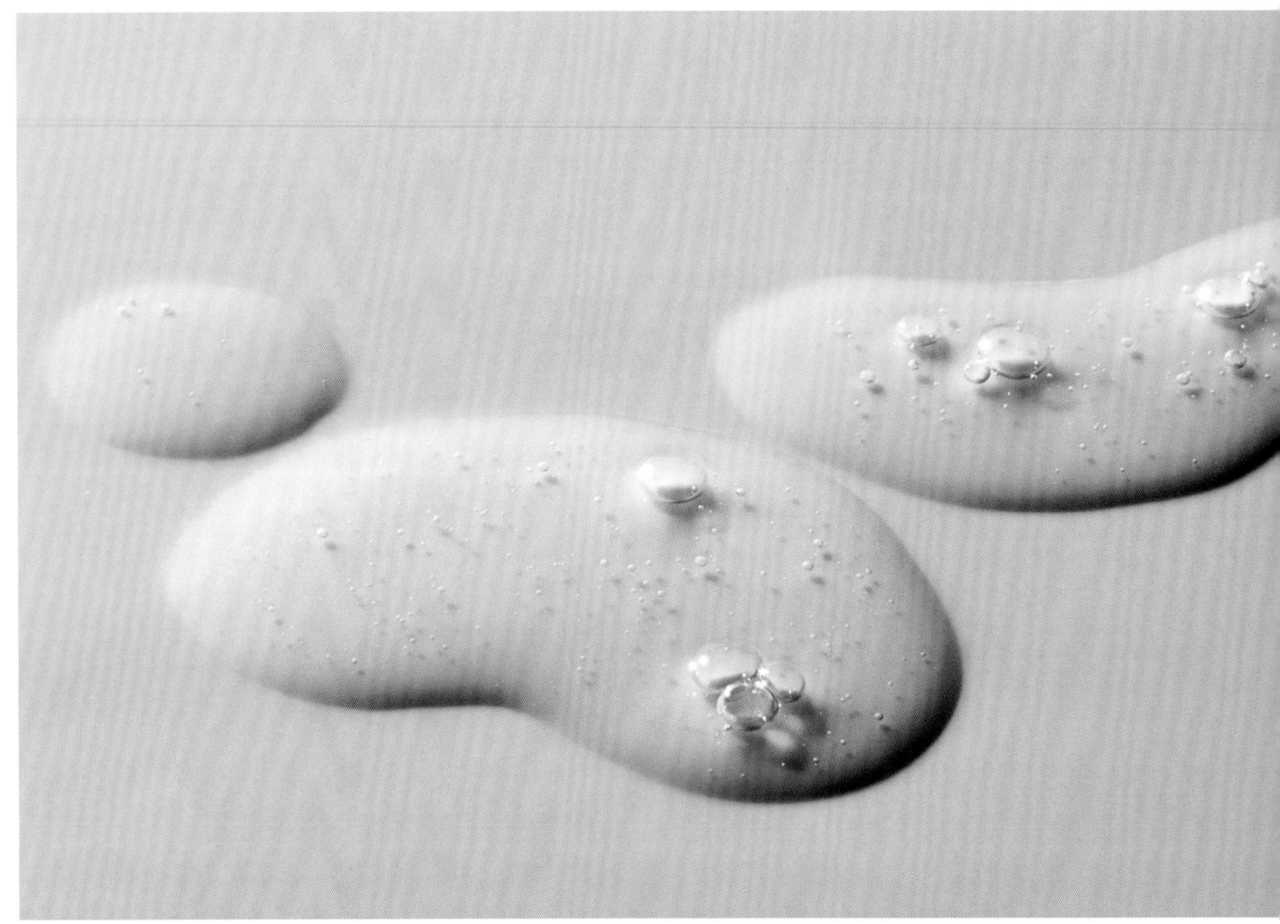

Moisturizing

Aloe vera gel is composed largely of water and, when applied topically, it helps to replenish the skin's moisture levels. Applying aloe vera extract to the skin has been shown to increase the water content of the stratum corneum (the outermost layer of skin). Aloe also contains polysaccharides, such as acemannan, which have humectant properties, attracting moisture to the skin and enhancing its ability to retain water. This helps improve the skin's moisture balance, making it feel softer and more supple. By enhancing the skin's hydration, aloe can also help reduce the appearance of dryness and flakiness.

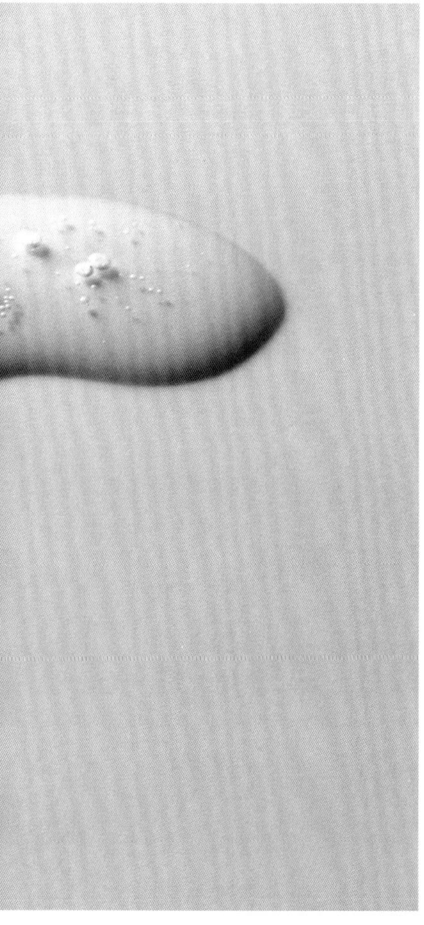

Soothing

In addition to its moisturizing properties, aloe vera is known for its calming effect on the skin. This is largely because it contains compounds such as glycoproteins, which reduce the sensation of irritation and inflammation. These glycoproteins help to calm redness, irritation, and discomfort in the skin. This makes aloe a common ingredient in products formulated for sensitive or sun-exposed skin.

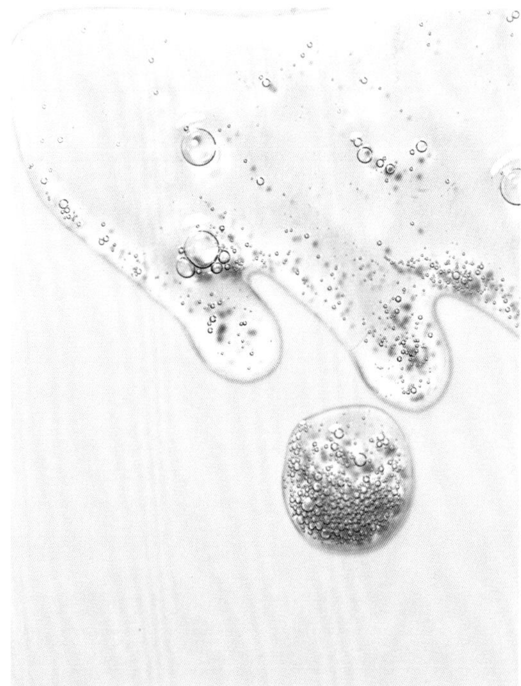

001 **INCI Names:** Alpha-Arbutin

002 **Common/ Other Names** α-arbutin, 4-hydroxyphenyl-alpha-D-glucopyranoside, hydroquinone-O-α-d-glucopyranoside, 4-hydroxyphenyl α-d-gluco-hexopyranoside

003 **Classification** Glycoside

Alpha-arbutin

004 **Primary Function** Uneven tone

005 **Phonetic Spelling** AL-fuh ar-BYOO-tin

006 **First Discovered** A. Kawalier, 1852

007 **Clinical Concentration(s)** 2–10%

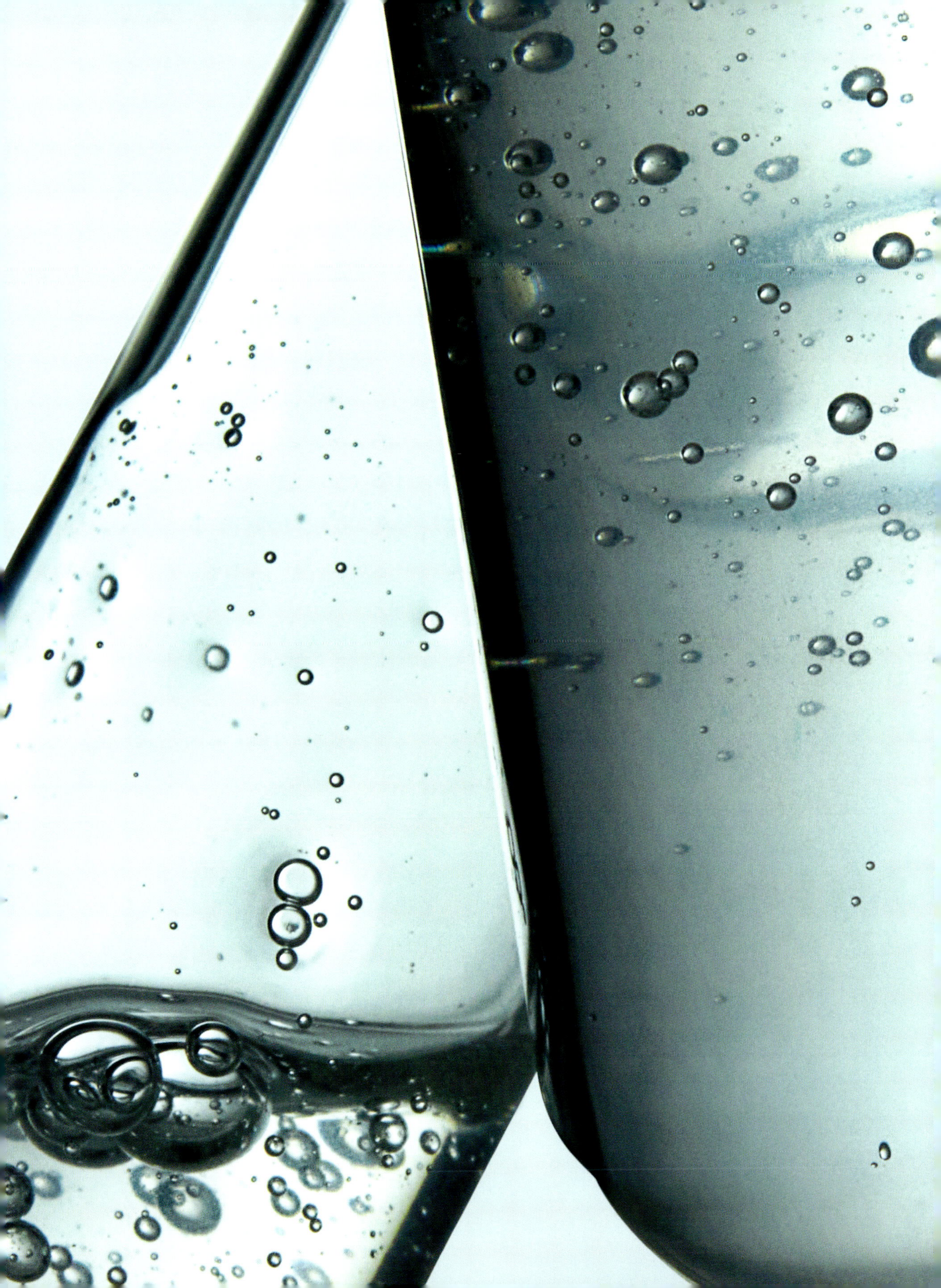

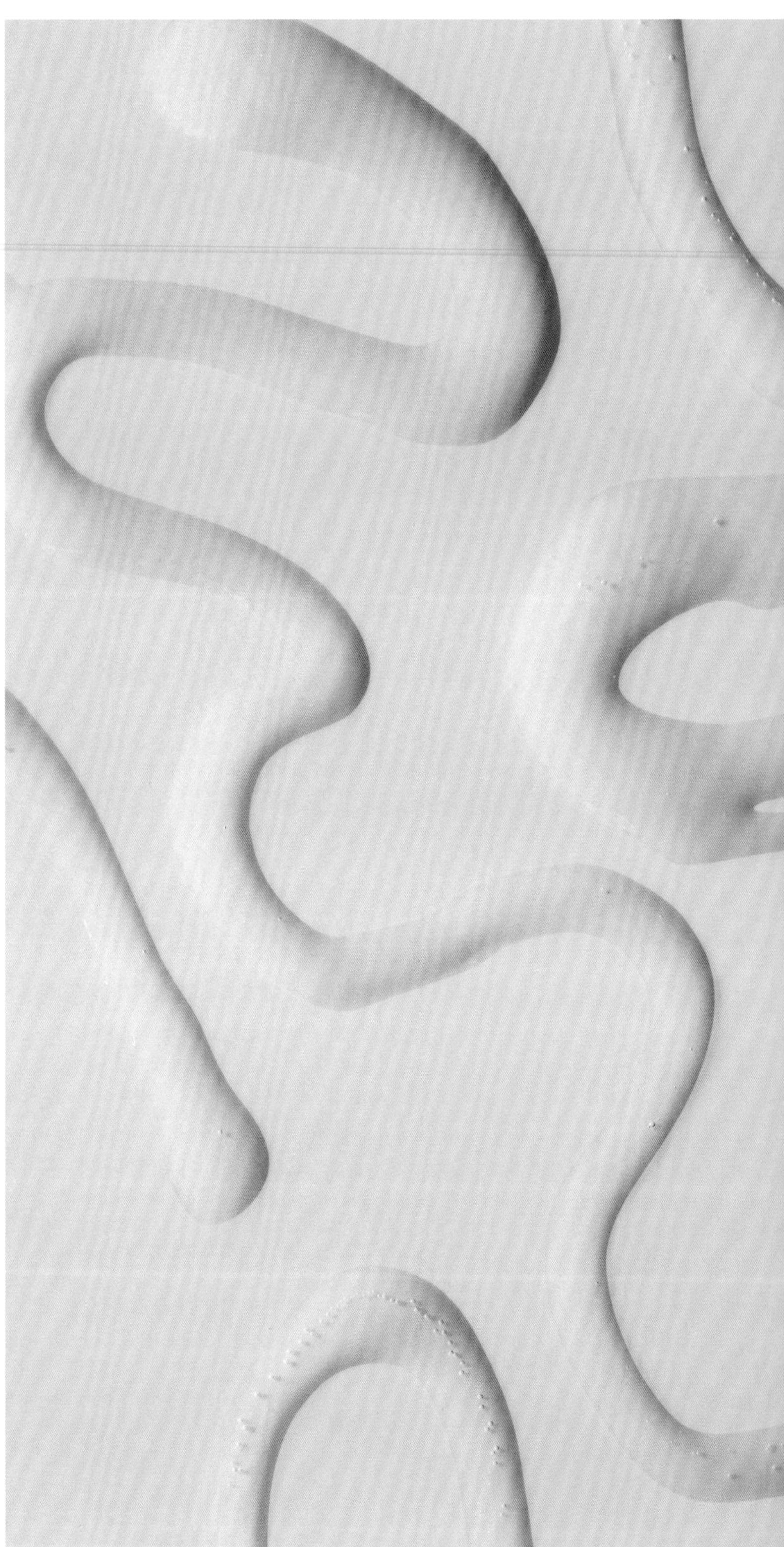

What it is

Alpha-arbutin (α-arbutin) is a naturally occurring derivative of hydroquinone, a compound known for its ability to target uneven skin tone. Chemically, α-arbutin is a glycosylated hydroquinone, meaning it has a hydroquinone molecule bound to a sugar molecule (D-glucose). While hydroquinone is an effective ingredient, it carries safety concerns. Alpha-arbutin offers a safer alternative due to its different chemical structure.

There are two isomers of arbutin: alpha-arbutin and beta-arbutin. The difference lies in the way the D-glucose molecule is attached to hydroquinone. Alpha-arbutin is not found naturally and is produced through enzymatic or microbial synthesis. In contrast, beta-arbutin (β-arbutin) occurs naturally in plants like bearberry, pear, and wheat, but is not as stable, making it less desirable for cosmetic applications.

What it's used for

Alpha-arbutin is a popular skincare ingredient due to its ability to address a range of pigmentation concerns and promote a brighter, more even complexion. Thanks to its ability to improve the appearance of dark spots, it is commonly found in formulations that target the look of sun spots, age spots, and post-blemish marks, and that promote a more radiant appearance. Less commonly, alpha-arbutin can also be used to address specific concerns like the sallowness and loss of elasticity associated with glycation, a process where sugar molecules bind to important structural proteins.

Mechanism of action

Alpha-arbutin is a powerful brightening ingredient that works by targeting tyrosinase, the key enzyme involved in the initial stages of melanin production in the skin. By attaching to the enzyme's active site, alpha-arbutin interrupts the process that leads to the formation of melanin, helping to visibly reduce the appearance of dark spots and uneven skin tone. Its potency surpasses that of its beta isomer, arbutin, making alpha-arbutin a superior choice for achieving a more radiant complexion. This difference in potency is attributed to the alpha-glucoside bond in alpha-arbutin having a greater affinity for tyrosinase's active site than the beta-glucoside bond in beta-arbutin.

Both isomers of arbutin also demonstrate a strong antioxidant capacity, which can begin to elucidate alpha-arbutin's ability to counteract the effects of glycation. Reactive oxygen species (ROS) play a significant role in promoting the formation of advanced glycation end products (AGEs), the harmful compounds that contribute to glycation-induced skin damage. Alpha-arbutin's ability to scavenge ROS, including hydroxyl radicals, and increase glutathione levels, inhibiting ROS production, could potentially mitigate the oxidative stress that drives AGE formation. This antioxidant action might help protect the skin from AGE-induced damage, indirectly contributing to firmer, more youthful-looking skin.

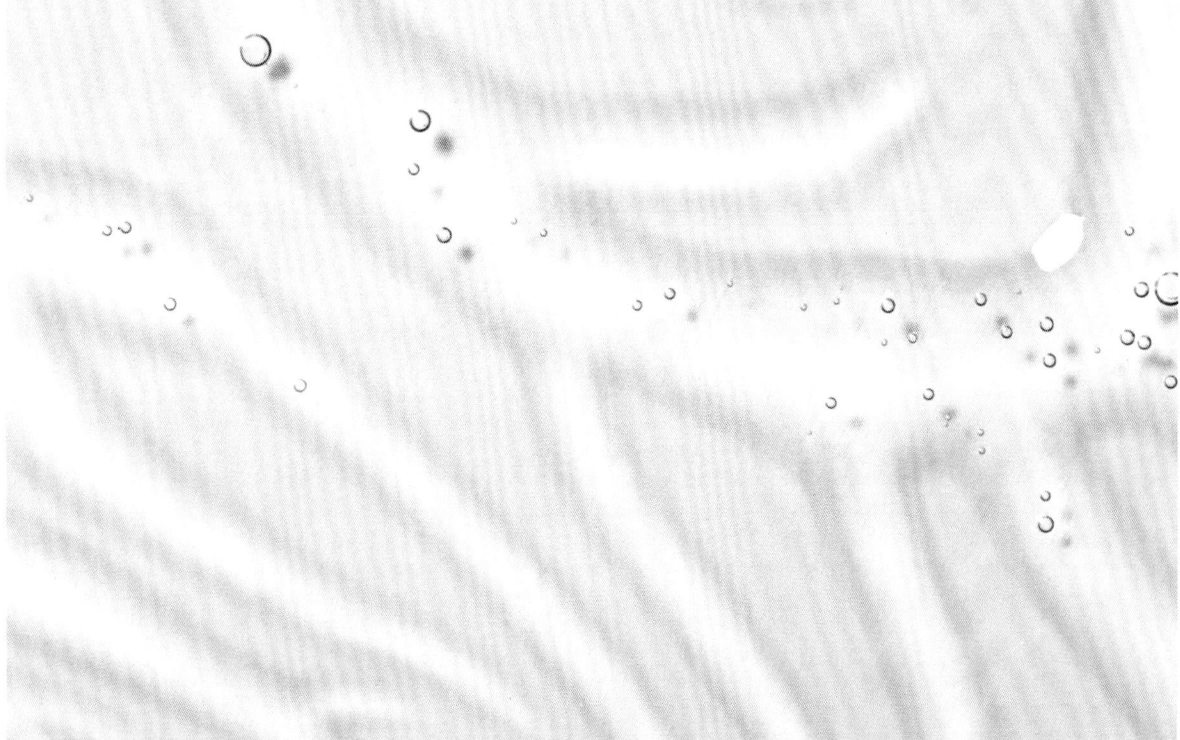

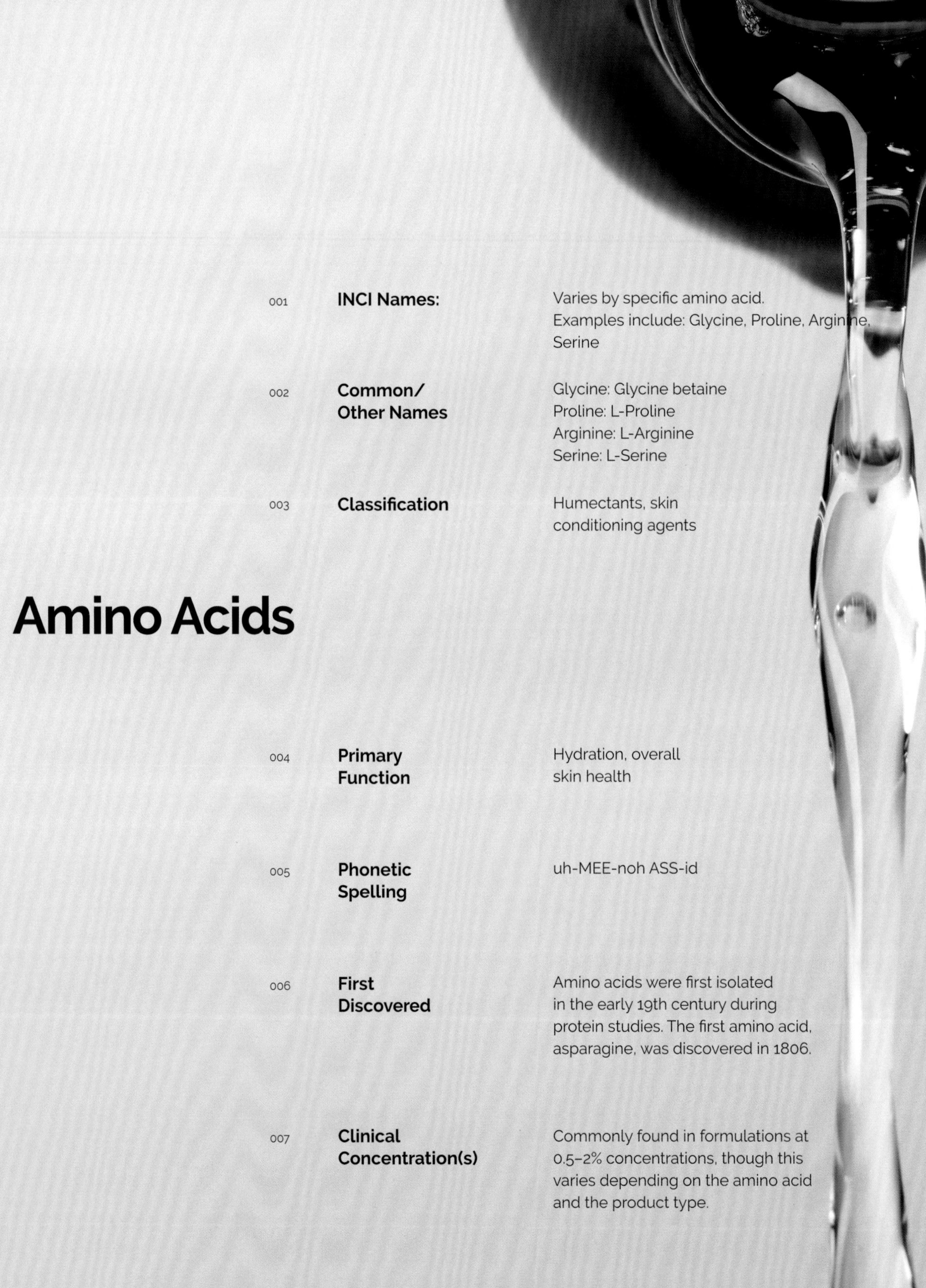

Amino Acids

001 **INCI Names:** Varies by specific amino acid. Examples include: Glycine, Proline, Arginine, Serine

002 **Common/ Other Names** Glycine: Glycine betaine
Proline: L-Proline
Arginine: L-Arginine
Serine: L-Serine

003 **Classification** Humectants, skin conditioning agents

004 **Primary Function** Hydration, overall skin health

005 **Phonetic Spelling** uh-MEE-noh ASS-id

006 **First Discovered** Amino acids were first isolated in the early 19th century during protein studies. The first amino acid, asparagine, was discovered in 1806.

007 **Clinical Concentration(s)** Commonly found in formulations at 0.5–2% concentrations, though this varies depending on the amino acid and the product type.

What it is

Amino acids are organic compounds that serve as the building blocks of proteins, essential to nearly all biological processes in the body. They are composed of carbon, hydrogen, oxygen, and nitrogen, and their structure includes an amino group ($-NH_2$), a carboxyl group ($-COOH$), and a side chain that varies between different amino acids. These compounds are critical for growth, repair, and maintenance of cells and tissues. In total, 20 standard amino acids are naturally found in the human body, categorized into essential (must be obtained through diet) and non-essential (produced by the body).

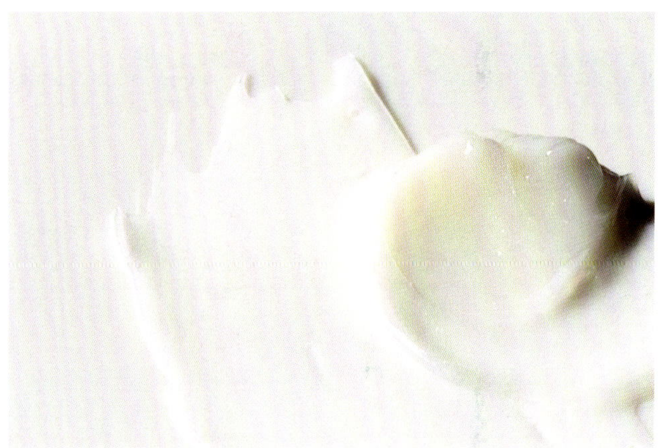

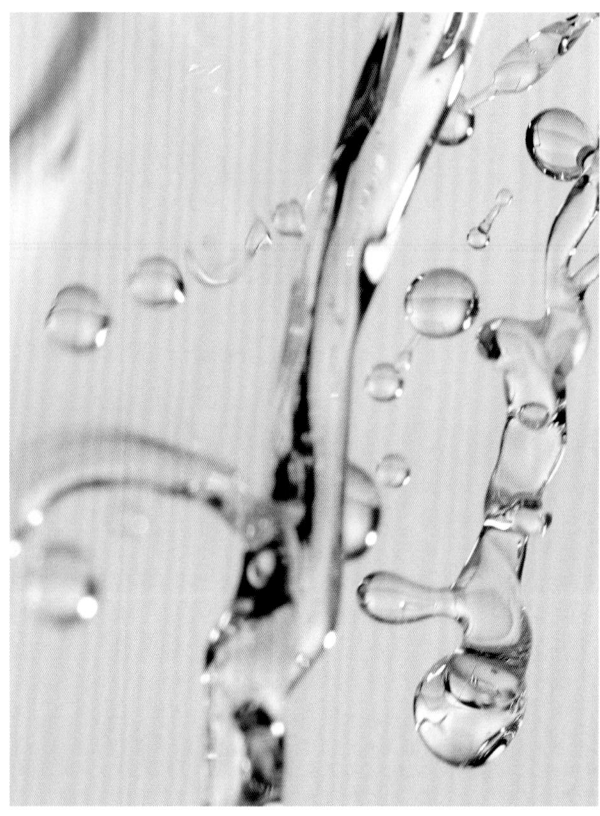

What it's used for

In skincare, amino acids play a vital role in maintaining skin health and hydration. Naturally present in the skin as part of the Natural Moisturizing Factors (NMF), they help retain water, support the skin barrier, and improve elasticity. Additionally, amino acids can contribute to collagen production and antioxidant protection. Their small molecular size allows them to penetrate the skin effectively, making them popular ingredients in hydrating and anti-aging products.

Mechanism of action

Amino acids in skincare work by mimicking and replenishing the skin's Natural Moisturizing Factors (NMF), which are crucial for maintaining optimal hydration levels. Their small molecular size allows them to penetrate the skin's outermost layers, where they attract and bind water molecules through their hydrophilic properties. This action enhances the skin's ability to retain moisture, keeping it hydrated and supple while supporting the skin barrier to reduce water loss.

Additionally, amino acids also provide the building blocks necessary for the production of proteins like collagen and elastin, which help improve the look of firmness and elasticity in the skin. Some amino acids also exhibit antioxidant properties, supporting the skin antioxidant responses and working synergistically with other antioxidants in your skincare routine. This combined effect of improved hydration, firmness and elasticity, and barrier support contributes to healthier, more resilient skin over time.

Argan Oil

001	**INCI Names:**	Argania spinosa kernel oil
002	**Common/ Other Names**	Argan oil
003	**Classification**	Plant oil, emollient
004	**Primary Function**	Hydration
005	**Phonetic Spelling**	AHR-guhn OYL
006	**First Discovered**	Argan oil has been used for centuries in Morocco for its cosmetic and medicinal properties. It began gaining significant commercial use in the global skincare industry around the early 2000s.
007	**Clinical Concentration(s)**	Up to 100%

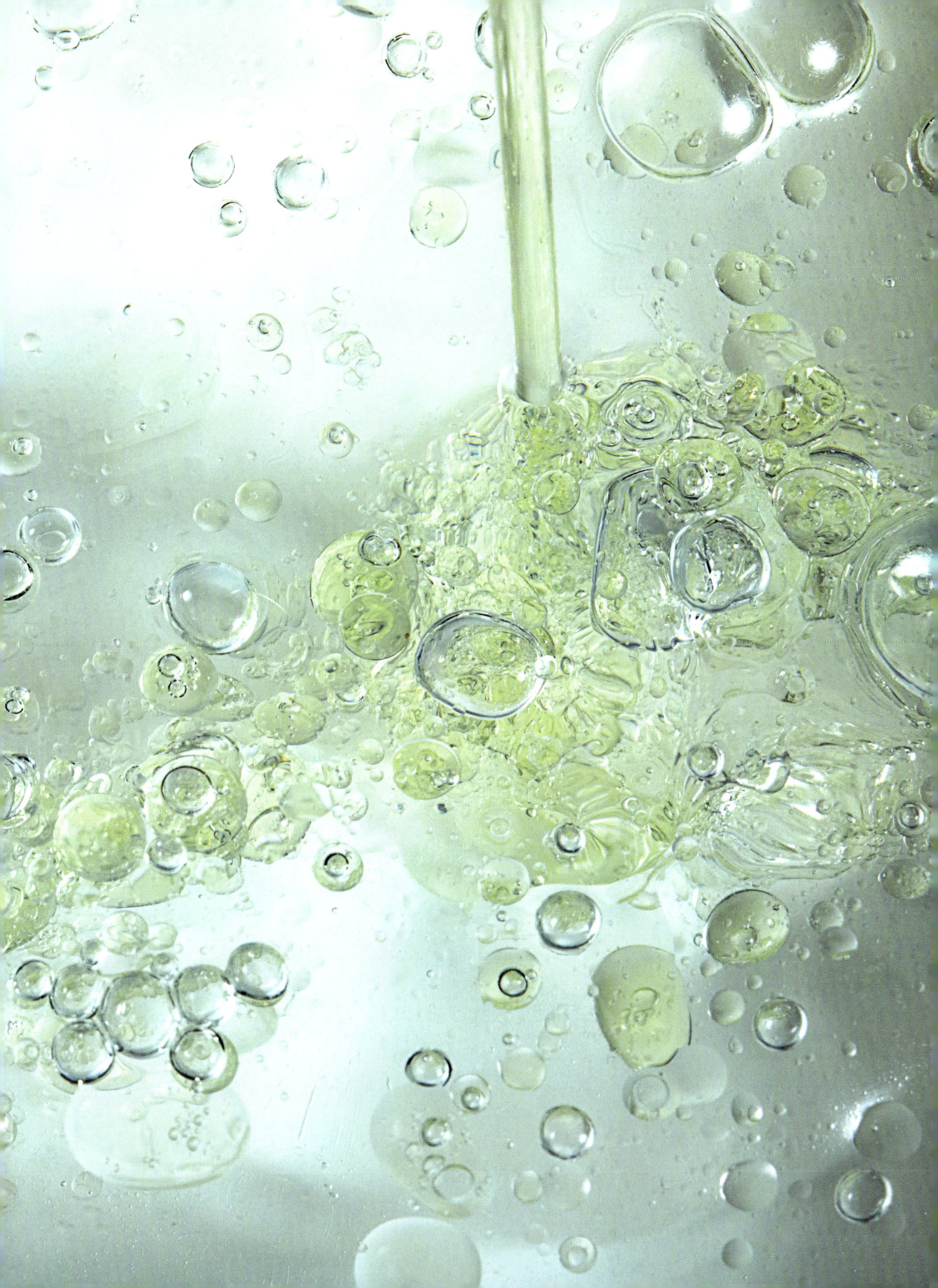

What it is

Argan oil, extracted from the nuts of the *Argania spinosa* tree native to Morocco, is a highly sought-after ingredient in skincare and haircare products due to its rich composition of essential fatty acids, antioxidants, and vitamin E.

What it's used for

This plant oil is celebrated for its nourishing properties, which make it an effective moisturizer and hydrator. It contains a high concentration of oleic acid, linoleic acid, and palmitic acid, which help to restore the skin's lipid barrier and lock in moisture, leaving the skin soft, smooth, and supple. Additionally, argan oil is known for its antioxidant properties, thanks to the presence of vitamin E and polyphenols, which help protect the skin from environmental damage and premature aging.

Its versatility makes it popular not only in skin moisturizers but also in hair treatments, where it helps improve elasticity, shine, and manageability. Argan oil's gentle, non-greasy texture makes it suitable for all skin types and it is often found in products designed to tackle issues such as dryness and hair frizz. Due to its nutrient-dense composition, argan oil remains a cornerstone of natural beauty and personal care products globally.

Mechanism of action

Argan oil works in cosmetics primarily through its rich content of fatty acids, particularly oleic and linoleic acids, which help to replenish and reinforce the skin's natural lipid barrier. This enhances moisture retention and protects the skin from dehydration. Argan oil can also contain antioxidants like vitamin E, which combat free radicals, reducing oxidative stress and promoting healthy-looking skin. Its soothing properties can calm irritated skin, while its ability to nourish and condition the hair is due to its high content of essential fatty acids and vitamins.

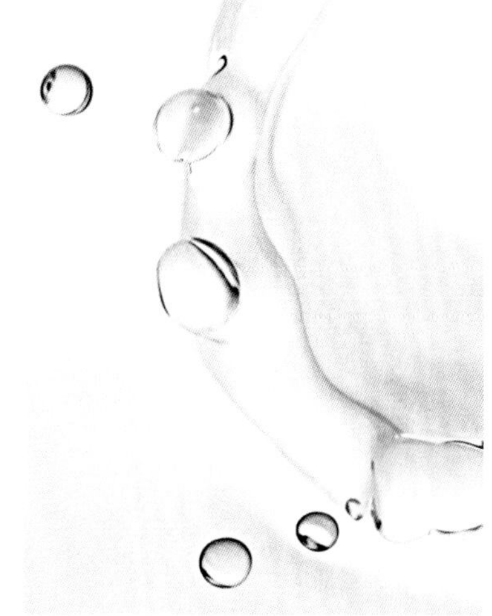

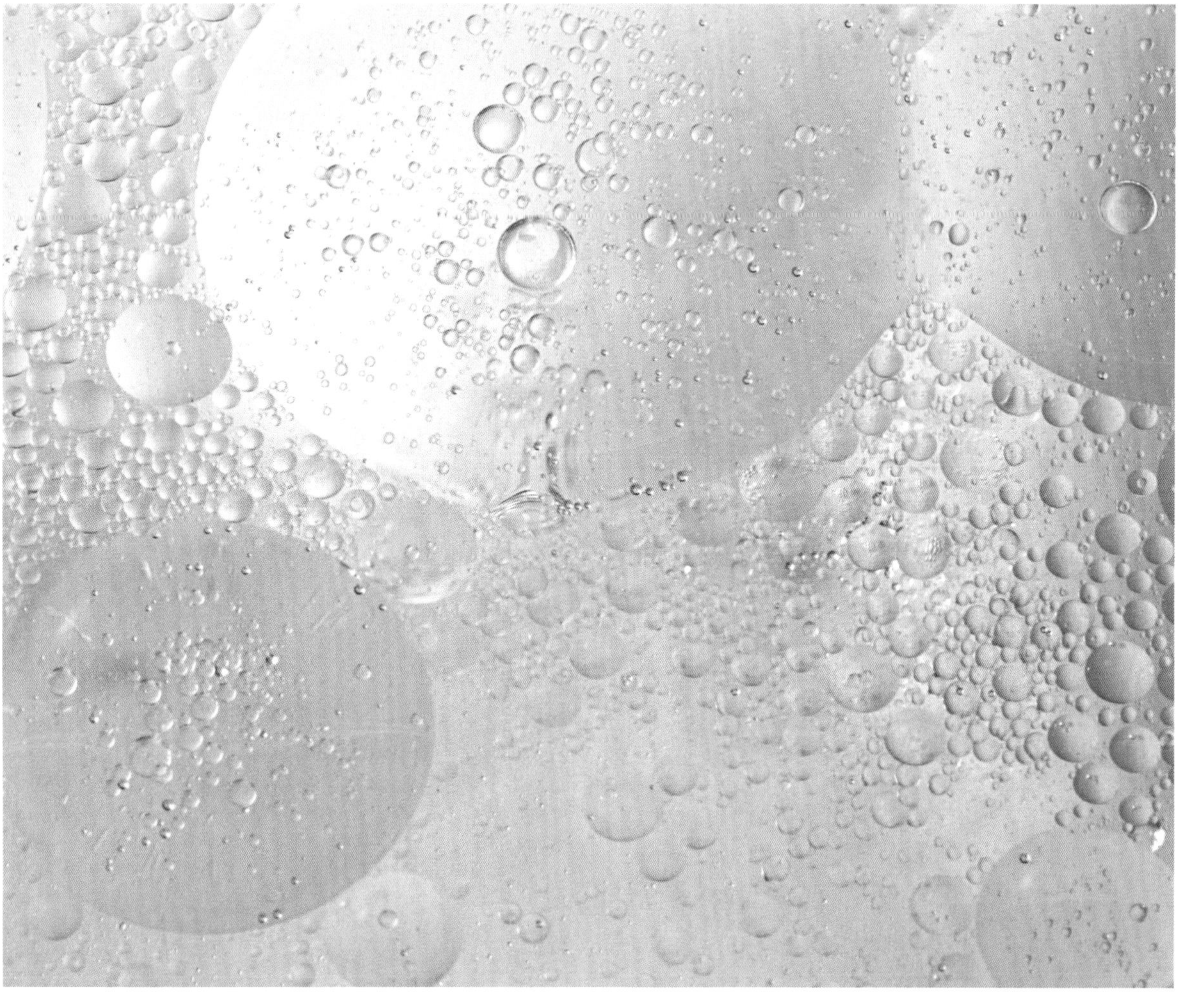

001 **INCI Names:** Acetyl Hexapeptide-8 (*Argireline*) & Acetyl Hexapeptide-8, Pentapeptide-18 (*Argirelox*)

002 **Common/ Other Names** Argireline™
Argirelox™

003 **Classification** Peptide

Argireline™ / Argirelox™

004 **Primary Function** Age support

005 **Phonetic Spelling** AR-juh-reh-leen (Argireline™), Ar-JEER-uh-loks (Argirelox™)

006 **First Discovered** Lubrizol, 2001

007 **Clinical Concentration(s)** 2–10%

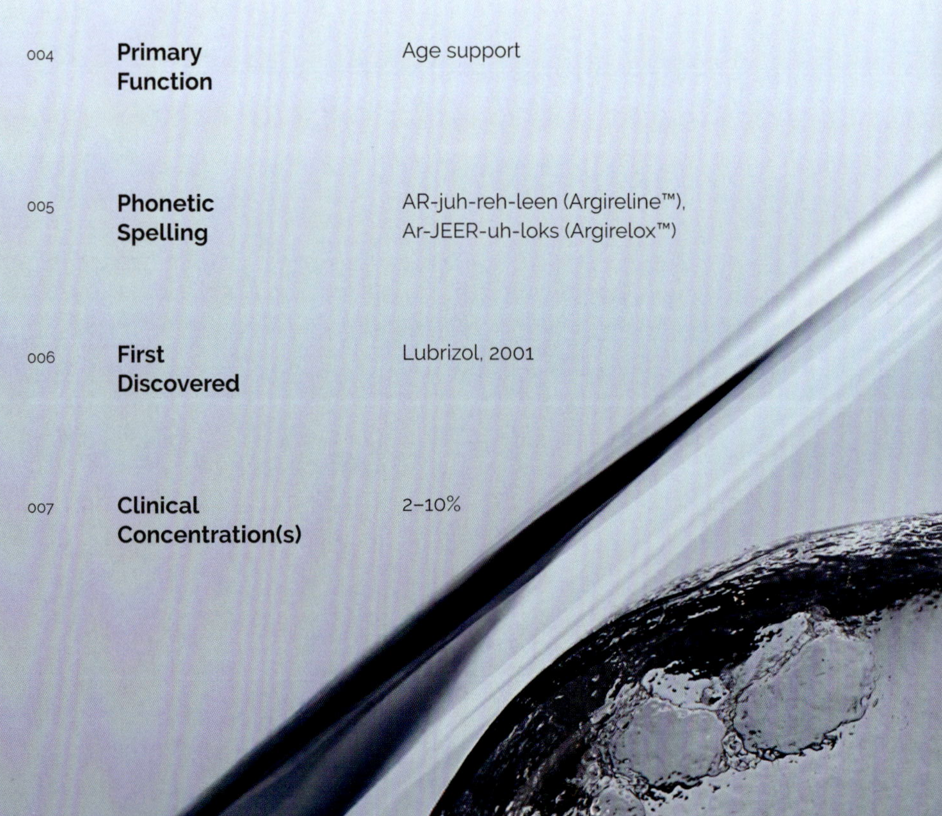

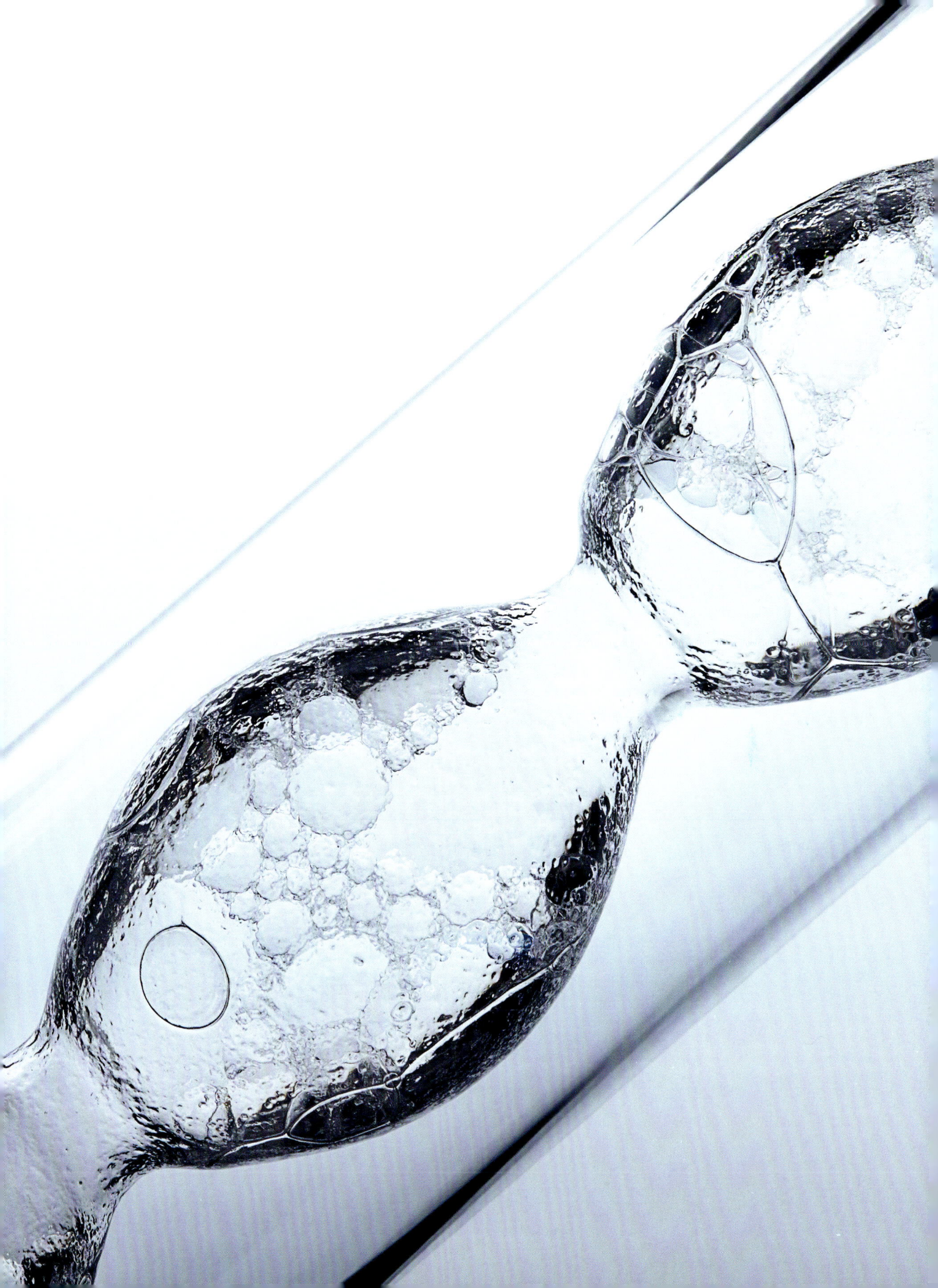

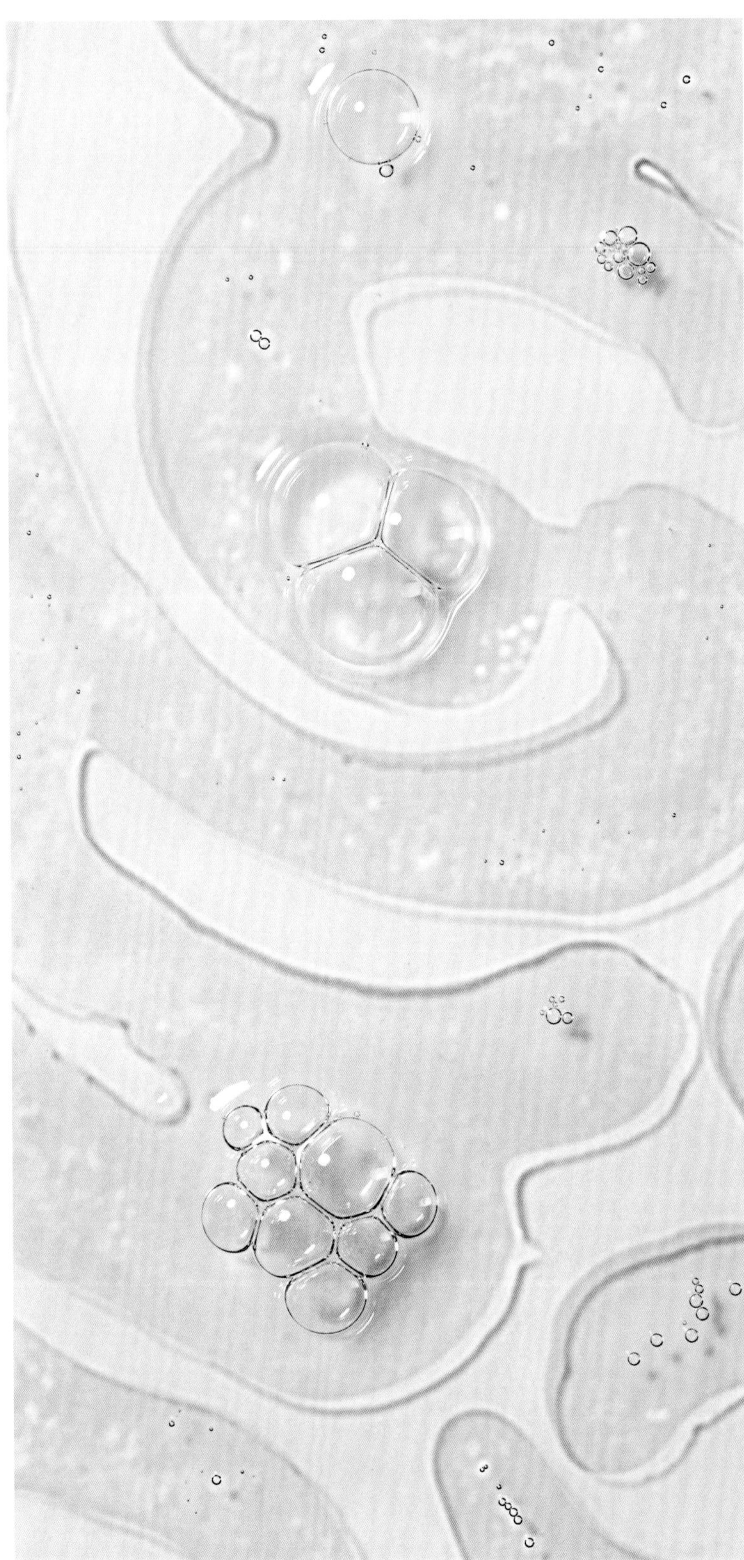

What it is

Argireline™ and Argirelox™ are both peptide complexes, with both containing Acetyl Hexapeptide-8, and Argirelox™ containing Pentapeptide-18 in addition. Peptides are small chains of amino acids that act by signaling molecules to target specific aspects of the skin. In the case of these two peptides, they are both classified as neurotransmitter peptides.

What it's used for

Argireline™ and Argirelox™ are innovative peptide-based ingredients used in skincare to address the visible signs of aging, such as fine lines and wrinkles. These advanced formulations work by targeting the appearance of expression lines that form as a result of repetitive muscle contractions.

Skincare products featuring Argireline™ or Argirelox™ are often included in formulations designed for daily use, offering a gentle, non-invasive approach to achieving smoother and more radiant-looking skin. Their compatibility with other active ingredients makes them versatile additions to multi-functional anti-aging routines, delivering visible results that help enhance skin's overall appearance.

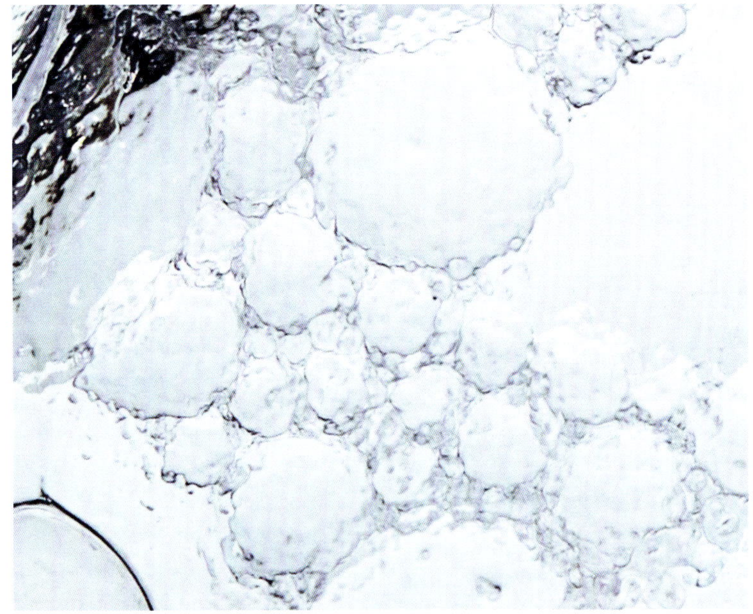

Mechanism of action

Repeated muscle contraction is one of the primary contributing factors that leads to the formation of fine lines and wrinkles over time. As a peptide, Acetyl Hexapeptide-8 is composed of amino acids that interact with the skin's surface, targeting areas prone to repetitive facial movements, such as around the eyes, forehead, and mouth. Its action helps to relax the visible effects of these dynamic movements, promoting a smoother and more youthful-looking appearance.

001	**INCI Names:**	Ascorbyl glucoside
002	**Common/ Other Names**	Vitamin C, ascorbic acid 2-glucoside, ascorbyl-2-glucoside, 2-O-α-D-glucopyranosyl-L-ascorbic acid
003	**Classification**	Antioxidant, Vitamin C derivative

Ascorbyl Glucoside

004	**Primary Function**	Antioxidant, uneven tone, signs of aging
005	**Phonetic Spelling**	uh-SKOR-bil GLOO-koh-side
006	**First Discovered**	N. Muto, S. Suga, K. Fujii, K. Goto & I. Yamamoto, 1990
007	**Clinical Concentration(s)**	2–10%

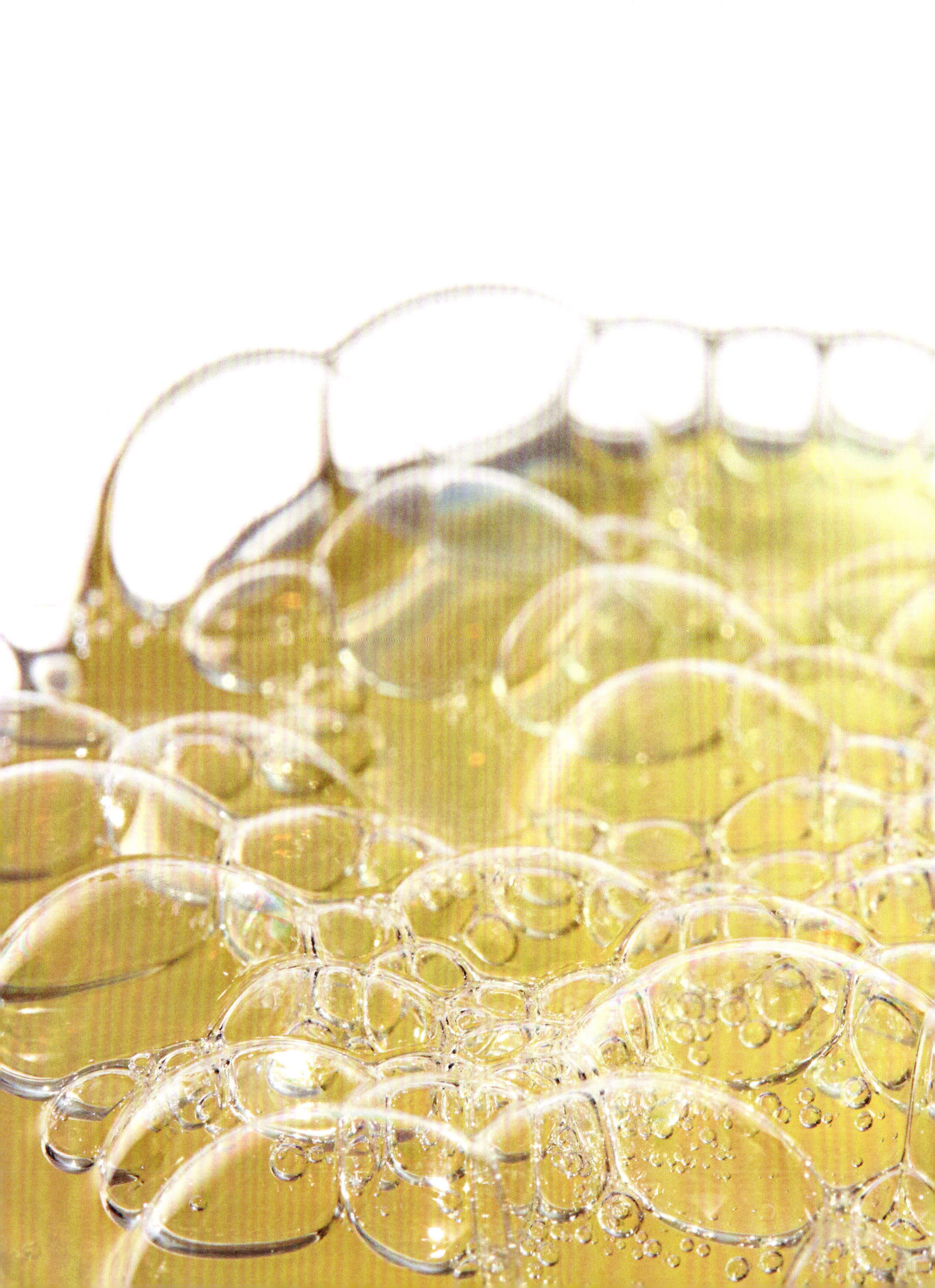

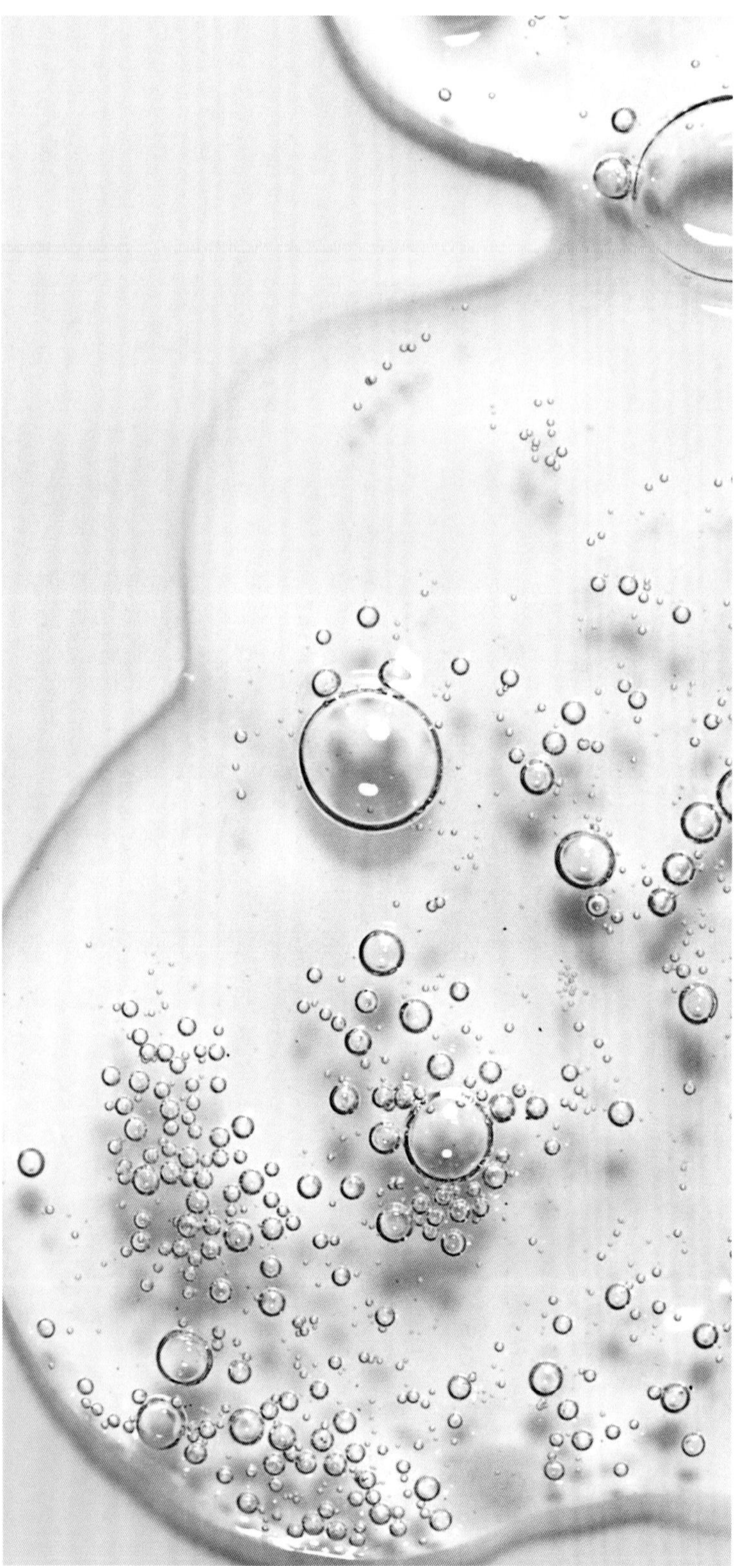

What it is

Ascorbyl glucoside is a chemically modified form of L-ascorbic acid (vitamin C). It is created through a process called biocatalytic transglucosylation, where a glucose molecule is attached to the ascorbic acid molecule. This modification enhances the stability of vitamin C, creating a water-soluble form of the molecule that is less prone to oxidation and degradation, allowing for easier formulation and longevity of the product.

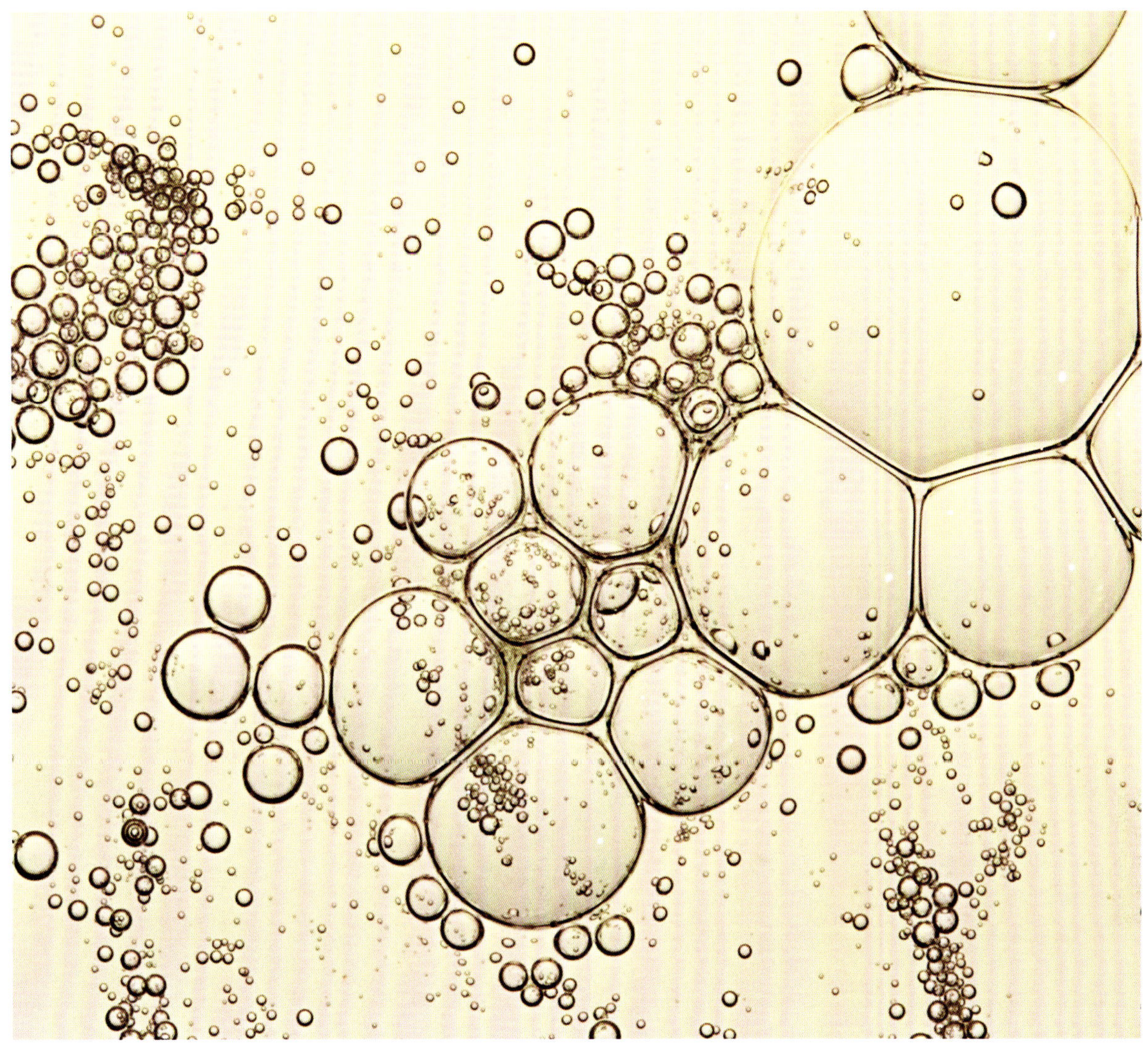

What it's used for

Ascorbyl glucoside must be broken down in the skin in order to release the active form of vitamin C (L-ascorbic acid). For this reason, ascorbyl glucoside is primarily used in skincare for its potential to provide the benefits of L-ascorbic acid in a more stable and deliverable form, as the bioactive end molecule is one and the same.

Much like L-ascorbic acid, it is included in formulations for its antioxidant properties, its ability to reduce the appearance of wrinkles and fine lines, and its effects on uneven skin tone, including age spots and sun spots.

Mechanism of action

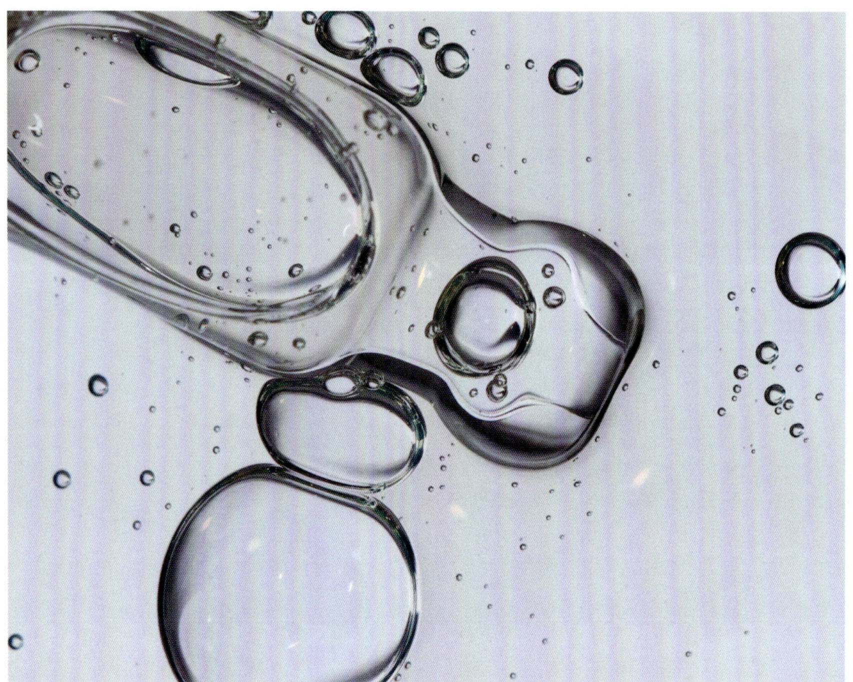

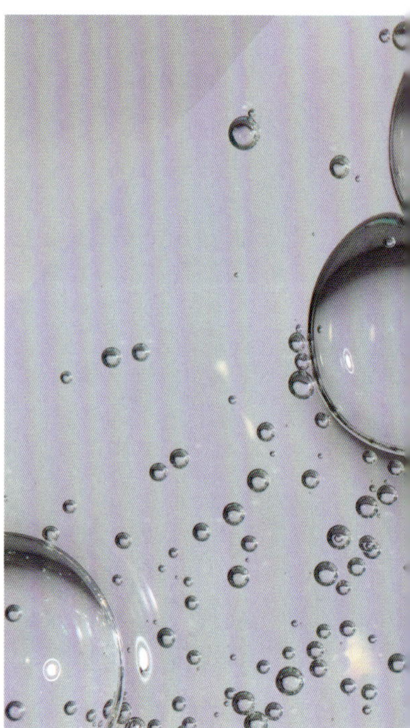

Ascorbyl glucoside can help to neutralize free radicals and their damaging effects, which can contribute to common concerns we associate with environmental stressors, like signs of aging and dullness. Although not as potent as L-ascorbic acid, it still contributes to the overall antioxidant capacity of skincare formulations.

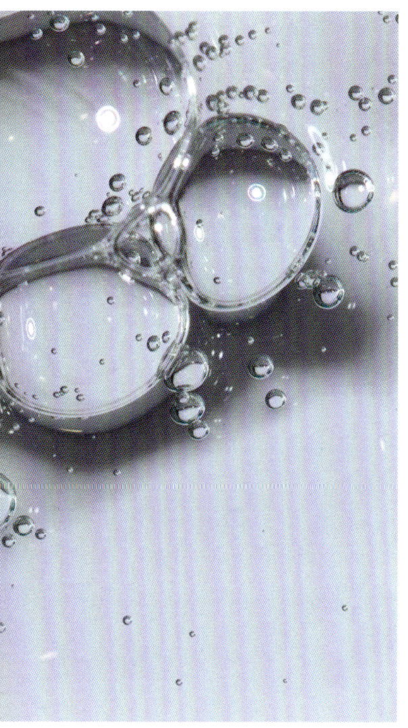

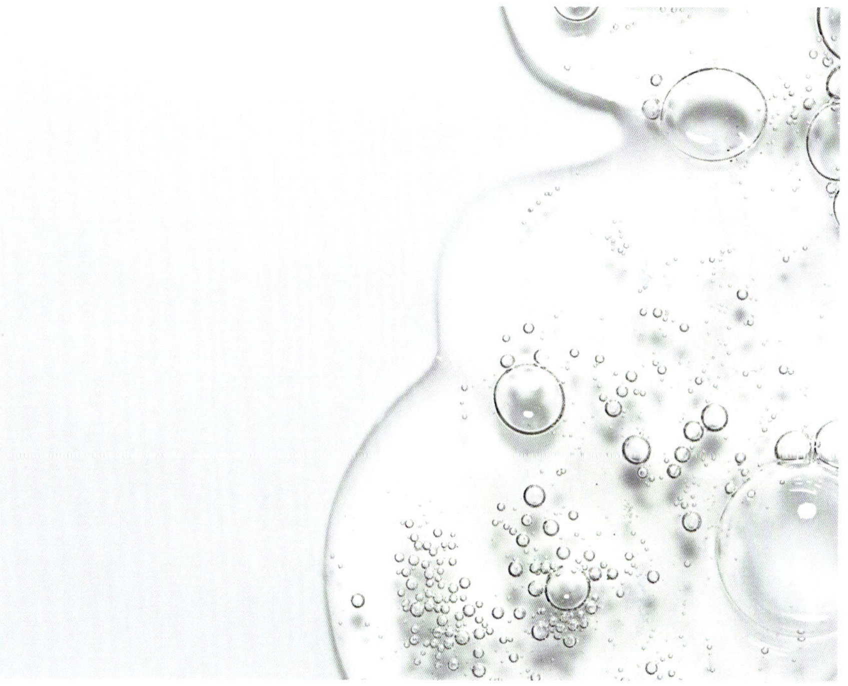

Much like L-ascorbic acid, ascorbyl glucoside has also been shown to support the skin's natural collagen, a key structural protein that maintains skin elasticity and firmness, and is directly associated with the appearance of fine lines and wrinkles.

While published literature assessing the effects of ascorbyl glucoside alone on uneven tone is lacking, it is known that ascorbic acid, and potentially ascorbyl glucoside after conversion, can inhibit tyrosinase activity. This inhibition can reduce melanin formation and may help improve the appearance of discoloration, making ascorbyl glucoside a popular choice for formulations designed for this purpose.

Azelaic Acid

001	**INCI Names:**	Azelaic acid
002	**Common/ Other Names**	Nonanedioic acid
003	**Classification**	Dicarboxylic acid, exfoliant
004	**Primary Function**	Exfoliation, soothing
005	**Phonetic Spelling**	az-uh-LAY-ik ASS-id
006	**First Discovered**	M. Nazzaro-Porro, 1978
007	**Clinical Concentration(s)**	10–20%

What it is

Azelaic acid is a naturally occurring dicarboxylic acid commonly used in skincare formulations. Found in grains like wheat, rye, and barley, it is known for its gentle exfoliating properties and its ability to address uneven skin tone and blemish-prone skin. Chemically, azelaic acid is an aliphatic, saturated dicarboxylic acid with the molecular formula $C_9H_{16}O_4$. It appears as a white, crystalline powder and is both water-soluble and oil-dispersible, which makes it versatile in cosmetic formulations.

One of the notable chemical properties of azelaic acid is its stability across a broad pH range, typically between 4 and 6, making it suitable for various skincare products. It is also non-comedogenic, meaning it does not clog pores, which contributes to its popularity in formulations for oily or blemish-prone skin.

What it's used for

Azelaic acid is a versatile ingredient in skincare known for its mild exfoliating action, helping to refine the skin's surface and unclog pores. This gentle exfoliation promotes a smoother texture and can help address common concerns such as post-blemish marks and uneven skin tone. Azelaic acid also has significant skin-calming properties, making it a great choice for reducing redness, irritation, and bumps. In addition, it provides antioxidant benefits, supporting healthier-looking skin by neutralizing free radicals that contribute to skin aging and damage.

Available in both prescription and over-the-counter formulations, azelaic acid offers flexibility in addressing a wide range of skin concerns. Its ability to even out skin tone, calm redness, and protect from environmental stressors makes it a popular choice in many skincare routines. Whether in higher concentrations for more targeted treatments or in lower concentrations for daily use, azelaic acid remains an effective option for those looking to improve skin clarity, tone, and overall skin health.

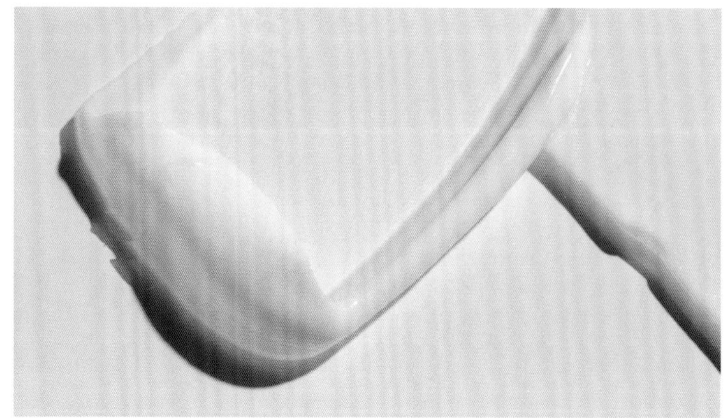

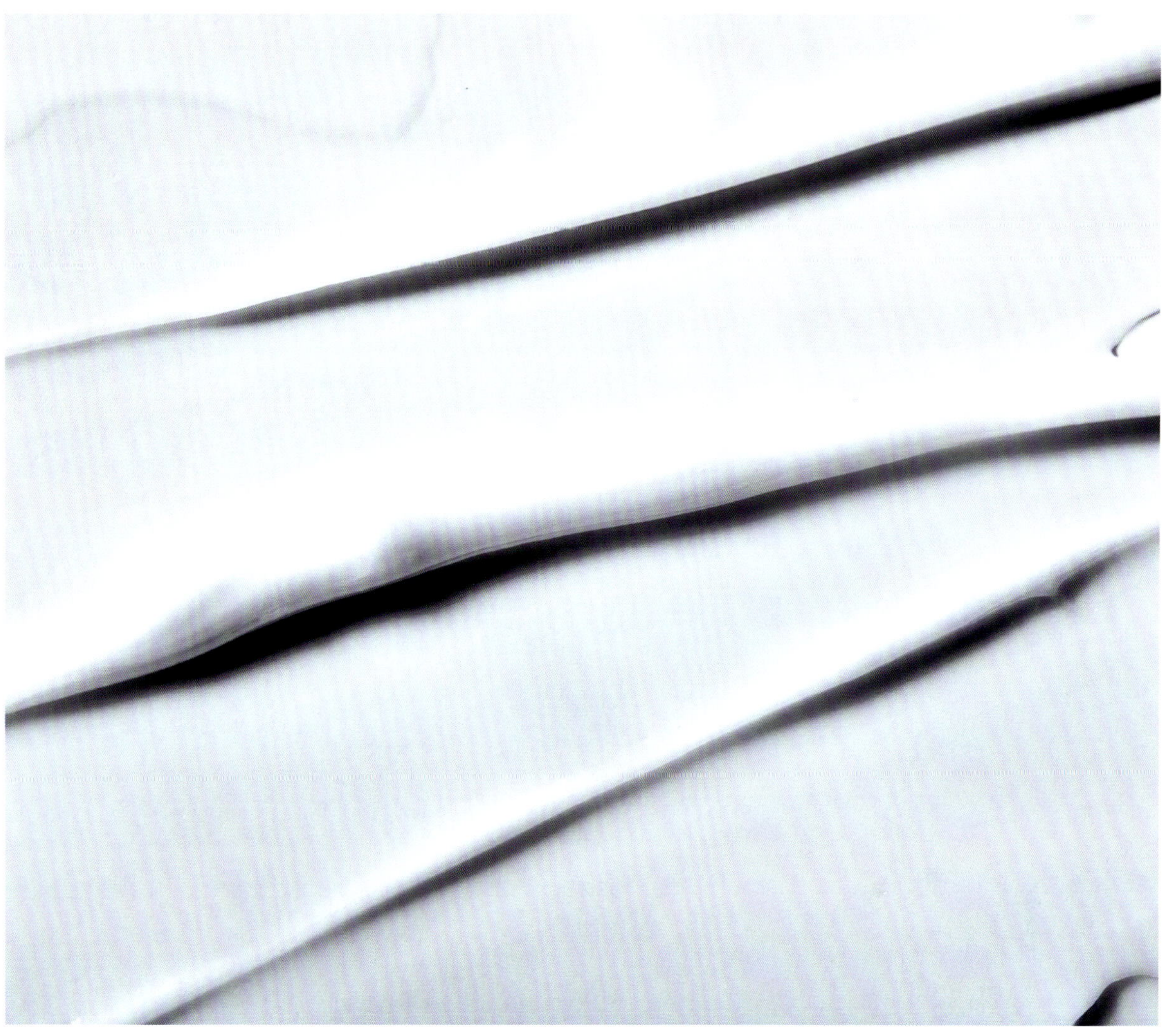

Mechanism of action

Azelaic acid works through several mechanisms that make it a powerful ingredient for improving the appearance and health of the skin. One of its primary actions is its mild exfoliating effect. By gently sloughing off dead skin cells, azelaic acid helps to promote skin cell turnover, which in turn helps unclog pores, refine the skin's texture, and reduce redness. This action is especially beneficial for those dealing with blemishes, blackheads, and post-blemish marks.

In addition to its exfoliating properties, azelaic acid is known for its ability to even out skin tone. It works by inhibiting the enzyme tyrosinase, which is involved in melanin production. By reducing melanin synthesis, azelaic acid helps fade dark spots and other types of discoloration, leading to a more uniform complexion.

Caffeine

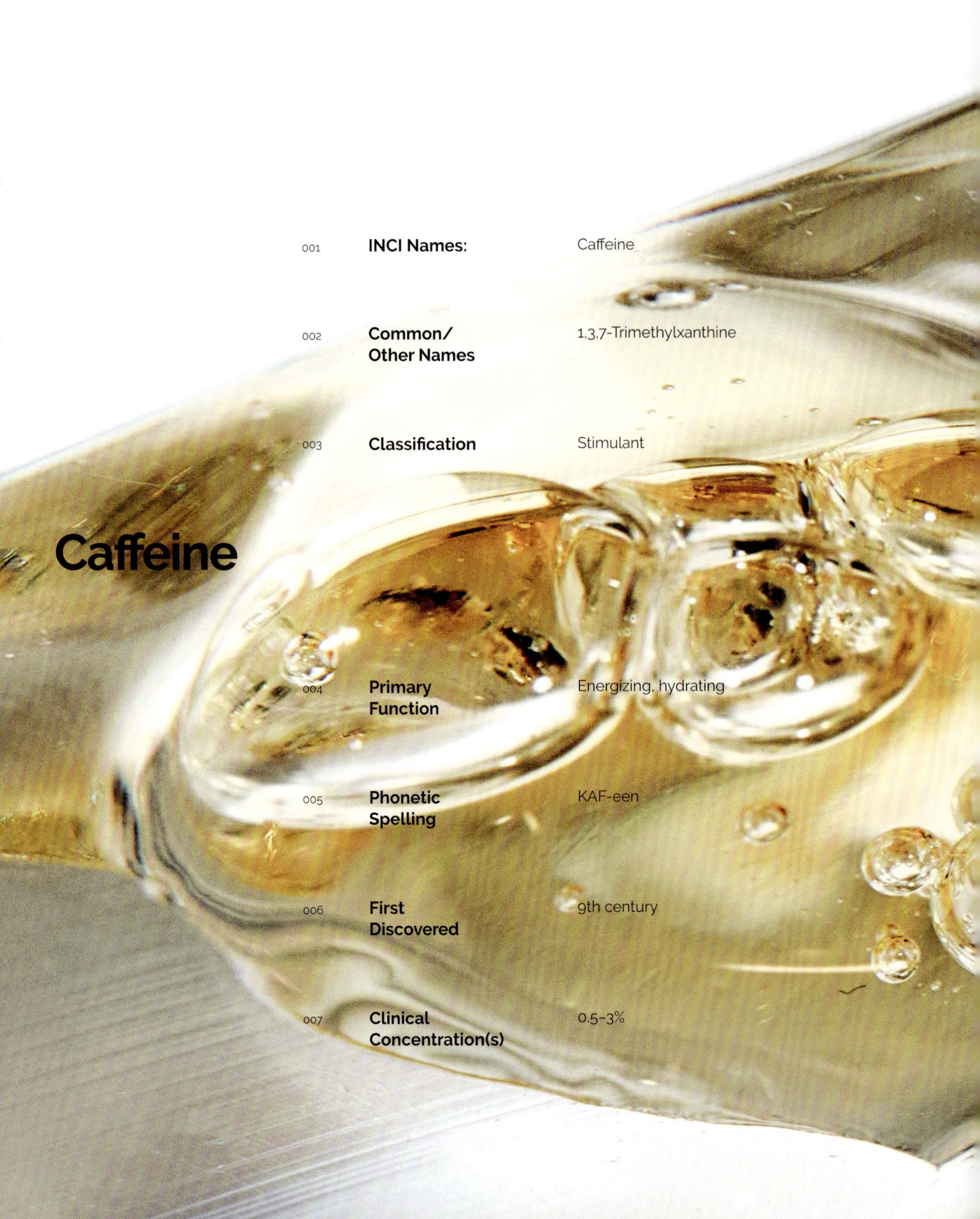

001	**INCI Names:**	Caffeine
002	**Common/ Other Names**	1,3,7-Trimethylxanthine
003	**Classification**	Stimulant
004	**Primary Function**	Energizing, hydrating
005	**Phonetic Spelling**	KAF-een
006	**First Discovered**	9th century
007	**Clinical Concentration(s)**	0.5–3%

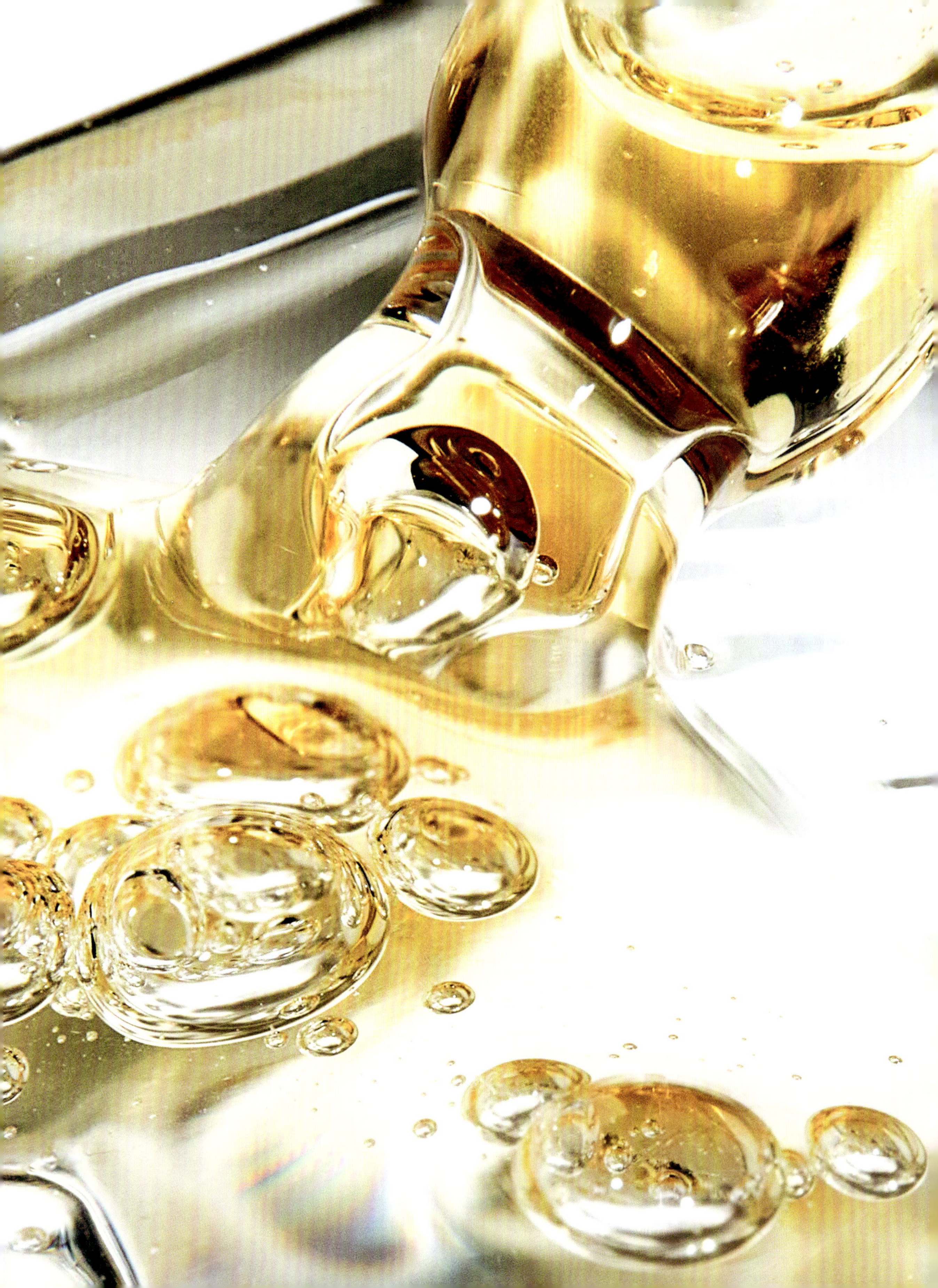

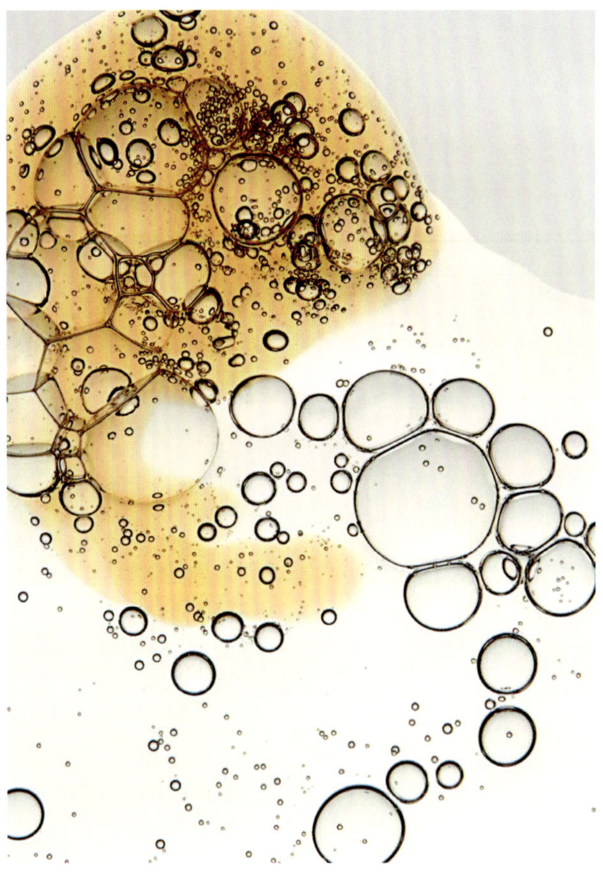

What it is

Caffeine is a naturally occurring compound found in coffee, tea, and over 60 plant species. Within these sources, it exists as part of a complex matrix of compounds. In plants, caffeine serves as a natural pesticide, protecting against herbivores and contributing to the plant's survival. It can be extracted from natural sources through a process that involves mixing plant material with solvents to selectively dissolve caffeine, then evaporating the liquid to concentrate the extract.

Alternatively, caffeine can be produced synthetically through chemical processes. These methods involve precursor ingredients undergoing a series of reactions to create caffeine, enabling large-scale production at a lower cost. This synthetic approach makes caffeine widely available for use in medicines, beverages, and skincare products. In its purified form, caffeine appears as a white, crystalline powder that is odorless with a slightly bitter taste.

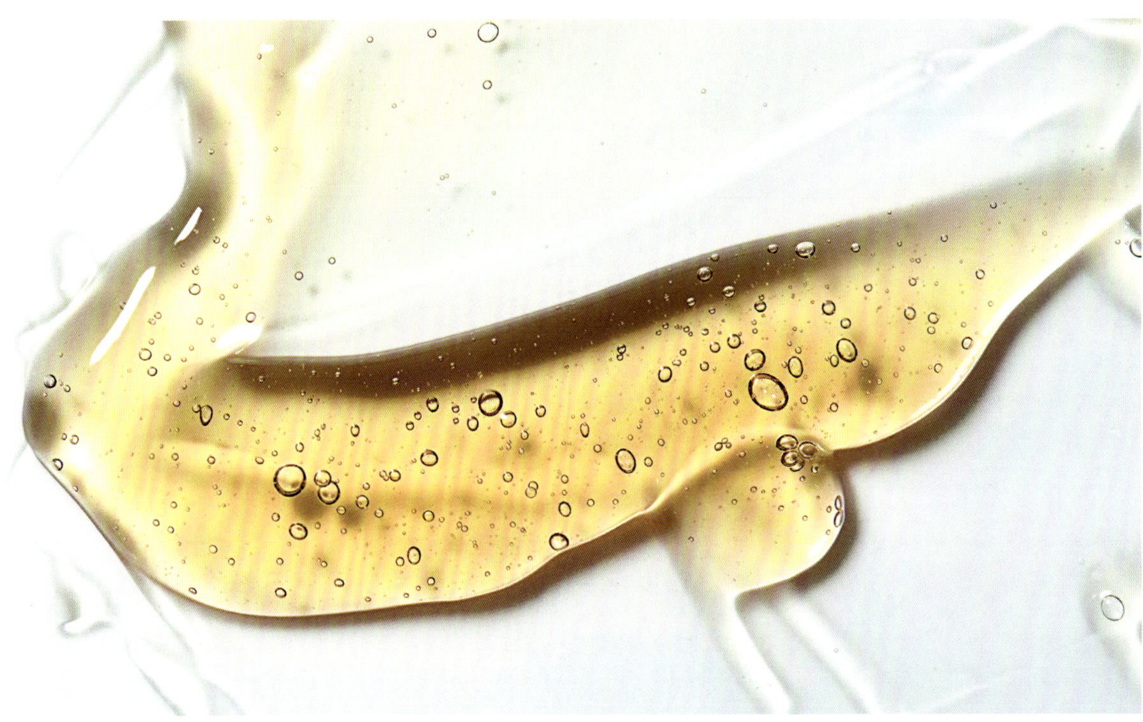

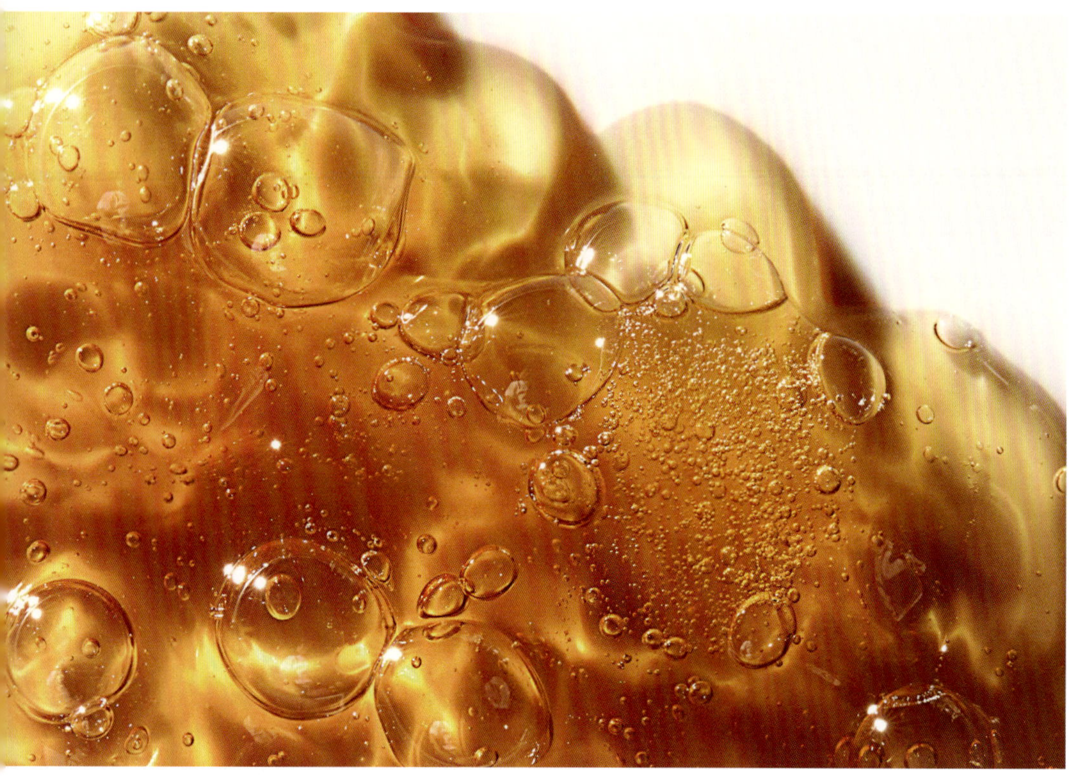

What it's used for

Caffeine is a natural stimulant celebrated for its ability to enhance alertness and reduce fatigue. Commonly consumed in beverages such as coffee and tea, caffeine is also found in edible products designed to boost energy and in pre-workout supplements. Its stimulating properties arise from its ability to block adenosine, a neurotransmitter associated with relaxation, thereby promoting a feeling of wakefulness and energy.

In the skincare industry, caffeine emerged as a sought-after ingredient in the late 20th century, gaining prominence with the introduction of caffeine-infused eye creams and gels. These formulations targeted concerns like puffiness and dark circles under the eyes, leveraging caffeine's ability to reduce water retention under the eye. Caffeine is also an antioxidant that neutralizes free radicals, protecting skin cells from oxidative damage and the development of premature signs of aging. When incorporated into sunscreen formulations, caffeine offers an added layer of defense against environmental aggressors like sun exposure and pollution. These innovations marked the beginning of caffeine's widespread use in skincare, which has since expanded to include facial treatments, sunscreens, haircare, and body care products.

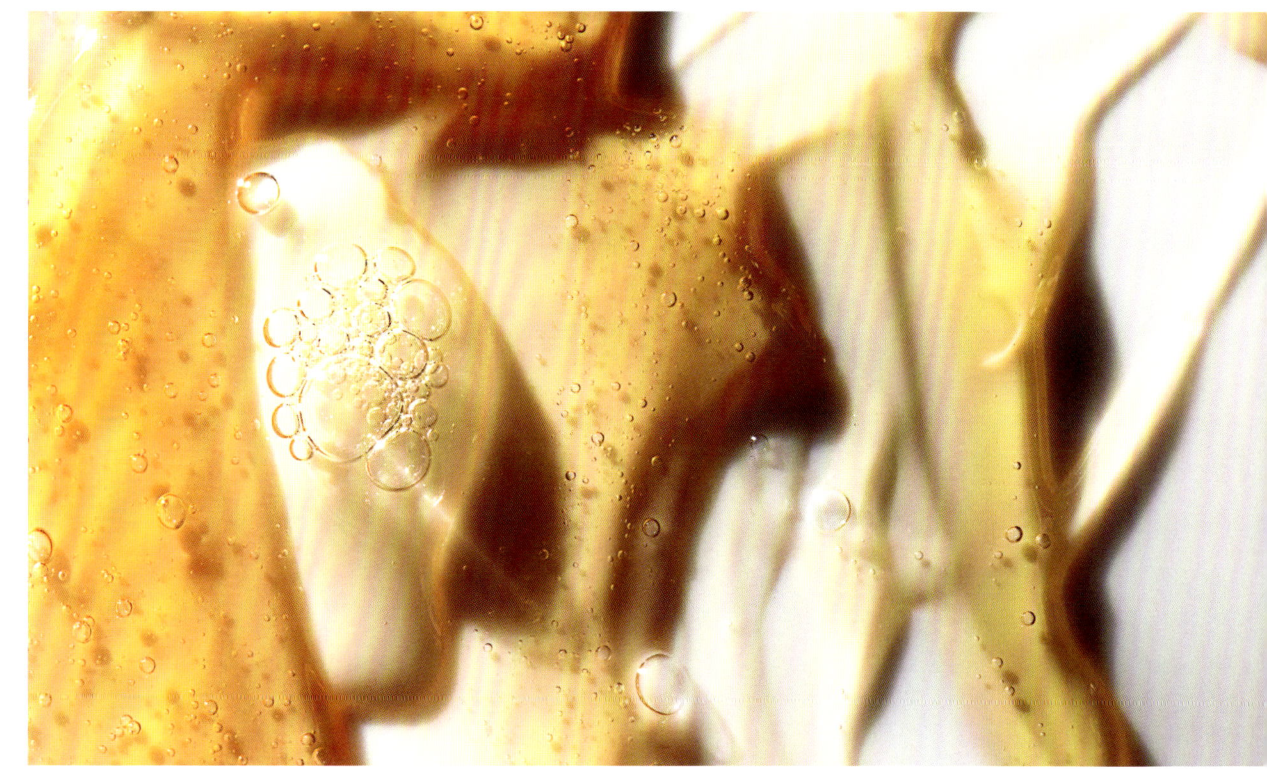

Mechanism of action

Caffeine is known for its ability to reduce the appearance of dark circles and puffiness under the eye through its work as a vasoconstrictor. Additionally, caffeine acts as an antioxidant, helping to protect the skin by neutralizing free radicals. By scavenging these free radicals, caffeine can help mitigate the damage caused by oxidative stress and environmental pollutants, further supporting skin brightening and preventing the appearance of premature signs of aging.

Centella Asiatica

001	**INCI Names:**	Centella asiatica
002	**Common/ Other Names**	Cica, gotu kola, tiger grass, Indian pennywort
003	**Classification**	Antioxidant
004	**Primary Function**	Antioxidant
005	**Phonetic Spelling**	sen-TEL-uh ay-see-AT-ih-kuh
006	**First Discovered**	Not known; traditional medicine herb
007	**Clinical Concentration(s)**	0.1–2%

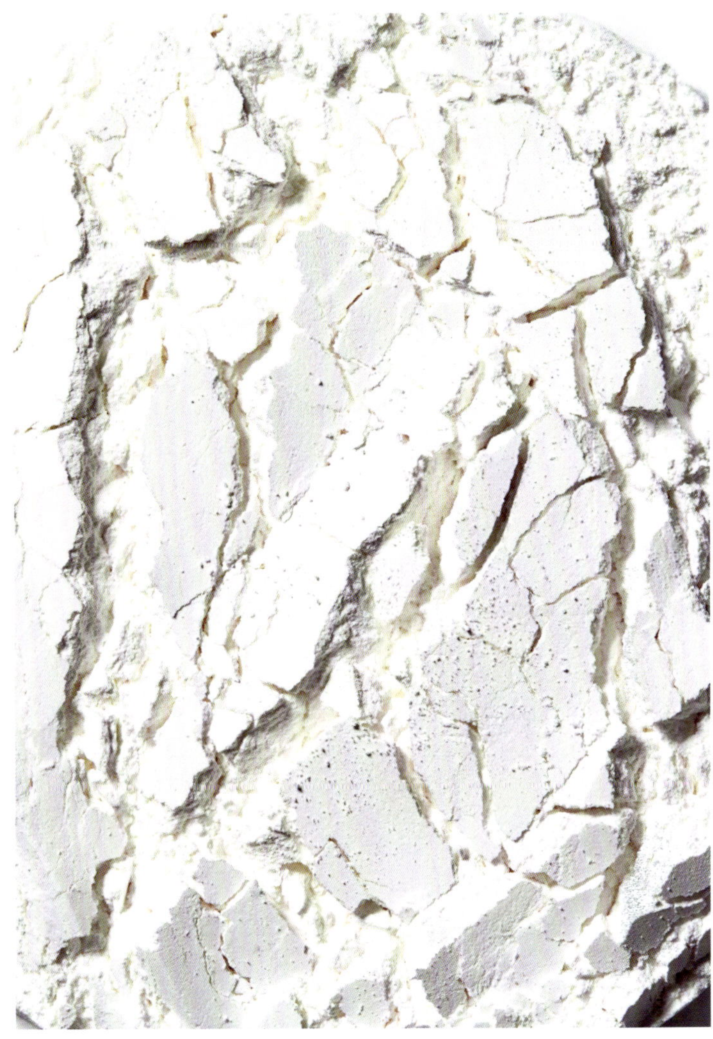

What it is

Centella asiatica, often referred to as gotu kola or tiger grass, is a small herbaceous plant from the Apiaceae family, long valued in traditional wellness practices across Asia. In skincare, it is prized for its rich composition of beneficial compounds, including triterpenoids such as asiaticoside, madecassoside, asiatic acid, and madecassic acid. These elements are complemented by flavonoids, phenolic acids, and triterpenic steroids, alongside a variety of vitamins, amino acids, and essential oils also present in this ingredient.

This intricate blend of naturally occurring compounds makes Centella asiatica a highly versatile ingredient in skincare. It is celebrated for its ability to soothe, calm, and help protect the skin barrier, with many formulations highlighting its antioxidant properties. This ingredient is often incorporated into products designed to leverage its plant-derived components to support skin resilience and balance.

What it's used for

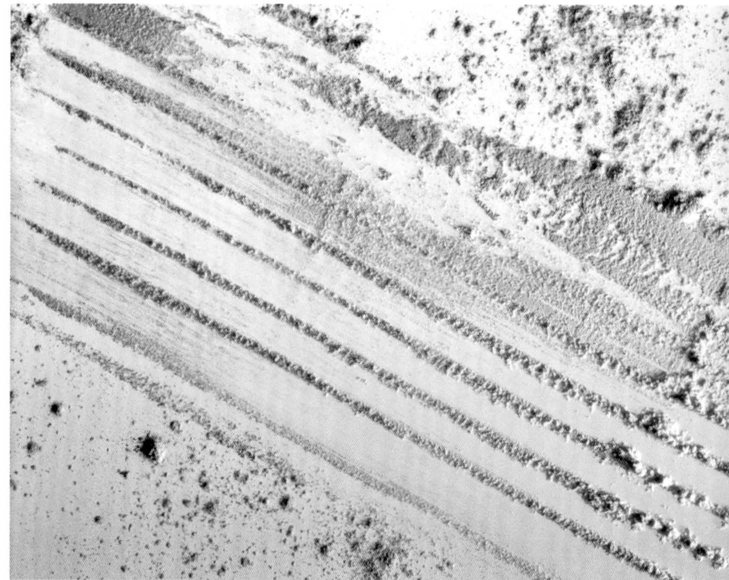

Centella asiatica is a botanical ingredient known for its soothing and hydrating properties, which can help comfort dry skin and leave it feeling refreshed. Its key components, such as asiaticoside and madecassoside, contribute to Centella's ability to calm visible redness and enhance the appearance of a more even skin tone. With its rich antioxidant composition, Centella asiatica helps reinforce the skin's natural barrier, enhancing its resilience against external stressors and environmental factors that may contribute to dryness, dullness, and visible signs of aging.

Its inclusion in cosmetics is particularly popular for enhancing hydration and promoting a smoother, more supple complexion. This multi-benefit ingredient is a favorite for products designed to target dryness or overall skin revitalization, making it a versatile choice for a variety of skincare needs.

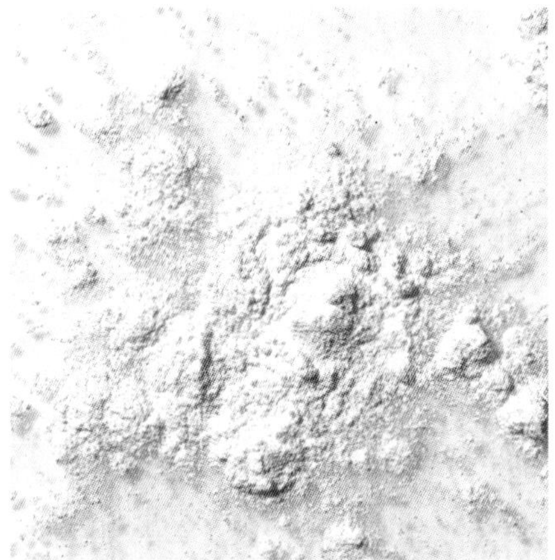

Mechanism of action

Centella asiatica works in skincare by stimulating the production of key components that maintain the skin's structure, including collagen type I. Its active compounds, including asiaticoside and madecassoside, help to promote the look of skin rejuvenation, calm irritation, and improve hydration. By supporting the skin's natural barrier, it enhances the skin's ability to protect itself from external environmental stressors, helping to reduce signs of aging and soothe sensitive or stressed skin.

Ceramides

001	**INCI Names:**	Ceramide NP, Ceramide AP, Ceramide EOP, etc.
002	**Common/ Other Names**	Ceramides
003	**Classification**	Emollient
004	**Primary Function**	Barrier repair, moisturization
005	**Phonetic Spelling**	SER-uh-midez
006	**First Discovered**	Michael Elias, 1980–90
007	**Clinical Concentration(s)**	0.5–2%

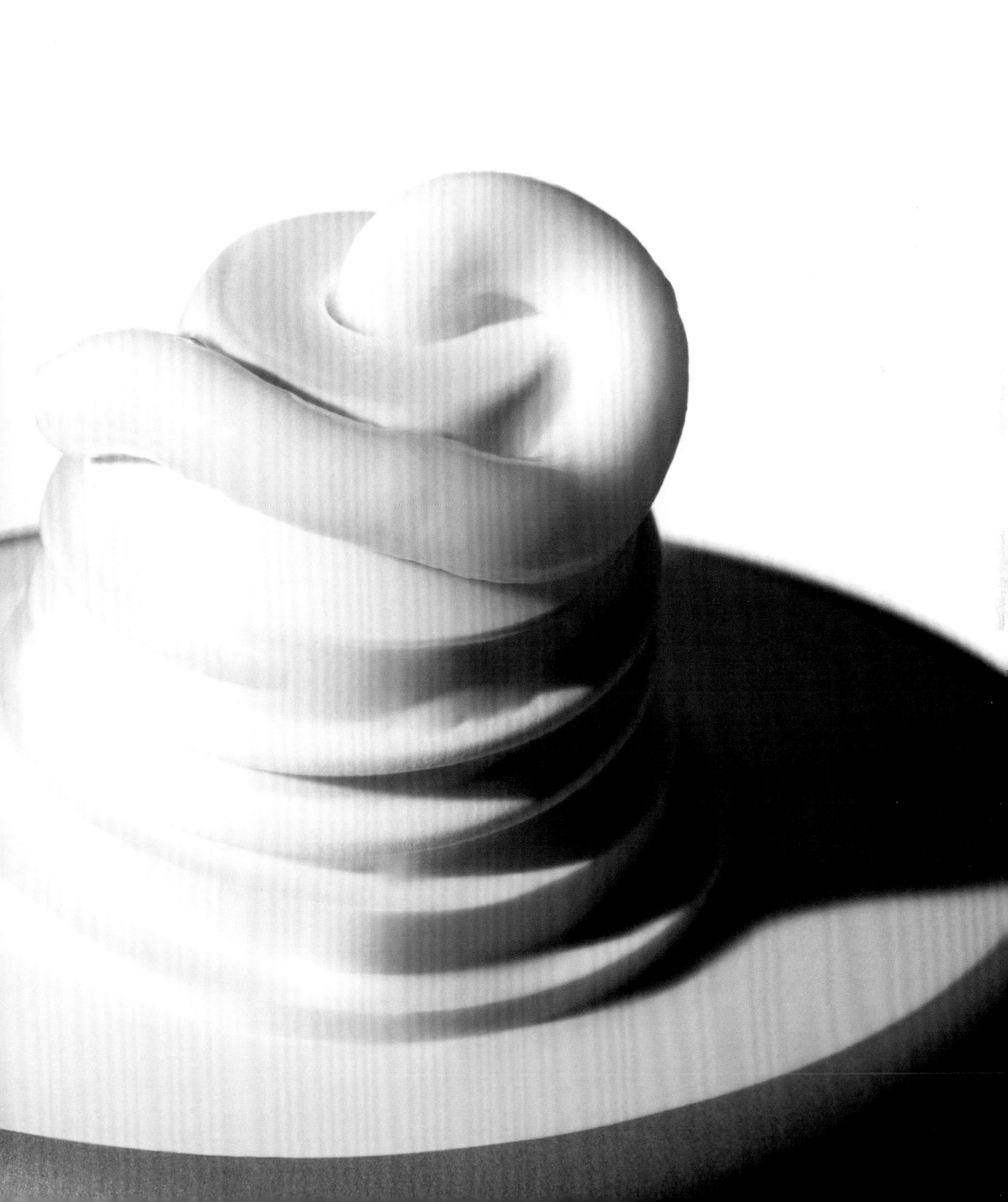

What it is

The word ceramide comes from the Latin word "cera" (wax). Ceramides are a heterogeneous family of waxy lipid molecules present in the stratum corneum of the epidermis. Structurally, they contain a sphingolipid backbone that fatty acids are connected to via amide linkage. There are 12 subclasses of ceramides, categorized by the types of constituent sphingosines and fatty acids. Ceramides are also present in high concentrations in our cell membranes, where they are integral components of sphingomyelin, a key lipid in the lipid bilayer.

What it's used for

Ceramides have the ability to hold water and are used in formulations for moisturizing and hydrating dry skin. They are also used to maintain the skin barrier, on the basis of studies that have indicated that ceramide synthesis is the initiating event for barrier repair following damage. By helping reinforce the skin barrier, ceramides have been shown to help reduce sensitivity and irritation, leading to a calmer and more even-toned complexion.

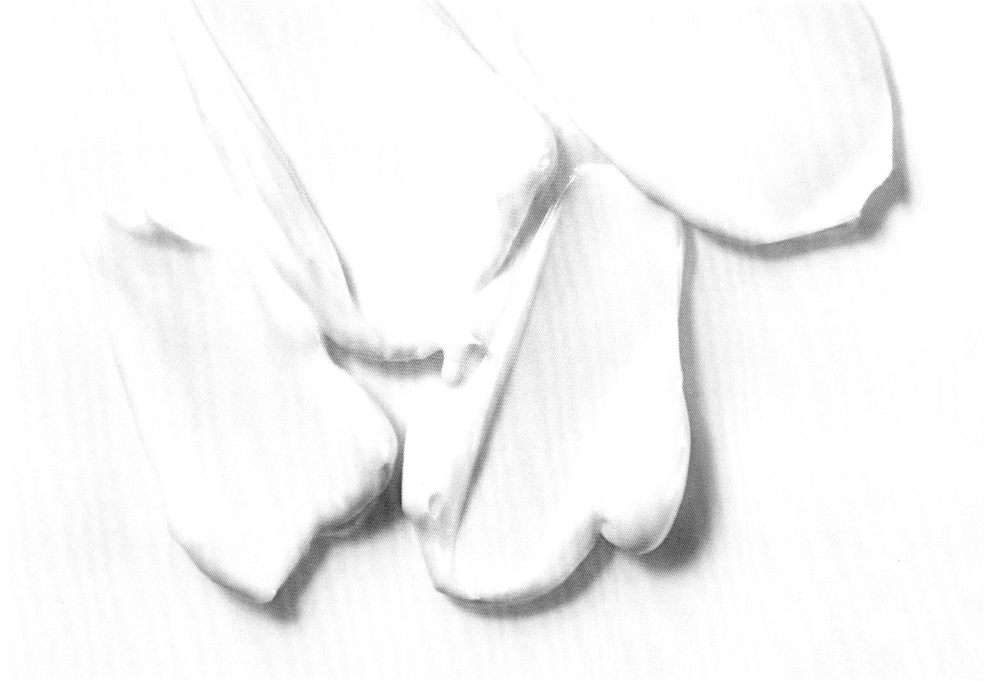

Mechanism of action

Ceramides are fundamental components of the skin's lipid matrix, which is additionally composed of fatty acids and cholesterol. This lipid matrix forms layers between the stratum corneum (the outermost layer of the skin). This arrangement, often described as "brick and mortar," forms the skin barrier. The components of the lipid matrix work to retain bound water, perform a moisturizing function, and maintain the strong bond between cells of the stratum corneum (corneocytes).

Studies have shown that ceramide-containing creams increase the lipid content of the stratum corneum, reduce transepidermal water loss (TEWL), and have a moisturizing effect. This is because added ceramides are thought to help strengthen the skin barrier, which aids in preventing moisture from evaporating. By enhancing this barrier, ceramides may create an occlusive effect that effectively traps moisture within the skin, leading to improved hydration and a more moisturized complexion.

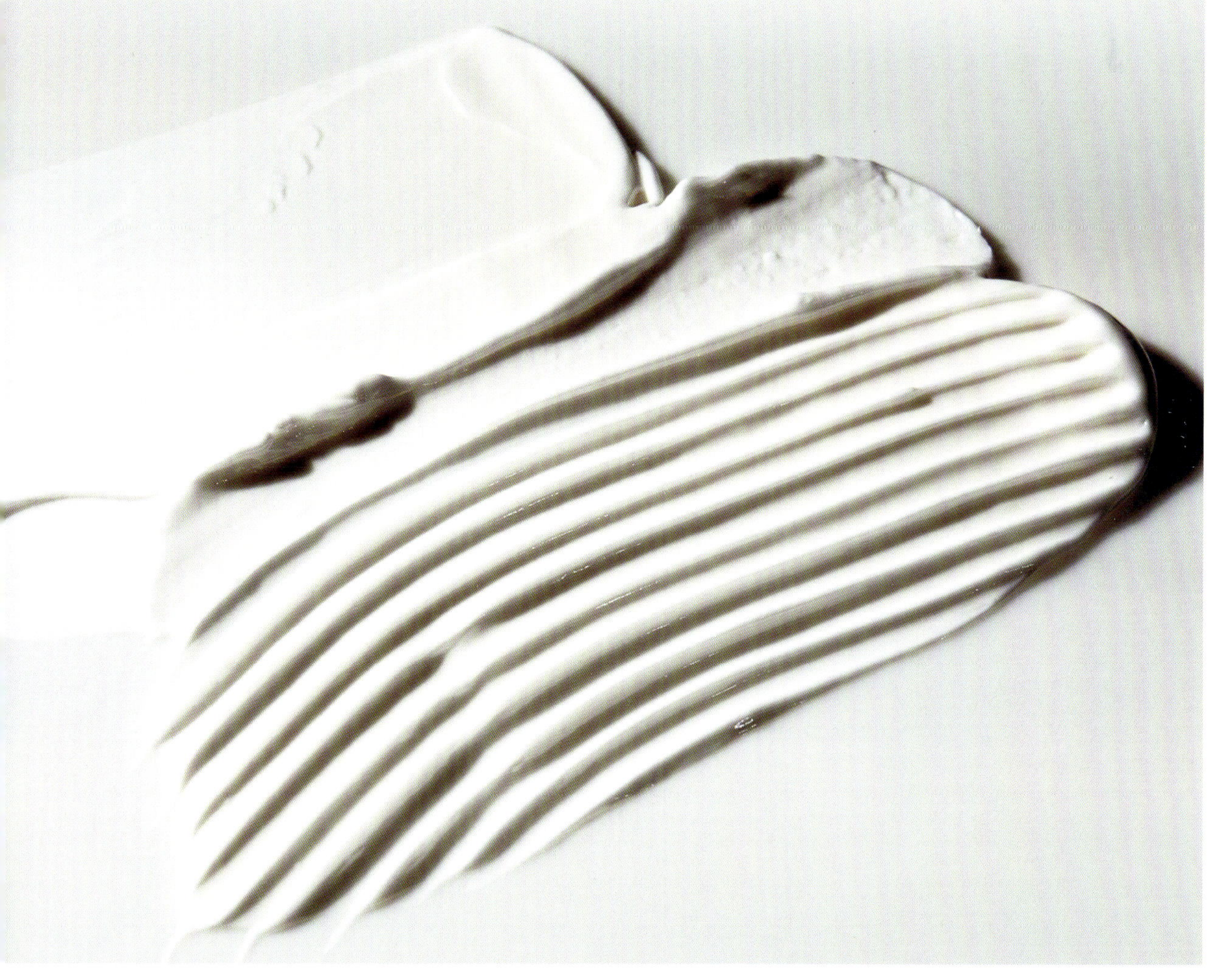

001	**INCI Names:**	Copper tripeptide-1
002	**Common/ Other Names**	Copper peptides
003	**Classification**	Signal peptides

Copper Peptides

004	**Primary Function**	Reparative and anti-aging
005	**Phonetic Spelling**	KAH-per PEP-tides
006	**First Discovered**	Loran Pickart, 1973
007	**Clinical Concentration(s)**	1–2%

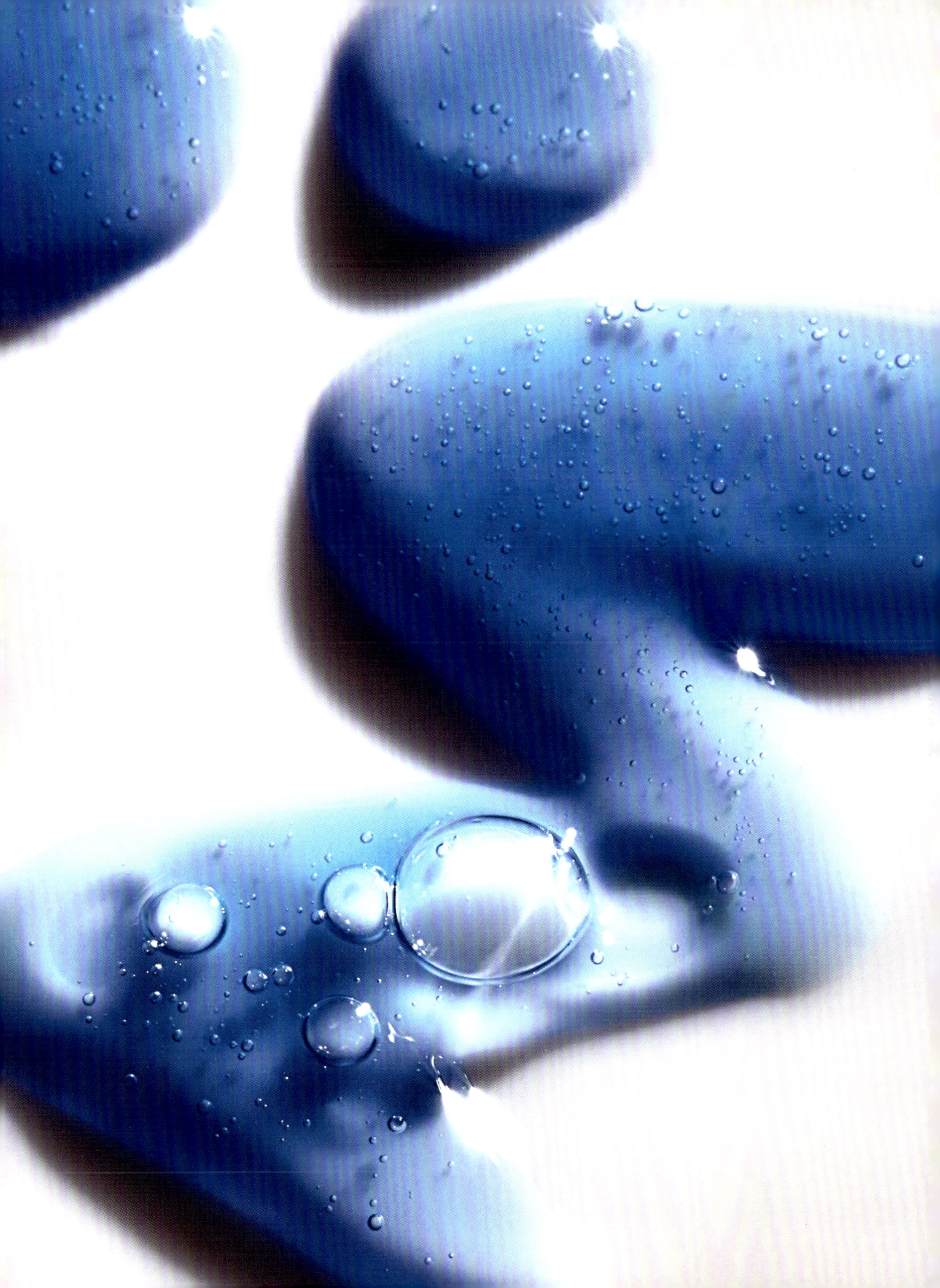

What it is

Copper peptides, often referred to as GHK-Cu, are small protein fragments that bind to copper ions, which are vital for maintaining healthy-looking skin. In cosmetics, copper peptides are valued for their ability to support the skin's natural processes, contributing to a smoother, more radiant, and youthful appearance. They are commonly used in formulations designed to improve the visible firmness and elasticity of the skin, as well as to promote a hydrated and resilient complexion.

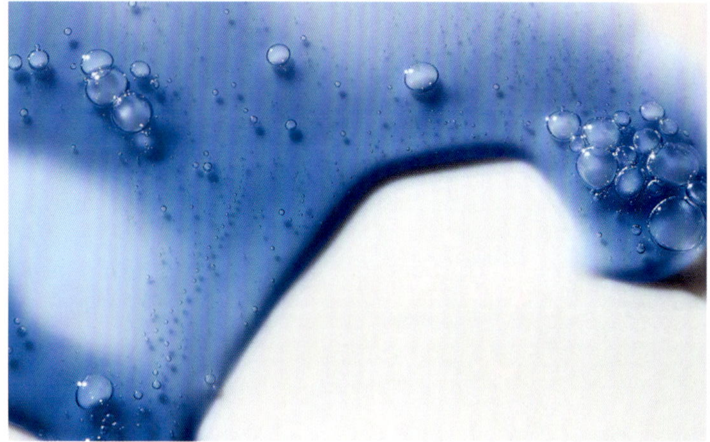

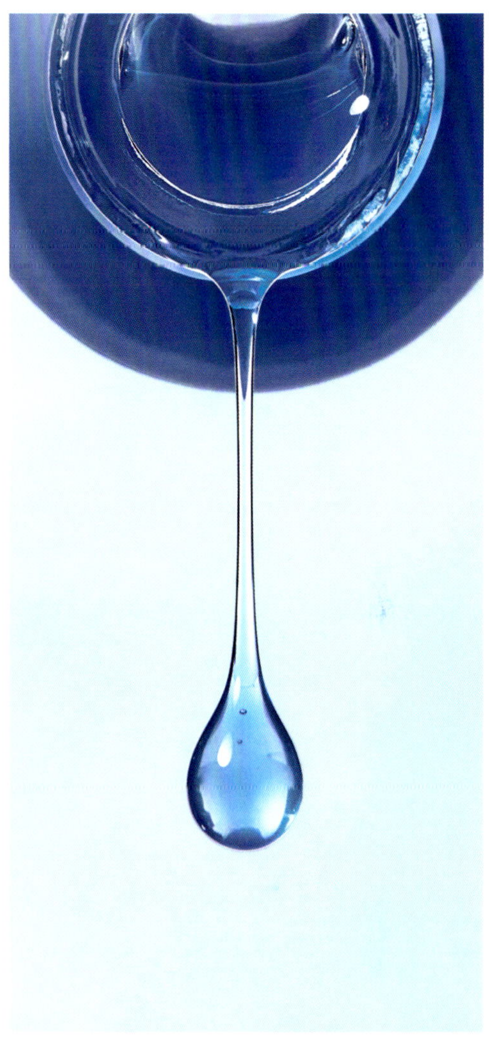

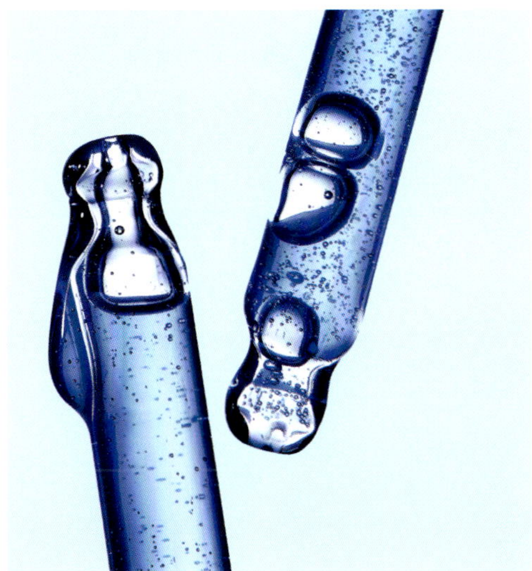

What it's used for

As part of their benefits, copper peptides help stimulate the production of glycosaminoglycans within the surface of the skin, helping maintain the skin's moisture levels and support its natural barrier. This contributes to a healthier look and feel. Over time, the natural presence of copper peptides in the skin decreases, which can contribute to the visible signs of aging. Incorporating copper peptides into a skincare routine can help improve the appearance of skin texture, enhance the look of firmness, and diminish the visibility of fine lines and wrinkles, which makes them a sought-after ingredient in anti-aging products.

Mechanism of action

Copper peptides, known for their anti-aging and skin-rejuvenating properties, have become a staple in advanced skincare formulations. These bioactive molecules, composed of copper ions and short chains of amino acids, engage in a multifaceted mechanism of action to enhance skin feel and appearance.

Collagen and elastin production

The primary function of copper peptides involves stimulating the production of collagen and elastin, essential proteins that maintain the skin's structural integrity and elasticity. Collagen provides the skin with its firmness and helps maintain its overall integrity, acting as a supportive framework. Elastin, on the other hand, allows the skin to stretch and rebound, contributing to its flexibility and resilience. Together, these proteins play a crucial role in maintaining a youthful, smooth, and plump appearance.

Hydration

Copper peptides also improve skin hydration by increasing the synthesis of glycosaminoglycans, such as hyaluronic acid. These molecules are vital for retaining moisture in the skin, enhancing its suppleness and resilience. By helping boost the skin's moisture content, copper peptides help to plump the skin, reduce the appearance of fine lines and wrinkles, and promote a more youthful appearance.

Antioxidant support

When applied topically, copper peptides function as antioxidants by neutralizing free radicals generated from daily environmental factors such as pollution and UV exposure.

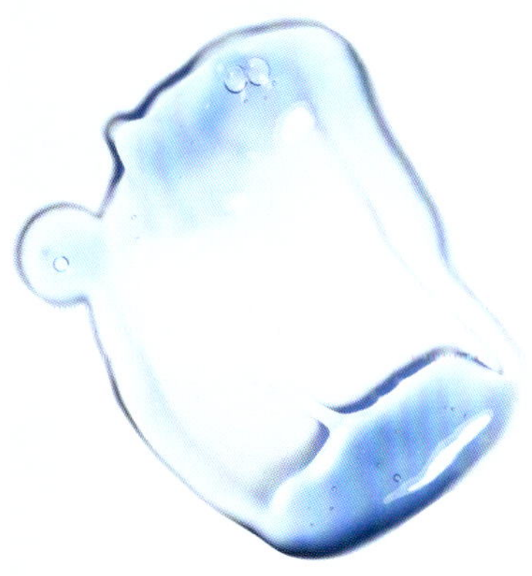

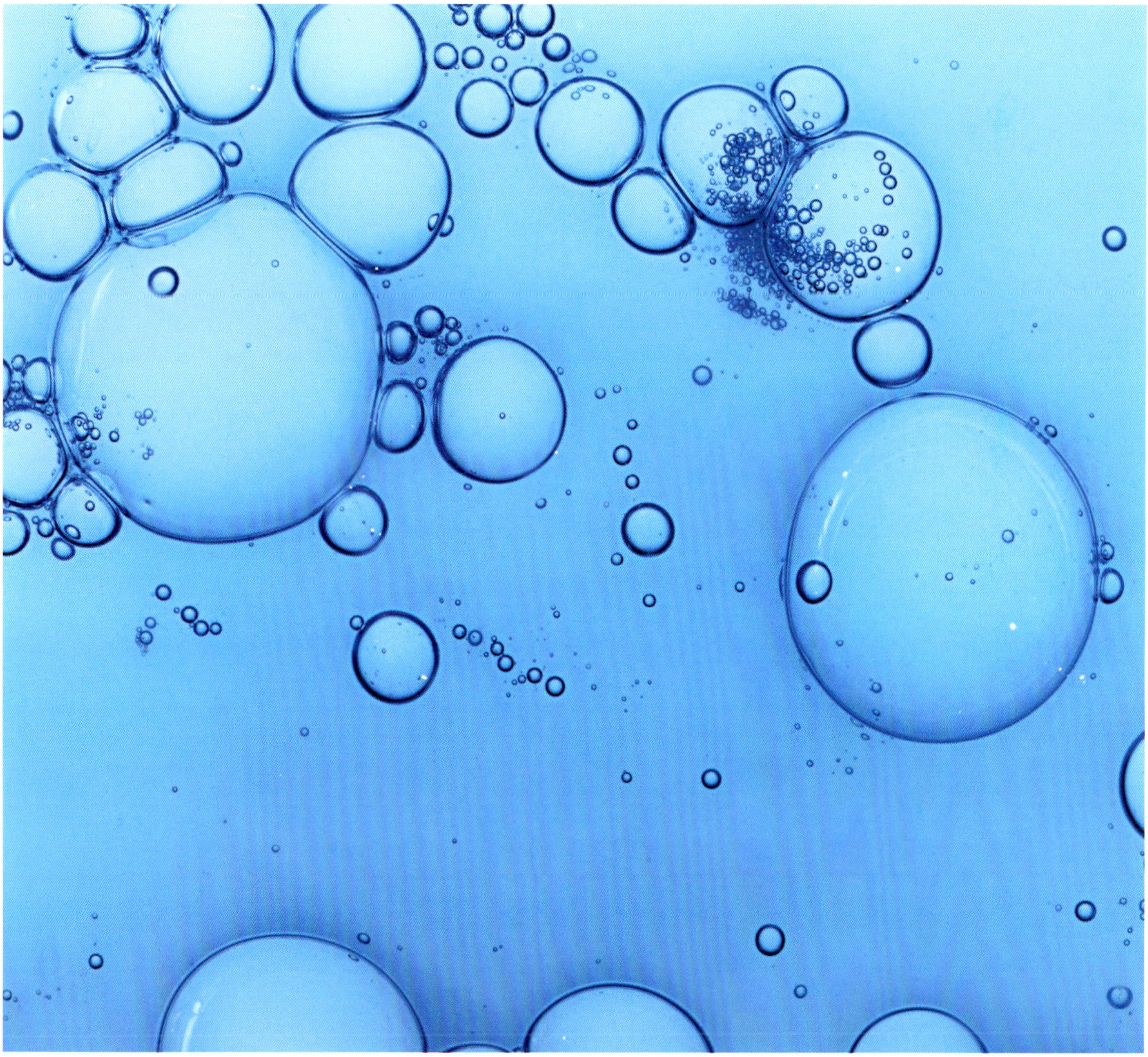

Glycerin

001	**INCI Names:**	Glycerin
002	**Common/ Other Names**	Glycerol
003	**Classification**	Humectant
004	**Primary Function**	Hydration
005	**Phonetic Spelling**	GLIH-suh-rin
006	**First Discovered**	Karl Wilhelm Scheele, 1779
007	**Clinical Concentration(s)**	2–10%

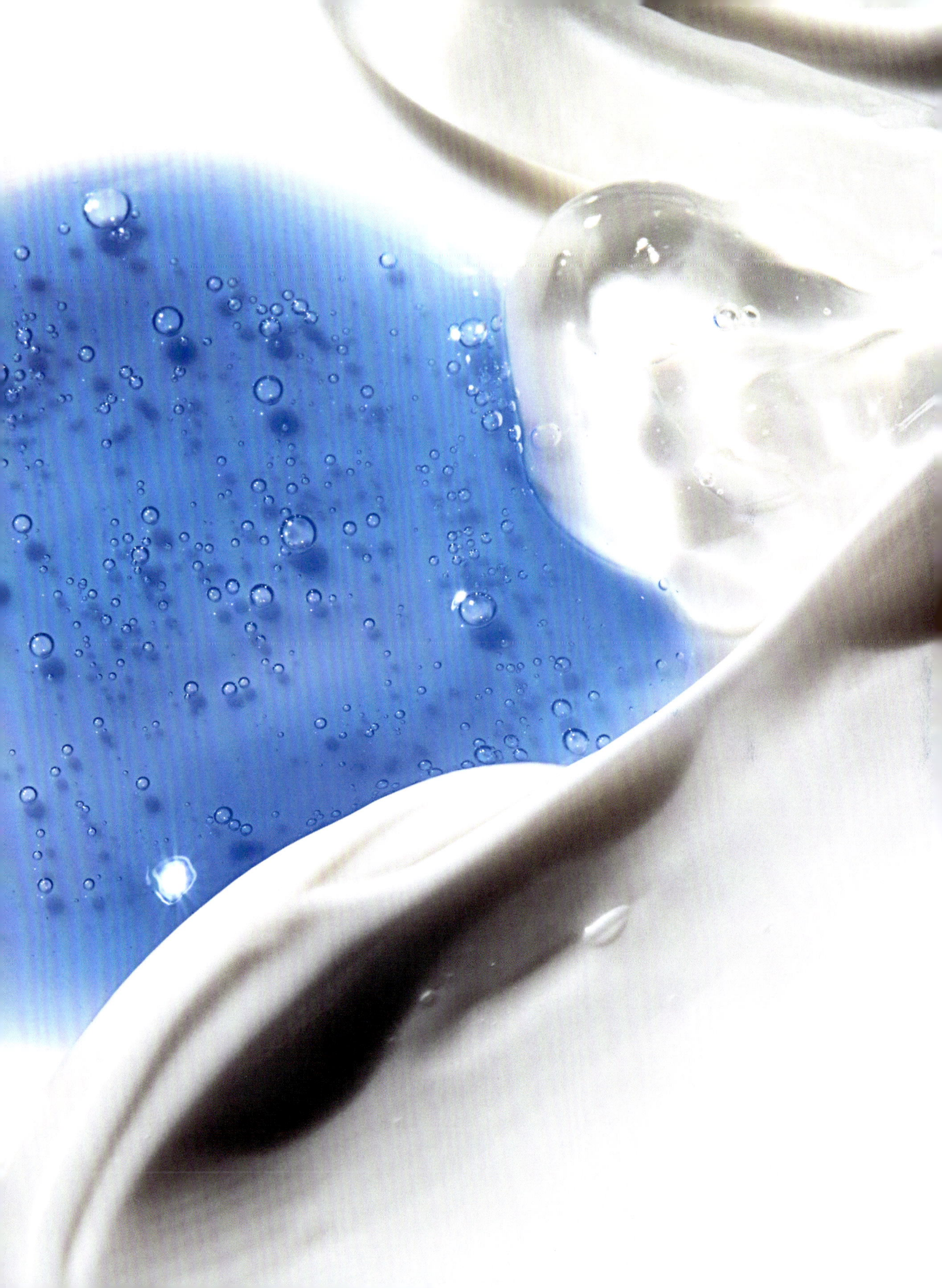

What it is

Glycerin, also known as glycerol, is a naturally occurring trihydroxy alcohol with the chemical formula $C_3H_8O_3$. It is a colorless, odorless, and viscous liquid that serves as one of the most widely used humectants in cosmetic formulations. Glycerin's hygroscopic nature enables it to attract and retain water, making it an effective hydrating agent in topical applications. Naturally derived from plant oils or animal fats through processes such as saponification, glycerin can also be synthesized industrially.

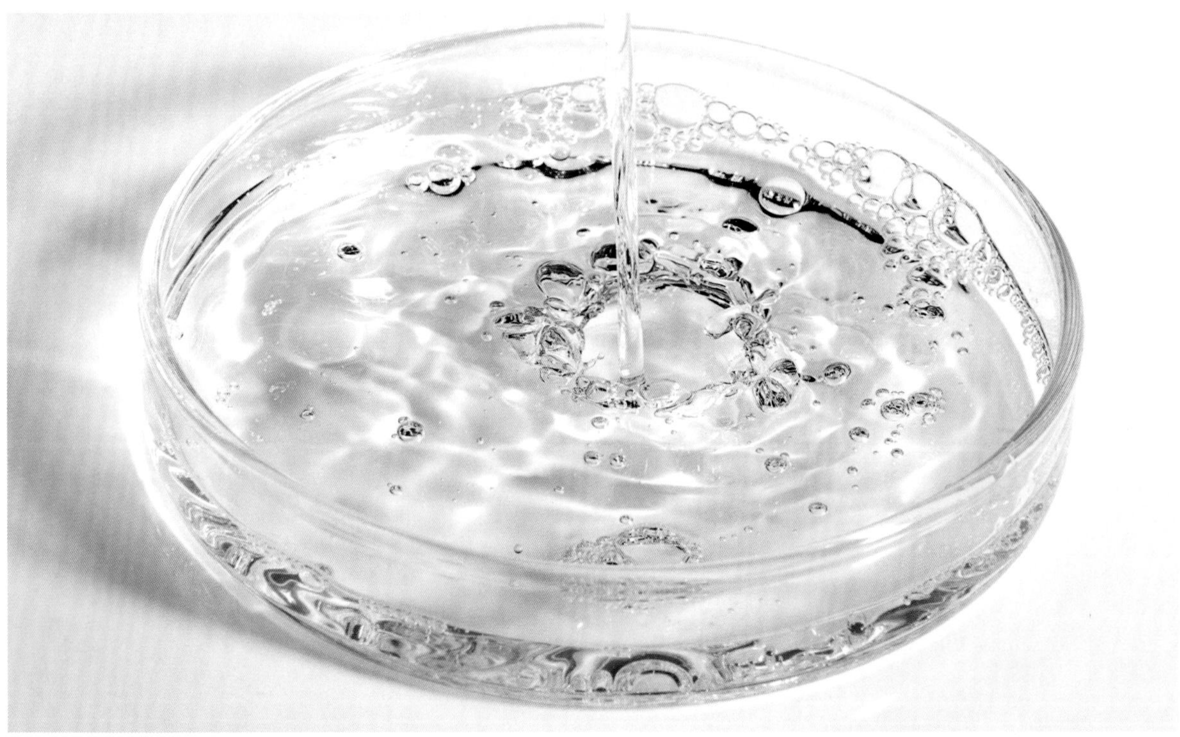

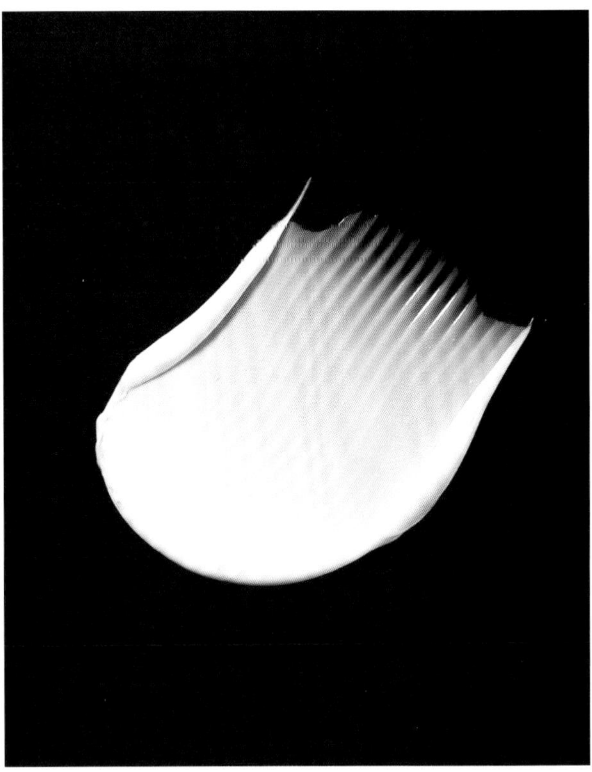

What it's used for

Glycerin is a highly effective humectant widely used in skincare due to its ability to draw water into the stratum corneum, the outermost layer of the skin. By enhancing hydration, glycerin helps maintain skin elasticity, smoothness, and a healthy appearance. It plays a key role in improving the skin barrier by reducing transepidermal water loss (TEWL), thereby supporting the skin's natural protective functions.

Beyond hydration, glycerin supports lipid organization within the stratum corneum, preventing disruptions that can lead to dryness. Its inclusion in formulations has also been shown to protect the skin from environmental stressors. Glycerin's gentle, non-irritating profile makes it suitable for dry skin types, reinforcing its reputation as a cornerstone ingredient in hydrating skincare formulations.

Mechanism of action

Research has identified potential pathways for glycerin's role in the skin, including its association with the aquaporin-3 transport channel and involvement in lipid metabolism within the pilosebaceous unit. Glycerin is widely recognized for its ability to enhance skin hydration, support a healthy skin barrier, and improve overall skin health. It has also been shown to help maintain lipid organization within the stratum corneum, protect against external stressors, and promote the natural processes of skin renewal.

Clinical studies have also demonstrated that glycerin can interact with aquaporins—membrane proteins in the skin—facilitating water transport and contributing to a plump, hydrated appearance.

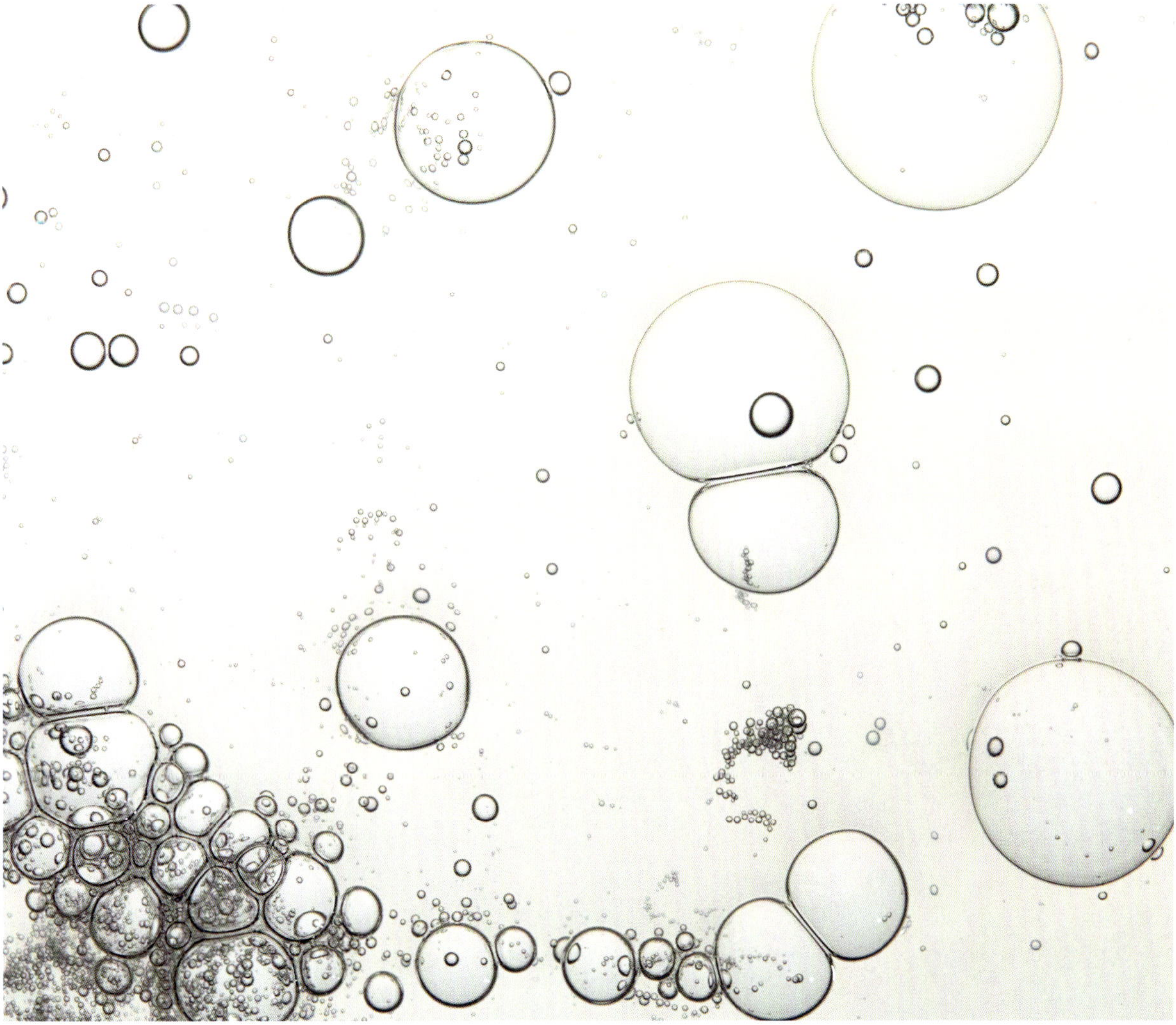

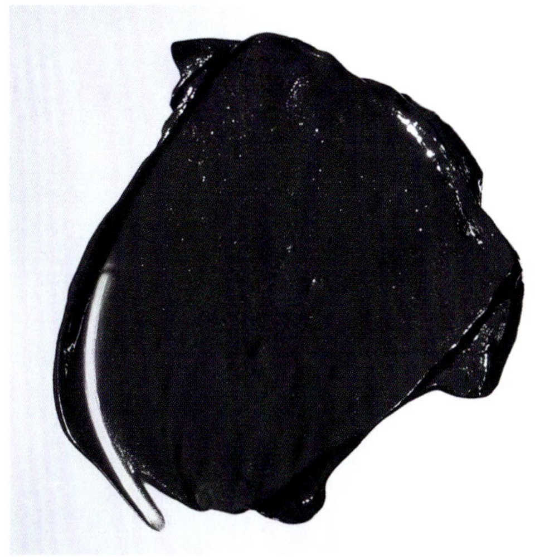

Glycolic Acid

001	**INCI Names:**	Glycolic acid
002	**Common/ Other Names**	Hydroxyacetic acid
003	**Classification**	Alpha hydroxy acid (AHA)
004	**Primary Function**	Exfoliation
005	**Phonetic Spelling**	GLY-koe-lik AS-id
006	**First Discovered**	Nicolas Sokoloff and Adolph Strecker, 1851
007	**Clinical Concentration(s)**	5–10%

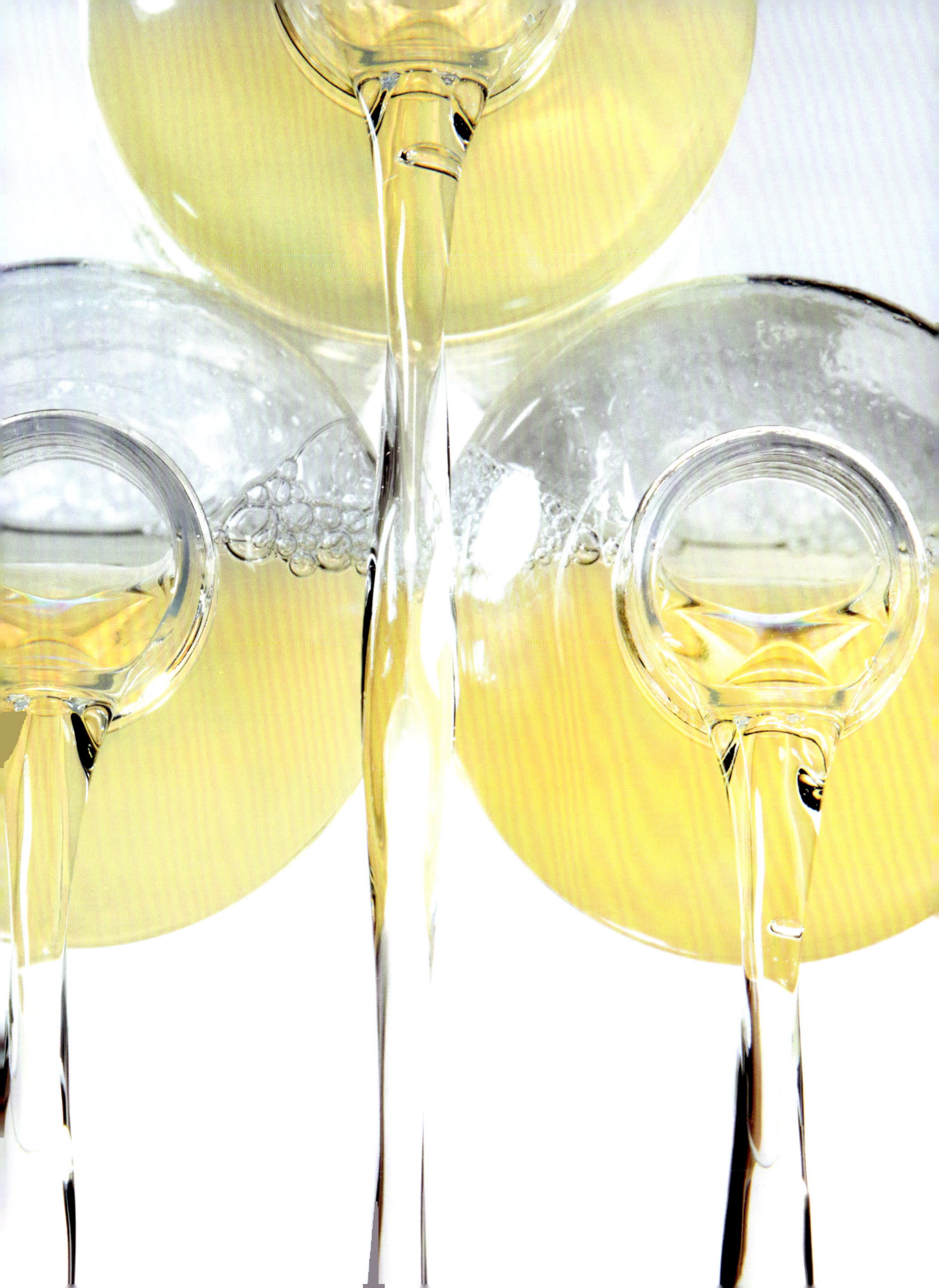

What it is

Hydroxy acids (HAs) are a category of organic acids that includes α-hydroxy acids (AHAs), β-hydroxy acids (BHAs), polyhydroxy acids (PHAs), and bionic acids. AHAs are organic carboxylic acids featuring a hydroxyl group attached to the α-position of the carboxyl group. Many AHAs are found in fruits, which is why they are often referred to as fruit acids. Glycolic acid, the smallest AHA, is derived from sugar cane and is the most commonly used HA in skincare products. The clinical concentrations for daily-use products are generally between 5% and 10%, while higher concentrations, ranging between 30 and 70%, are used in more intensive treatments and professional settings.

What it's used for

Hydroxy acids (HAs) have been a staple in cosmetics and dermatology for over 50 years. Their effectiveness in clinical applications is influenced by factors such as pH, concentration, formulation, and duration of use. Previously available only by prescription, HAs are now commonly found in a wide range of over-the-counter skincare products and cosmetics. Glycolic acid is extensively used in exfoliants, anti-aging treatments, moisturizers, peels, and products aimed at improving the look of uneven skin tone, radiance, and skin texture.

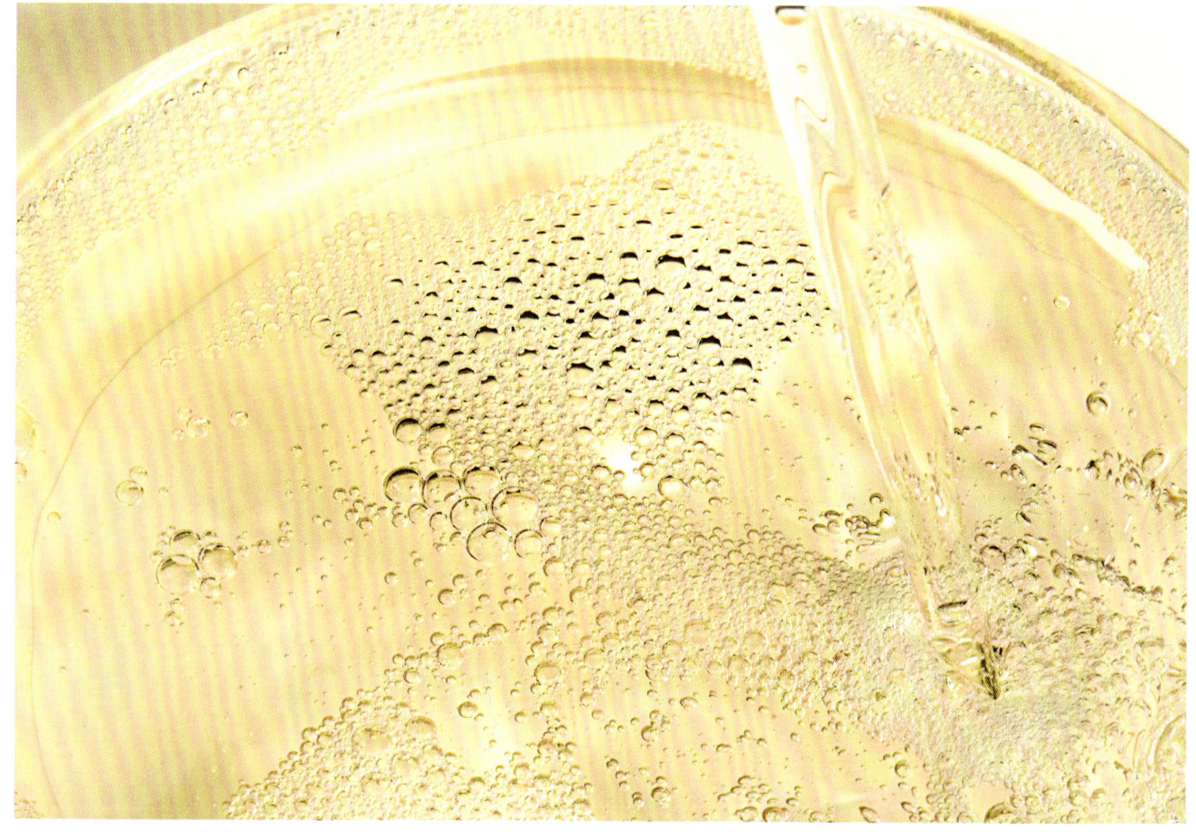

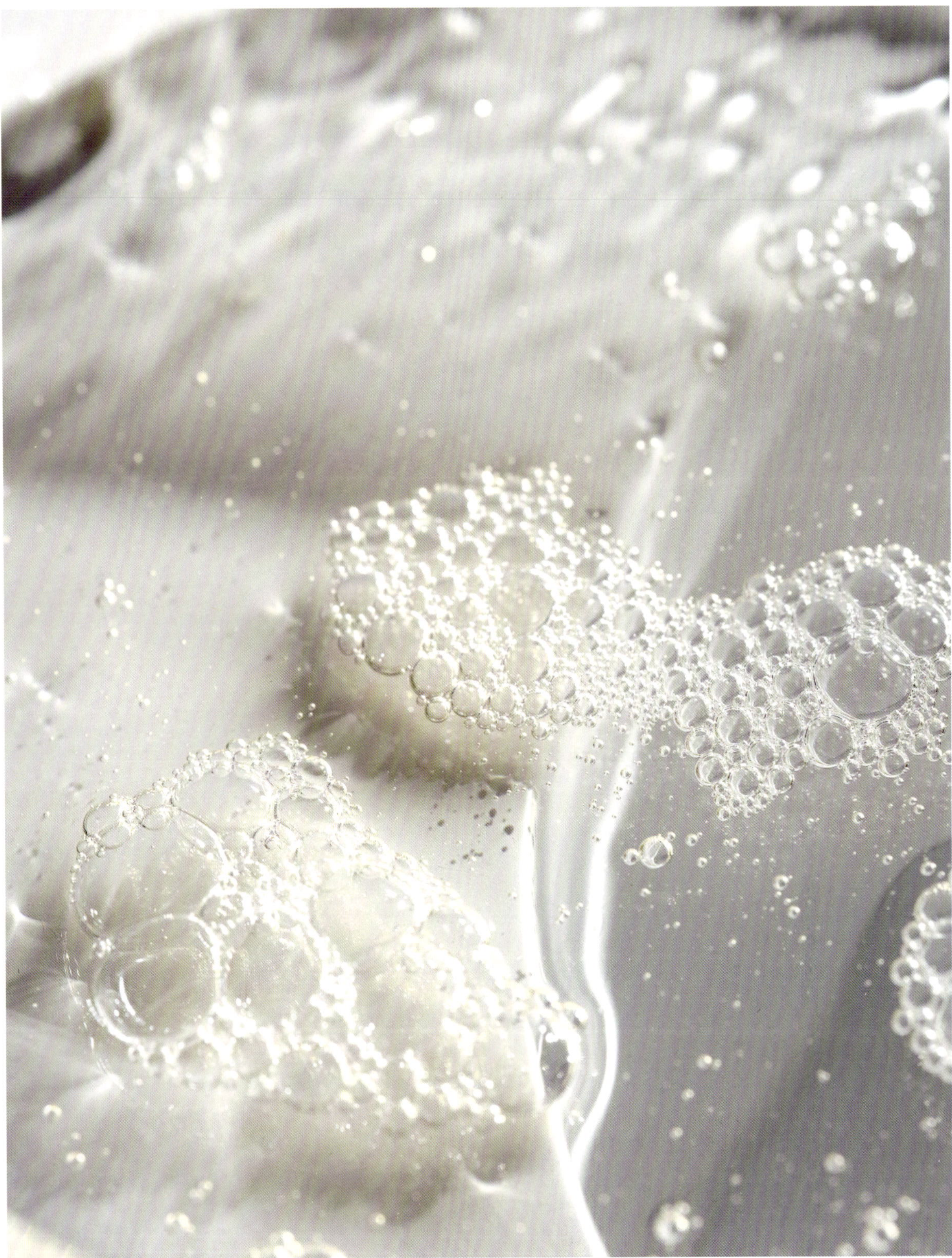

Mechanism of action

Glycolic acid, similar to other AHAs, is soluble in water and primarily acts on the skin's surface. It exfoliates the outer layer of the epidermis and encourages cell turnover. It works by gently dissolving the bonds between dead skin cells on the surface of the skin, helping to reveal fresher, smoother skin underneath. This exfoliation process helps to improve skin texture, remove dead skin buildup, and promote a brighter, more even-looking complexion. Regular use of glycolic acid can help reduce the appearance of fine lines, wrinkles, and uneven skin tone, leaving the skin looking renewed and radiant.

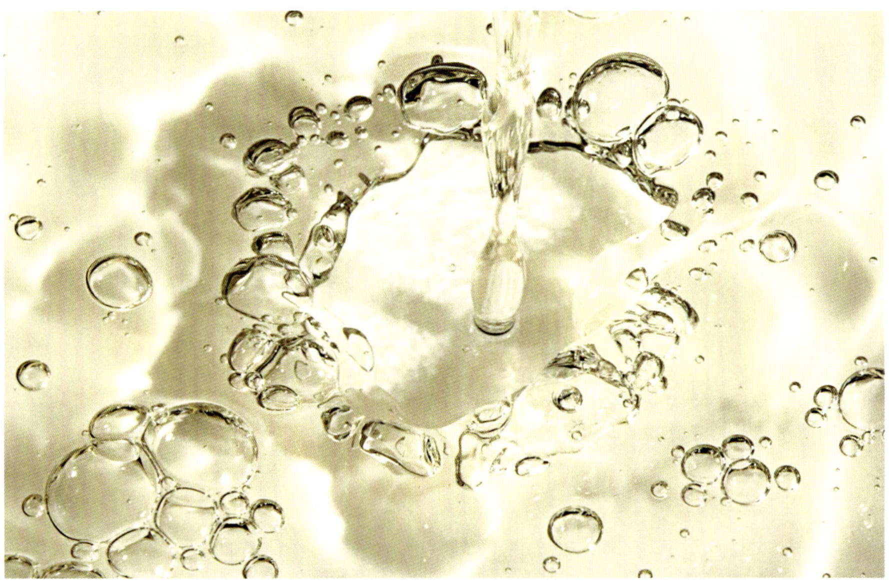

Hyaluronic Acid

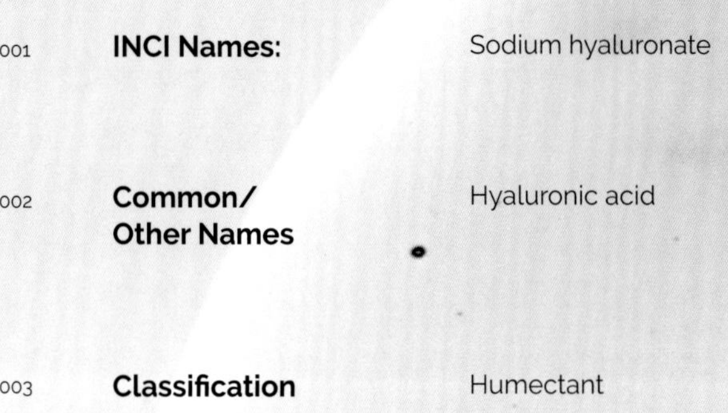

001	**INCI Names:**	Sodium hyaluronate
002	**Common/ Other Names**	Hyaluronic acid
003	**Classification**	Humectant
004	**Primary Function**	Hydration
005	**Phonetic Spelling**	HY-uh-loo-RON-ik AS-id
006	**First Discovered**	Karl Meyer, 1934
007	**Clinical Concentration(s)**	0.1–2%

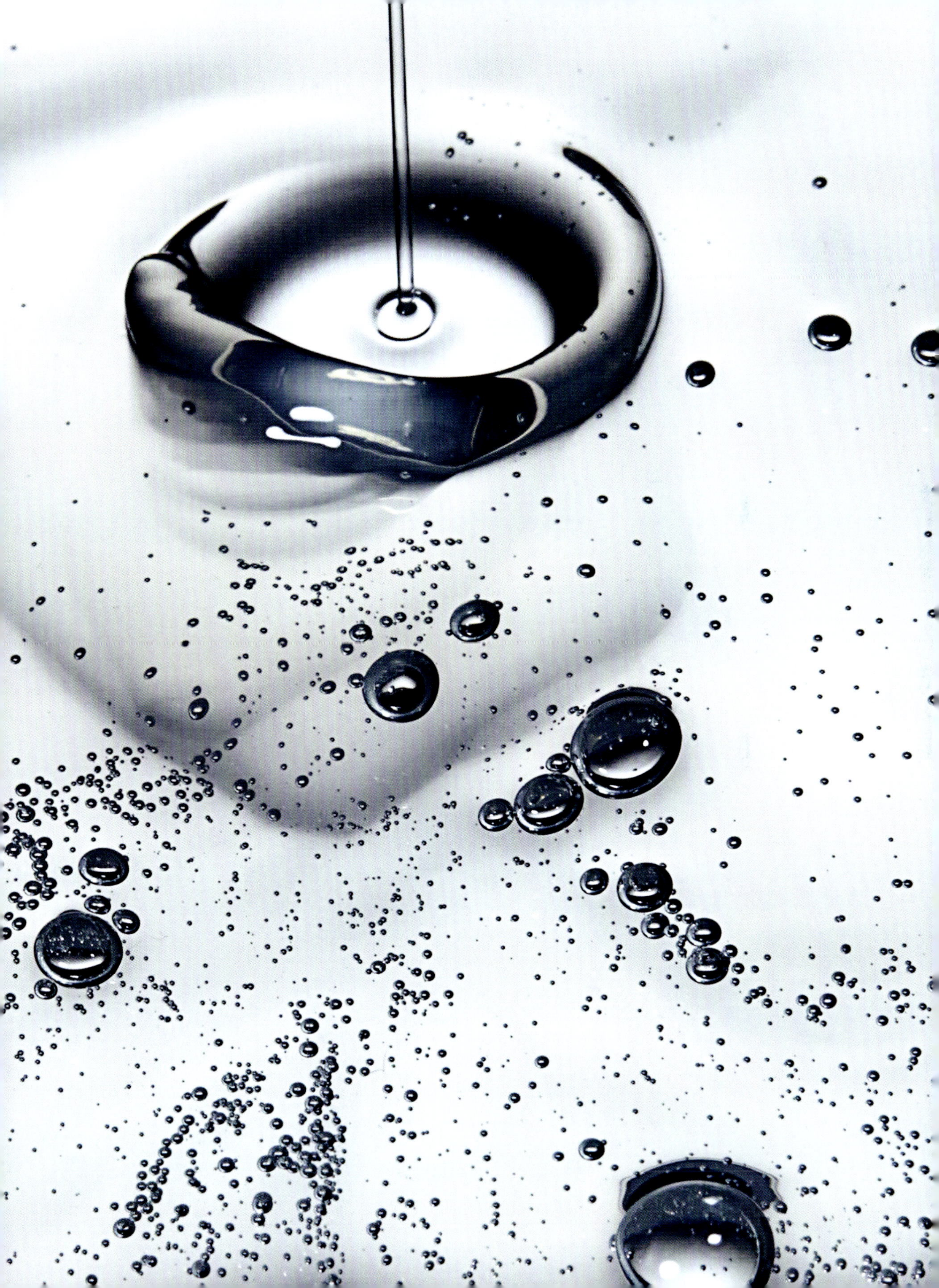

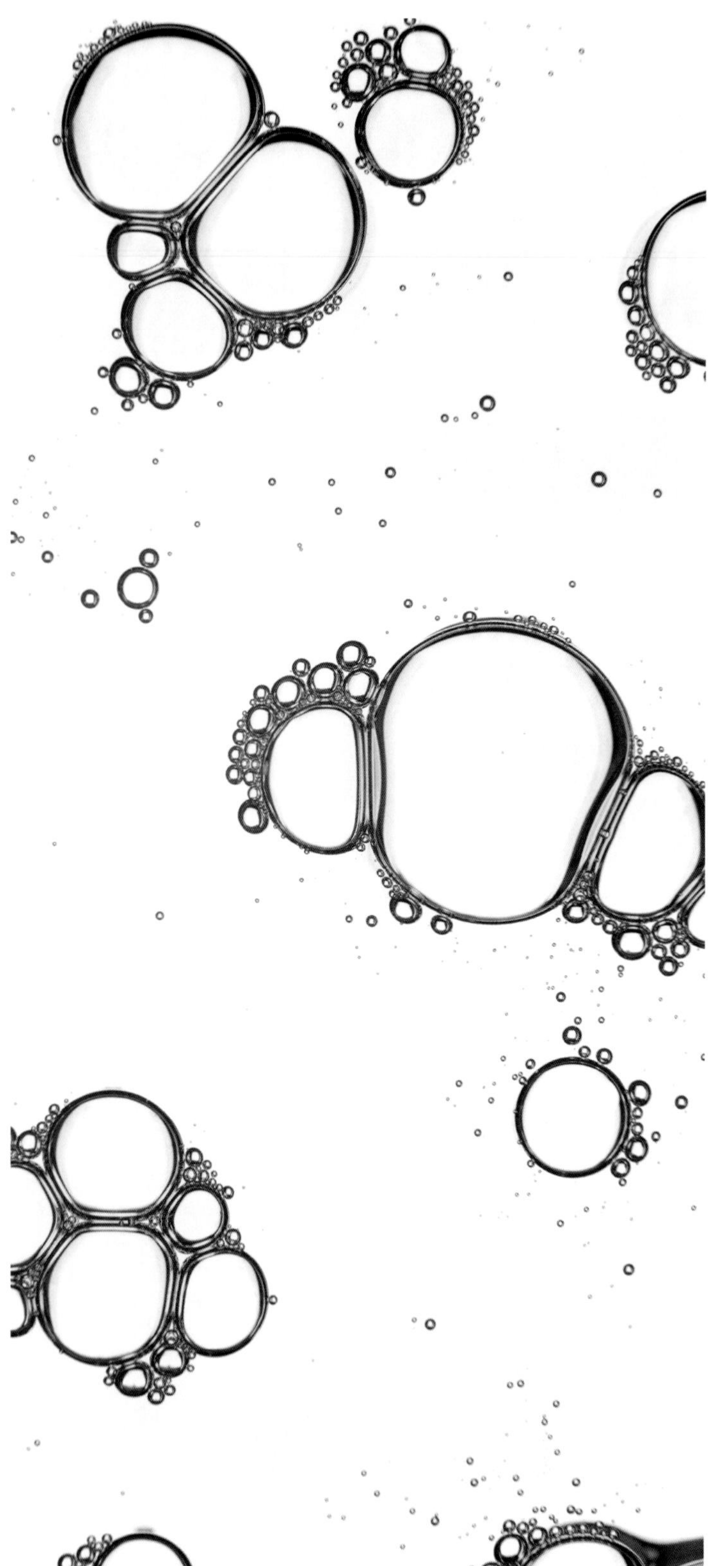

What it is

Hyaluronic acid (HA) is a naturally occurring glycosaminoglycan found in the skin, known for its exceptional ability to attract and hold moisture. This powerful hydrating ingredient helps to visibly plump and smooth the skin, supporting a refreshed and youthful look. As we age, the natural levels of HA in our skin gradually decline, which can contribute to the dryness and lack of suppleness often associated with aging. When applied topically, HA helps to lock in moisture by forming a lightweight, breathable layer on the skin's surface, leaving it feeling soft, hydrated, and rejuvenated.

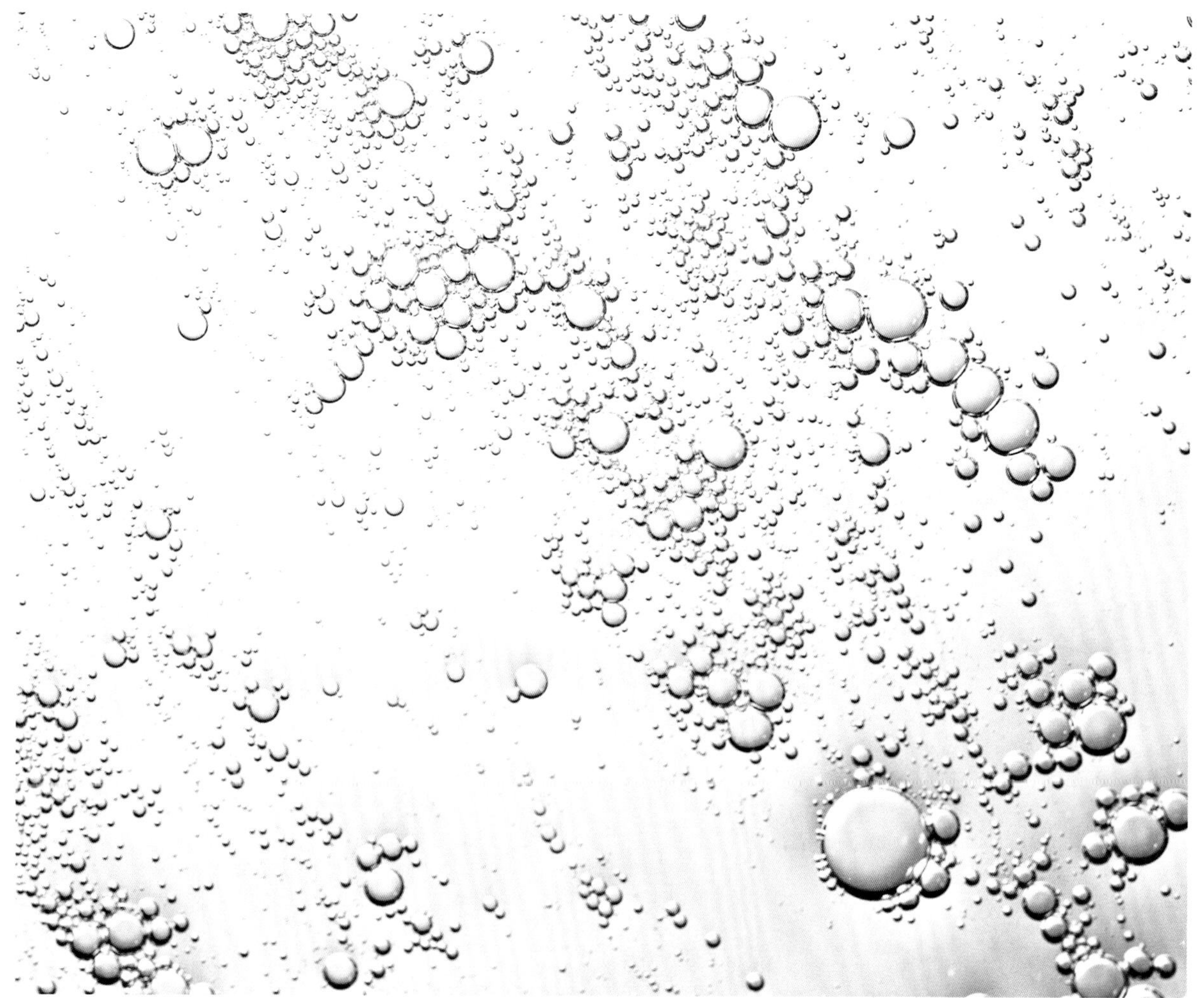

What it's used for

In skincare formulations, hyaluronic acid is celebrated for its humectant properties, attracting and retaining moisture within the skin. This hydration not only improves skin texture and appearance but also enhances the skin's barrier function, protecting it against environmental aggressors and preventing transepidermal water loss (TEWL). By maintaining optimal hydration levels, hyaluronic acid helps to reduce the appearance of fine lines and wrinkles, contributing to a smoother and more radiant-looking complexion.

Mechanism of action

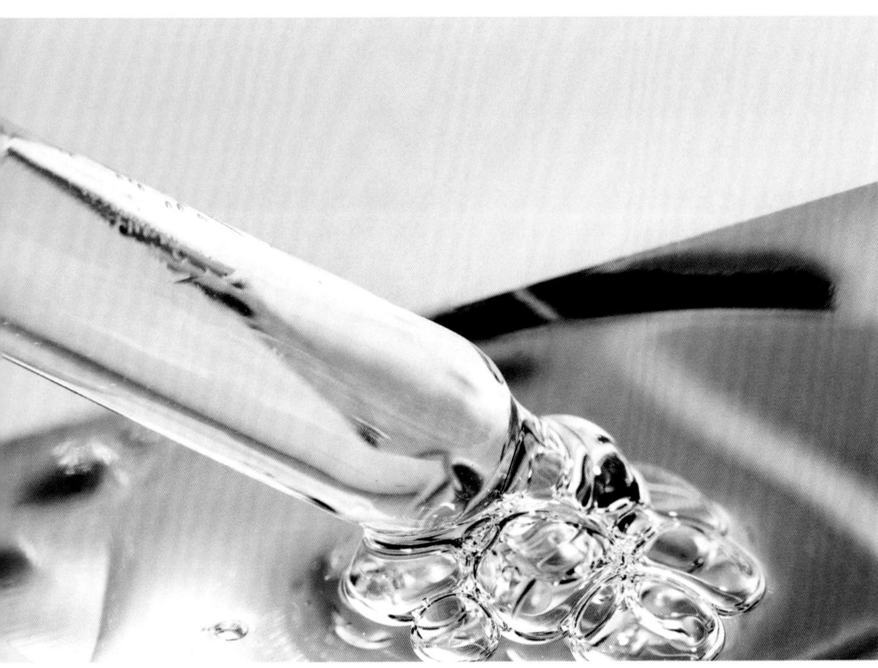

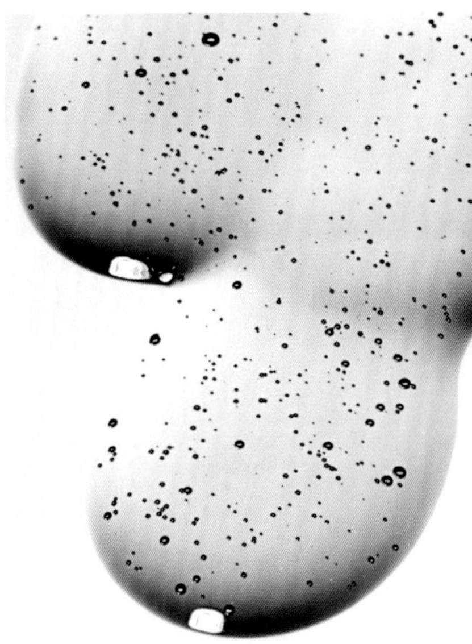

When applied topically, HA forms a viscoelastic film on the skin's surface, enhancing hydration by drawing moisture from moisture rich areas to drier areas on the stratum corneum (the outermost layer) .This increased hydration not only plumps up the skin, making it appear smoother and more youthful, but also strengthens the skin barrier, reducing transepidermal water loss (TEWL) and protecting the skin from environmental aggressors.

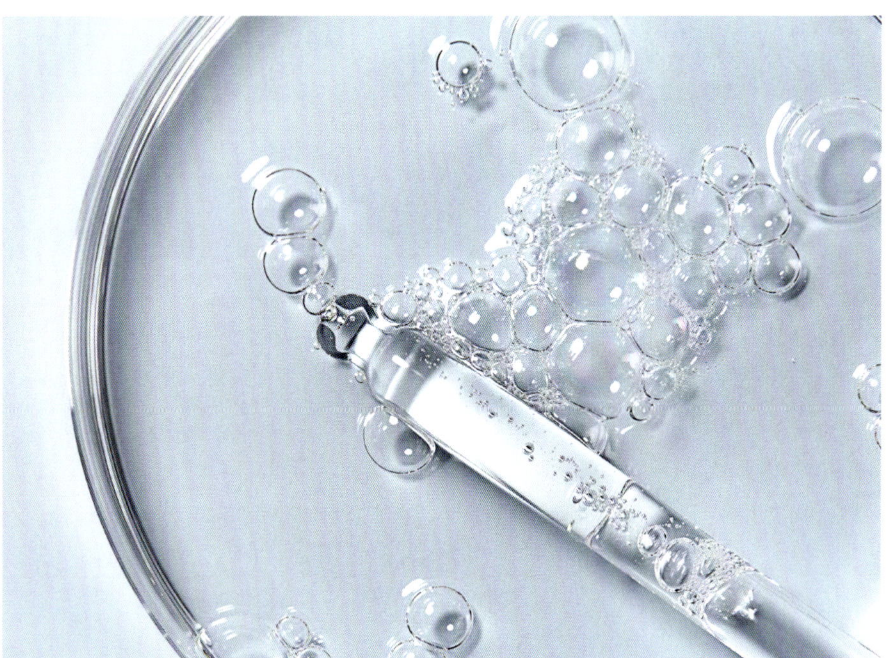

The benefits of HA are further amplified by using it in various molecular weights. High-molecular-weight HA sits on the skin's surface, providing a film-forming effect that locks in moisture and enhances the skin's appearance by smoothing fine lines. Medium-molecular-weight HA penetrates slightly deeper, delivering hydration to the upper layers of the epidermis for improved elasticity and visible radiance. Low-molecular-weight HA is designed to penetrate even deeper into the skin, delivering hydration where it is needed most and supporting a longer-lasting plumping effect. Together, these different molecular weights work synergistically to provide multi-level hydration, ensuring the skin looks and feels deeply moisturized, balanced, and revitalized.

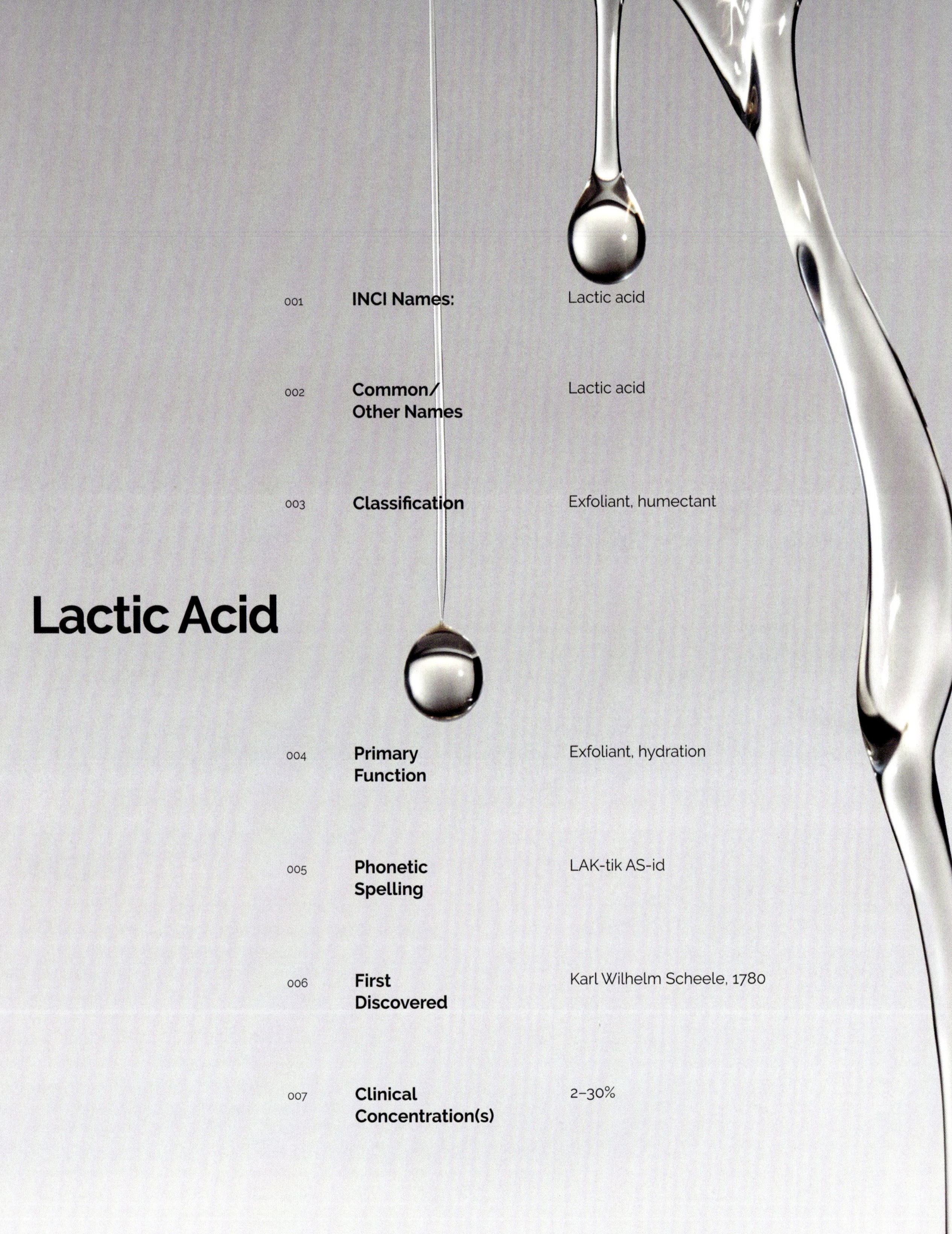

Lactic Acid

001	**INCI Names:**	Lactic acid
002	**Common/ Other Names**	Lactic acid
003	**Classification**	Exfoliant, humectant
004	**Primary Function**	Exfoliant, hydration
005	**Phonetic Spelling**	LAK-tik AS-id
006	**First Discovered**	Karl Wilhelm Scheele, 1780
007	**Clinical Concentration(s)**	2–30%

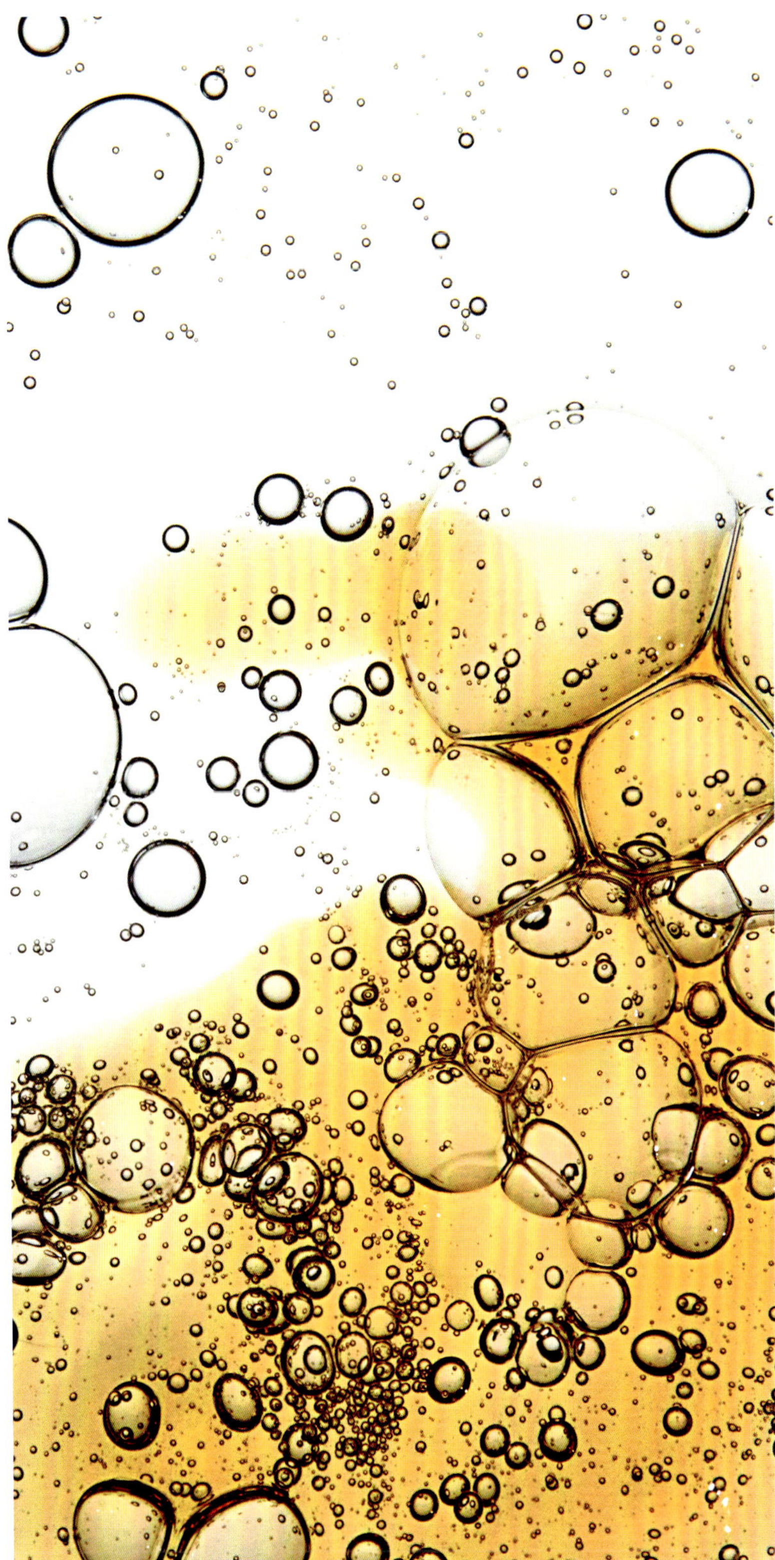

What it is

Lactic acid is a mild alpha hydroxy acid (AHA) commonly used in skincare for its exfoliating and hydrating properties. As a chemical compound, lactic acid is an organic acid derived from milk or synthetically produced, with the formula $C_3H_6O_3$. It is a water-soluble compound that belongs to the class of carboxylic acids, characterized by a hydroxyl group (-OH) attached to the carbon atom adjacent to the carboxyl group (-COOH).

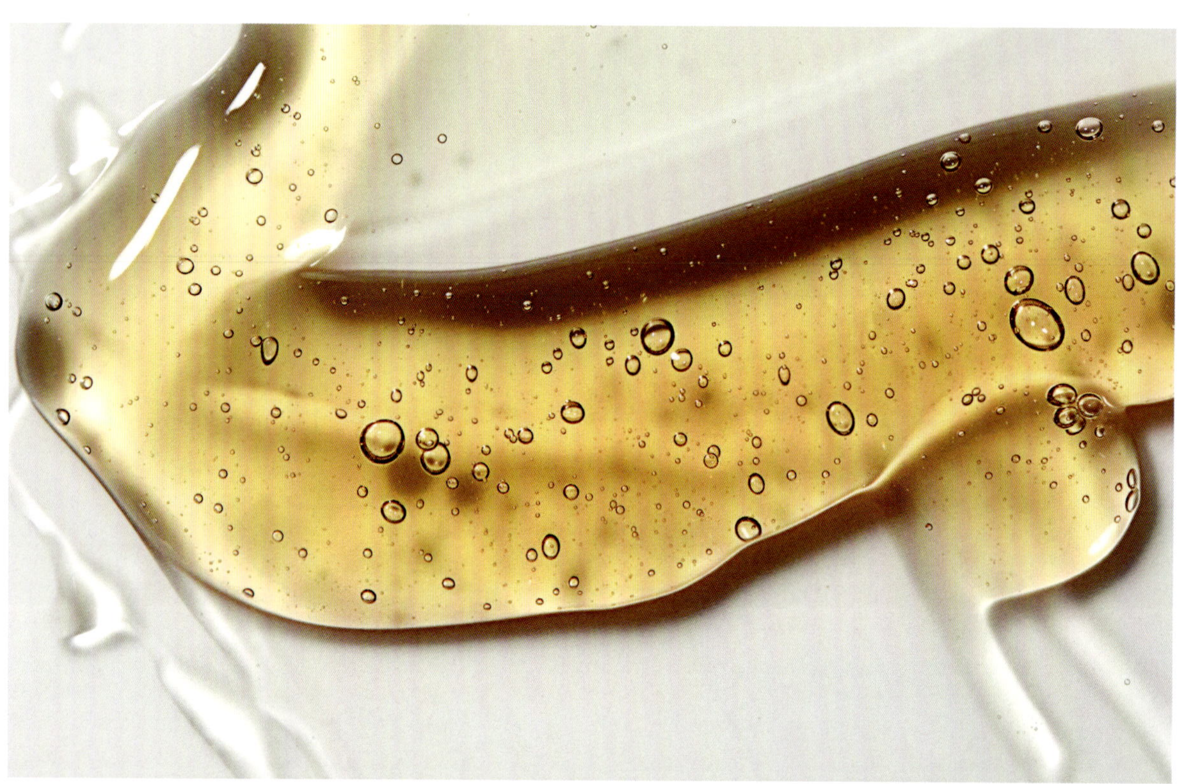

What it's used for

Lactic acid is widely used in skincare for its exfoliating and hydrating properties. It works by breaking down the bonds between dead skin cells on the surface of the skin, promoting their exfoliation and revealing the healthier-looking skin beneath. This process can help improve skin texture, making it appear smoother and more radiant.

In addition to its exfoliating benefits, lactic acid is a humectant and draws moisture into the skin to help keep it hydrated. Lactic acid is often found in serums, creams, and peels, and its concentration can vary depending on the desired effect. Lower concentrations are typically used in daily skincare products for gentle exfoliation, while higher concentrations can be used in professional treatments for more targeted results.

Mechanism of action

As a cosmetic ingredient, lactic acid works primarily through its action as an alpha hydroxy acid (AHA), which helps to exfoliate the skin by breaking down the bonds between dead skin cells. This process, known as keratolysis, encourages the exfoliation of the outer layer of the epidermis, leading to a smoother and more even skin texture. By facilitating the removal of these dead skin cells, lactic acid helps to improve congestion and enhance the penetration of other skincare ingredients. This exfoliation process also stimulates cell turnover, promoting the regeneration of new skin cells and contributing to a fresher, more youthful complexion.

Additionally, lactic acid attracts and retains moisture in the skin due to its humectant properties. It works by increasing the skin's Natural Moisturizing Factors (NMF), which are essential for maintaining skin hydration and barrier function. By drawing water into the skin and enhancing its ability to retain moisture, lactic acid helps to improve skin elasticity and suppleness. This hydrating effect is particularly beneficial for individuals with dry or dehydrated skin, as it helps to restore and maintain an optimal level of moisture, resulting in a healthier and more resilient skin barrier.

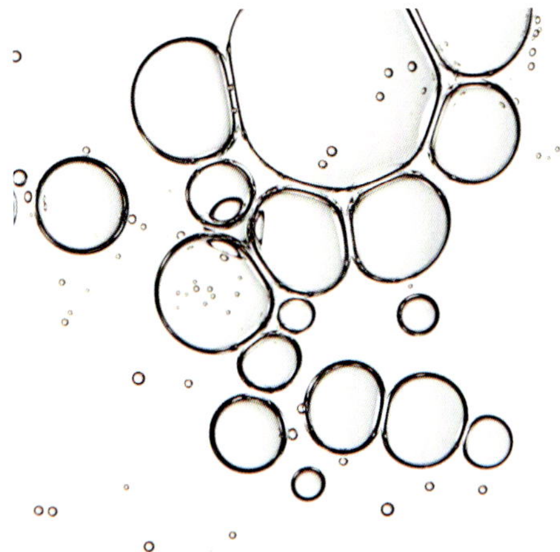

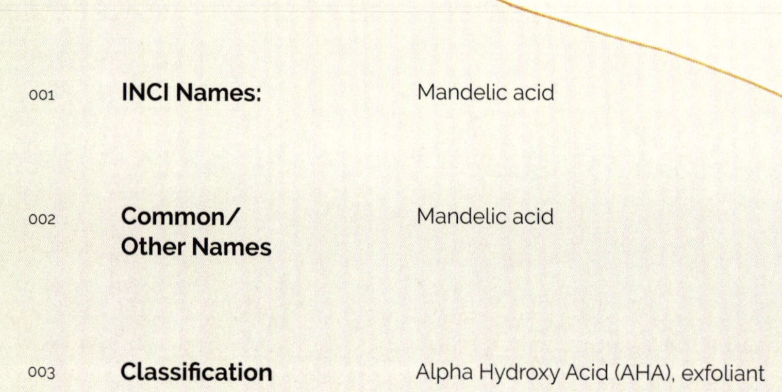

001	**INCI Names:**	Mandelic acid
002	**Common/ Other Names**	Mandelic acid
003	**Classification**	Alpha Hydroxy Acid (AHA), exfoliant

Mandelic Acid

004	**Primary Function**	Exfoliation
005	**Phonetic Spelling**	man-DEL-ik AS-id
006	**First Discovered**	Ferdinand Ludwig Winckler, 1831
007	**Clinical Concentration(s)**	5-10% in topical cosmetics, 20-40% in professional peels and treatments

What it is

Mandelic acid is an alpha hydroxy acid (AHA) derived from bitter almonds, known for its gentle yet effective exfoliating properties. Mandelic acid is particularly favored for its larger molecular structure, which allows for slower penetration into the skin, making it less irritating compared to other AHAs like glycolic acid. This slower absorption can reduce the risk of irritation, making mandelic acid more suitable for those with sensitive skin.

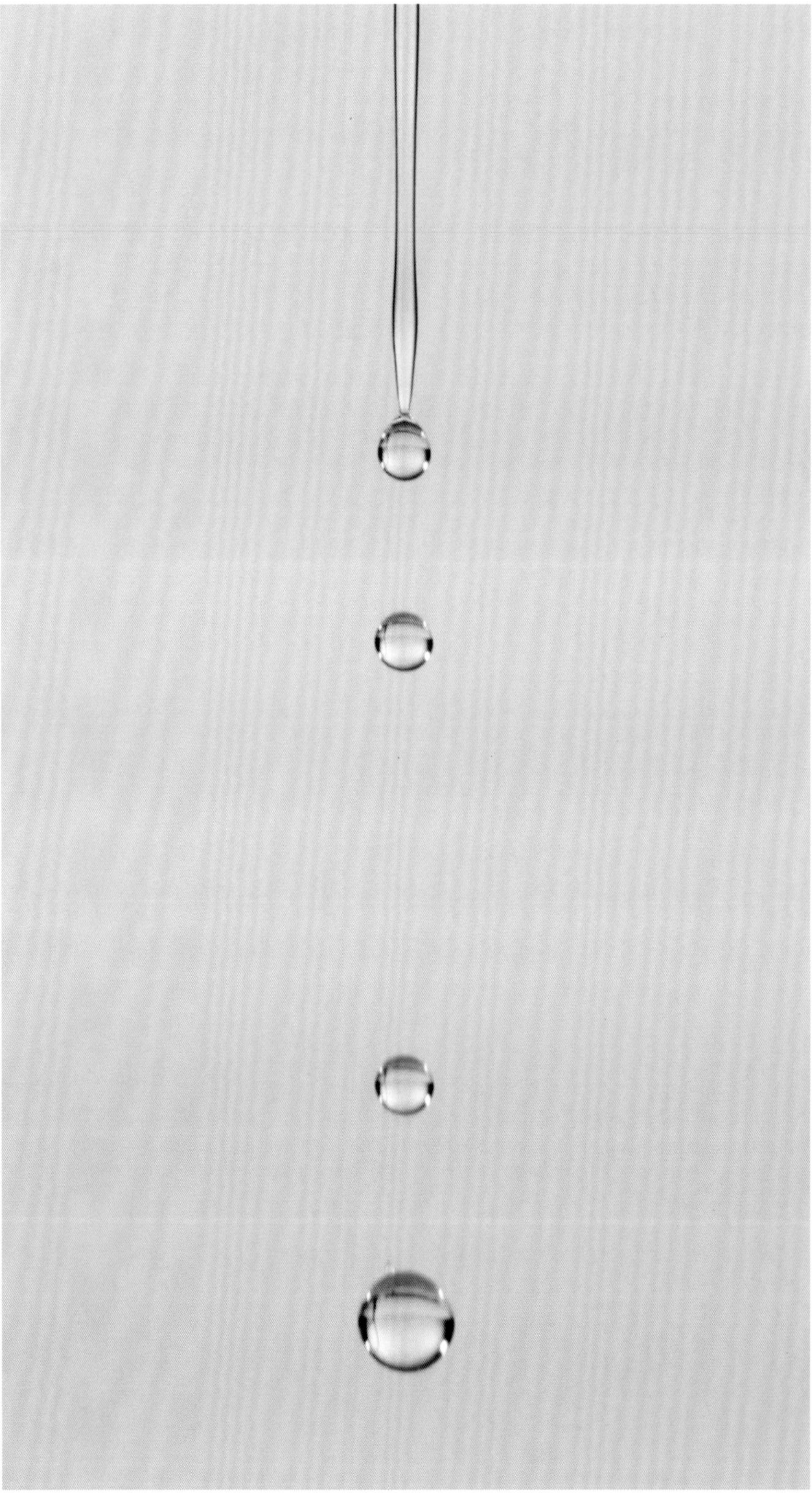

What it's used for

Mandelic acid is commonly used in skincare for its gentle exfoliating properties, promoting cell turnover and revealing smoother, brighter skin. It is often included in formulations designed to address concerns such as uneven skin tone, texture, and dark spots.

In addition to its exfoliating action, mandelic acid can help reduce the appearance of blemishes. Its ability to target surface-level concerns such as blemishes, fine lines, and dark spots makes it a versatile ingredient in both anti-aging and blemish-control products.

Mandelic acid is also less likely to cause irritation compared to other AHAs like glycolic acid, making it suitable for those with more reactive skin types. The combination of exfoliation and soothing benefits makes it a key ingredient in gentle yet effective skincare routines.

Mechanism of action

Mandelic acid functions primarily through its action as an AHA, which helps to exfoliate the skin by breaking down the intercellular bonds that hold dead skin cells together. This action promotes cell turnover, allowing newer, healthier skin cells to surface and promoting a more even complexion. Mandelic acid's larger molecular structure allows for slower penetration and minimizes the risk of irritation, making it a gentler option for exfoliation. As a result, mandelic acid effectively removes dead skin cells, smoothens the skin's texture, and helps in improving skin tone without causing significant irritation.

Beyond its exfoliating properties, mandelic acid also reduces the presence of sebum on the skin, which, in combination with its ability to help clear clogged pores, reduces the appearance of blemishes. Its dual action makes it a valuable ingredient for treating blemish-prone skin while simultaneously addressing dark spots and promoting a more even complexion.

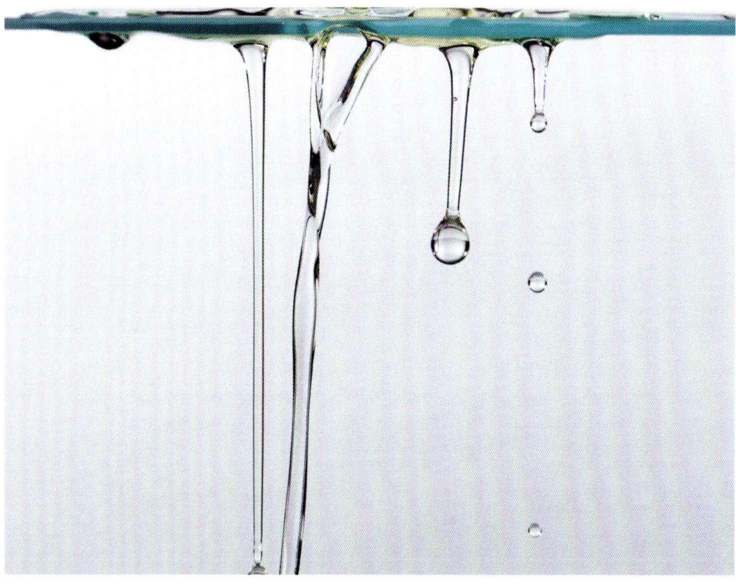

Matrixyl 3000™ & Matrixyl Synthe'6™

001	**INCI Names:**	Palmitoyl Tripeptide-1, Palmitoyl Tetrapeptide-7 (*Matrixyl 3000™*), Palmitoyl Tripeptide-38 (*Matrixyl Synthe'6™*)
002	**Common/ Other Names**	Matrixyl 3000™. Matrixyl Synthe'6™
003	**Classification**	Synthetic peptides
004	**Primary Function**	Anti-aging, reducing appearance of fine lines and wrinkles
005	**Phonetic Spelling**	MAT-riK-siL/ MAT-riK-siL Sin-TH
006	**First Discovered**	Sederma Inc., early 2000s
007	**Clinical Concentration(s)**	2–10%

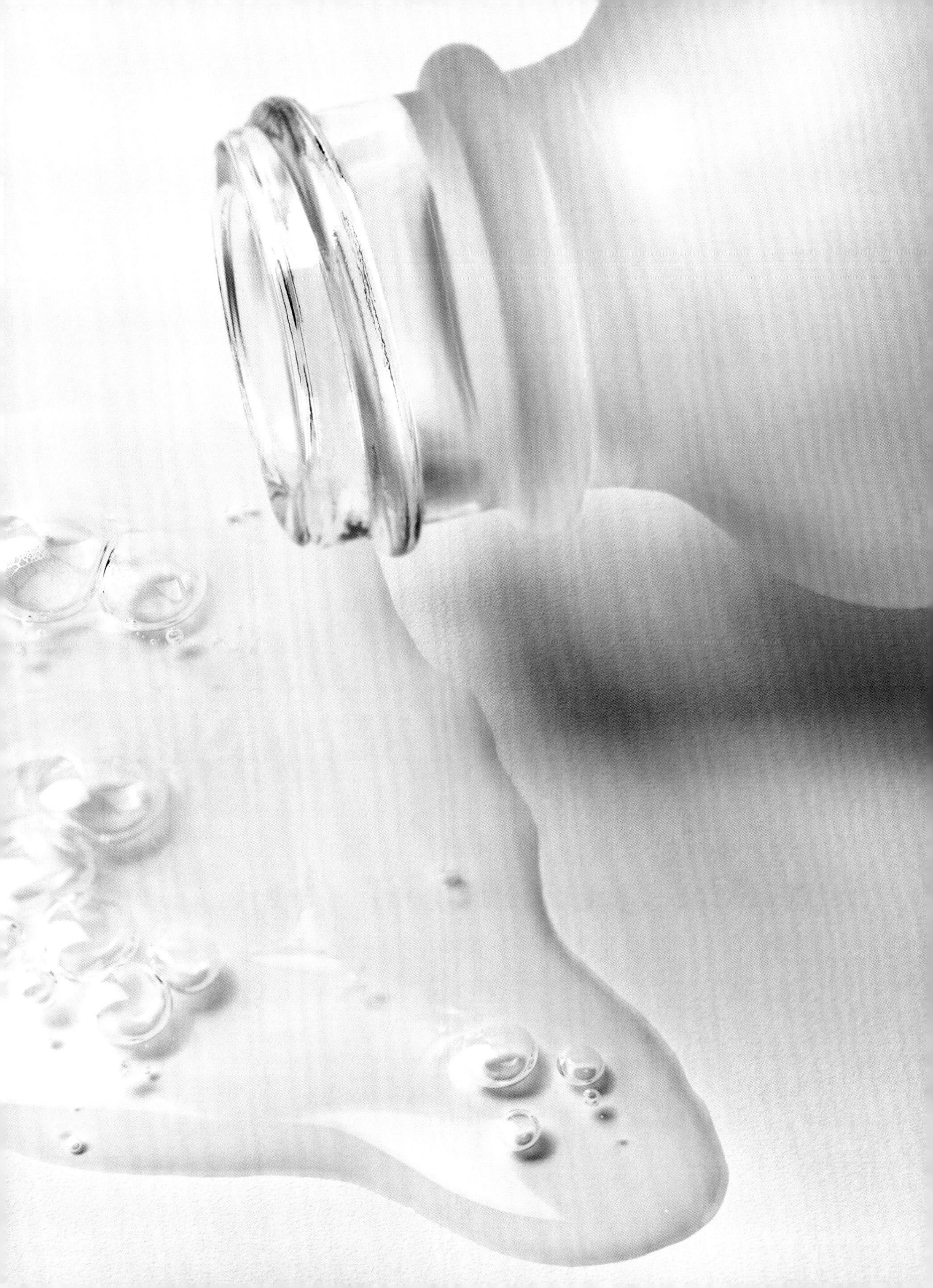

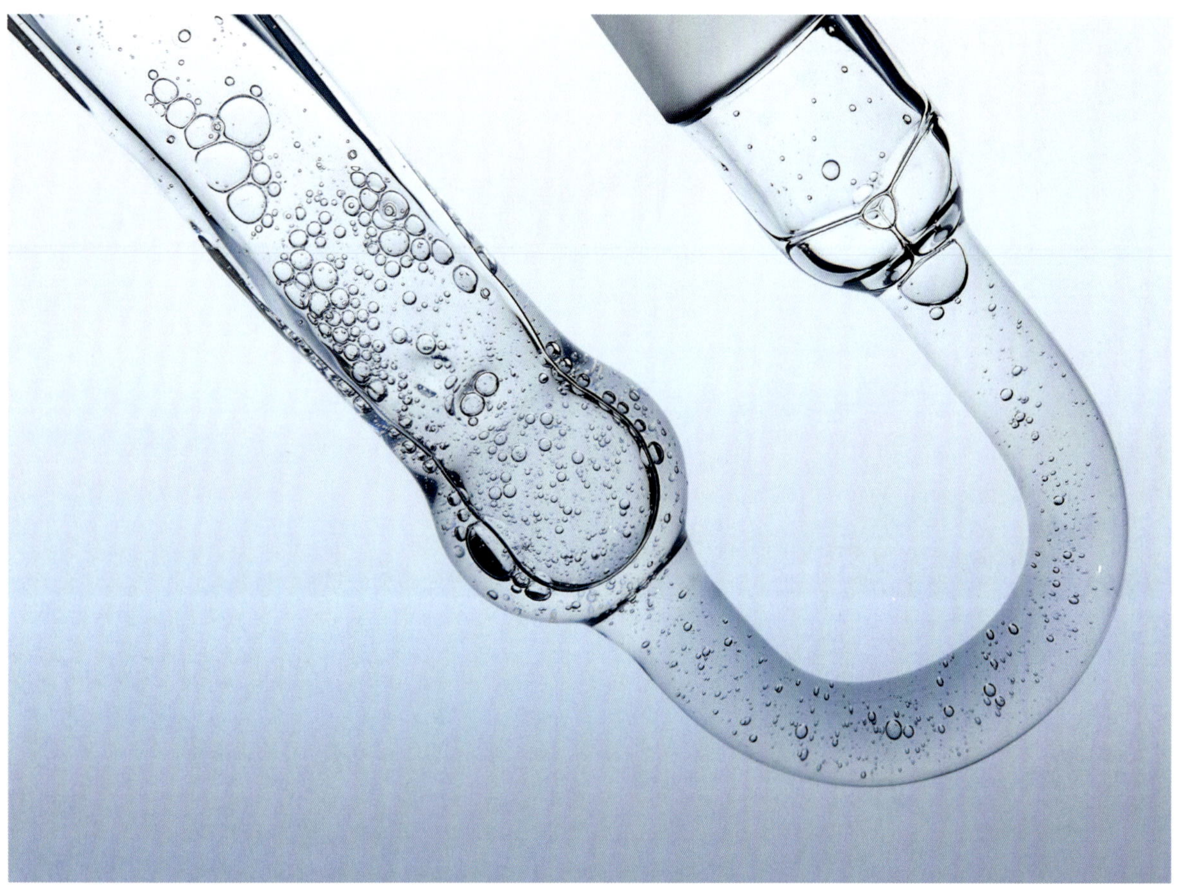

What it is

Matrixyl 3000™ is composed of two matrikines, palmitoyl tripeptide-1 and palmitoyl tetrapeptide-7. These peptides mimic naturally occurring signaling molecules in the skin and are designed to stimulate extracellular matrix components such as collagen and elastin. This stimulation helps to reduce the appearance of wrinkles and improve skin elasticity by promoting repair processes within the skin's dermal matrix.

Matrixyl Synthe'6™, on the other hand, features palmitoyl tripeptide-38, which is targeted at enhancing the synthesis of six major skin components, including collagen types I, III, and IV, as well as fibronectin, hyaluronic acid, and laminins.

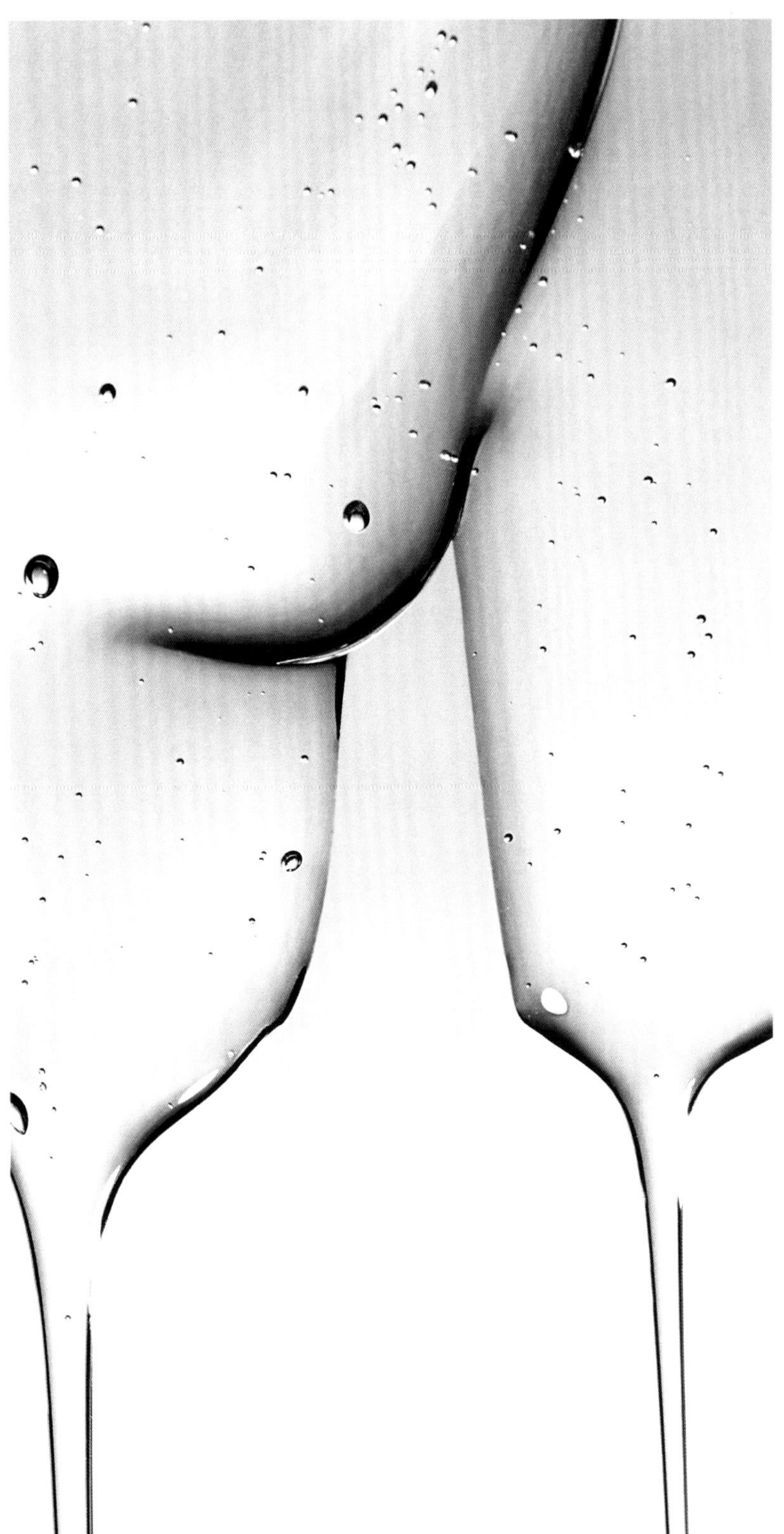

What it's used for

Matrixyl 3000™ and Matrixyl synthe'6™ are commonly used in skincare formulations for their anti-aging benefits. Their key peptides function together to stimulate the production of collagen, thereby reducing the appearance of visible fine lines and wrinkles. They also encourage skin regeneration and the production of elastin, which helps to improve the overall texture and firmness of the skin.

Mechanism of action

Matrixyl 3000™ and Matrixyl Synthe'6™ are peptide blends that help to promote smoother, firmer, and more youthful-looking skin. The two peptides of Matrixyl 3000™ work together to support the skin's natural rejuvenation processes. By boosting the skin's production of essential proteins like collagen and elastin, these peptides help improve the appearance of skin texture, reduce the appearance of fine lines, and enhance elasticity.

Matrixyl Synthe'6™, a more advanced peptide complex, encourages the production of six key skin components, including collagen and hyaluronic acid, which are important for maintaining the skin's elasticity and hydration. Matrixyl Synthe'6™ helps improve areas where fine lines and wrinkles form, helping to make the skin appear thicker and improve overall skin health.

Both complexes leverage the power of peptides to communicate with skin cells, supporting a refreshed, revitalized look and improving the overall appearance of the skin.

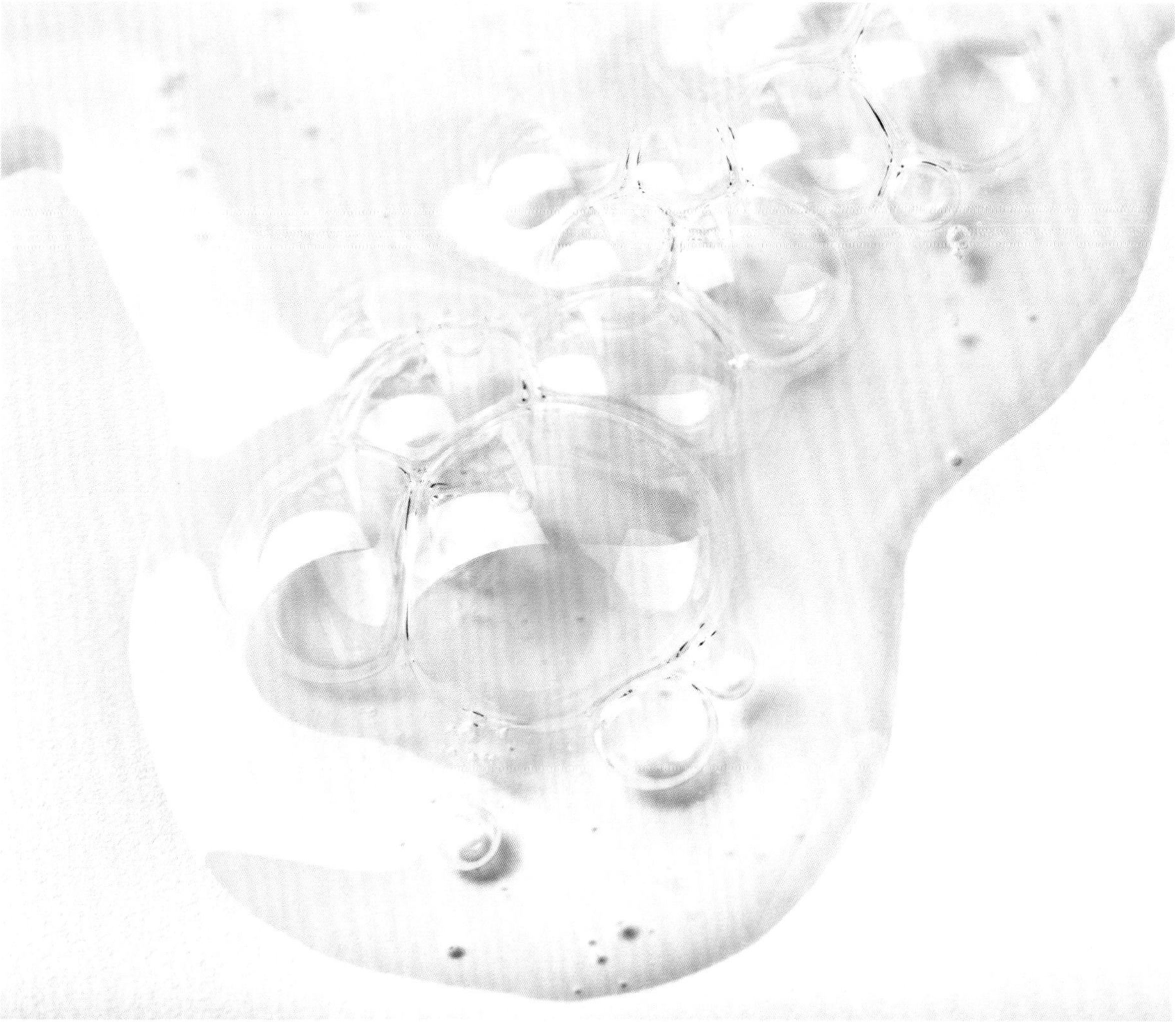

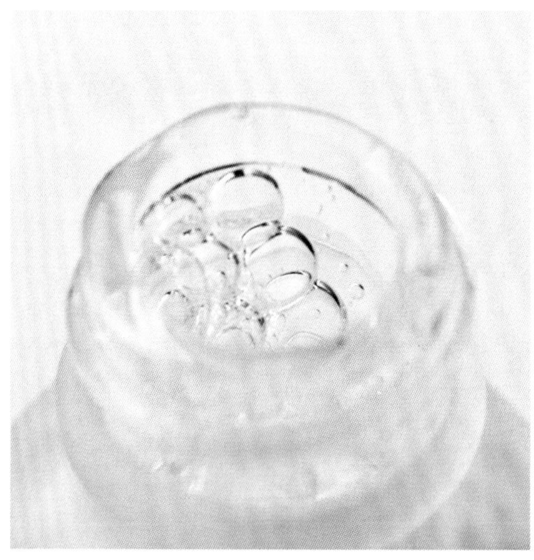

NAG

001	**INCI Names:**	N-acetyl glucosamine
002	**Common/ Other Names**	NAG
003	**Classification**	Peptide
004	**Primary Function**	Dark spots and uneven tone
005	**Phonetic Spelling**	en-uh-SEE-tul GLOO-koh-sah-meen
006	**First Discovered**	Early 20th century during studies of chitin, a structural component in crustaceans and fungi
007	**Clinical Concentration(s)**	2–4%

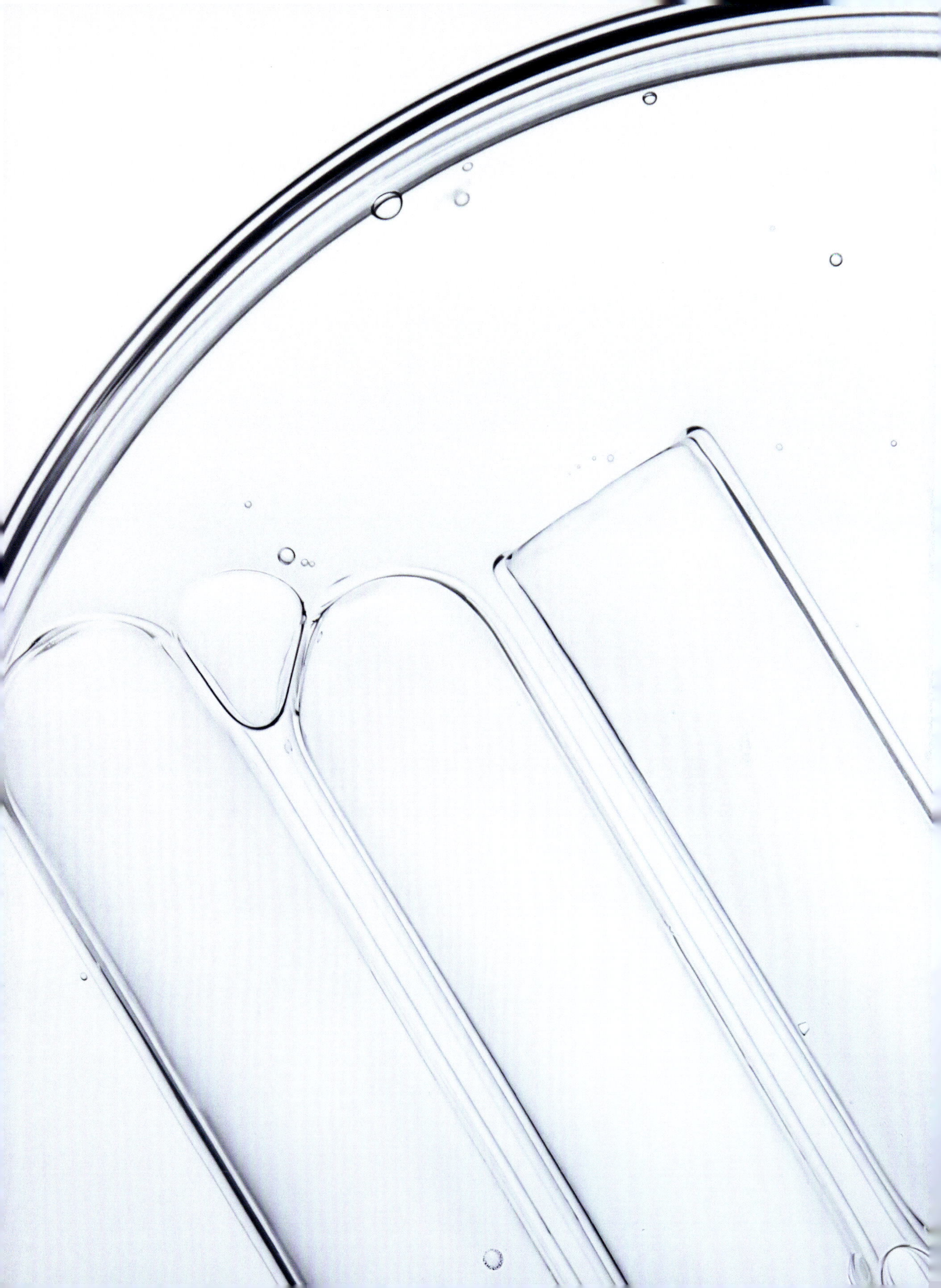

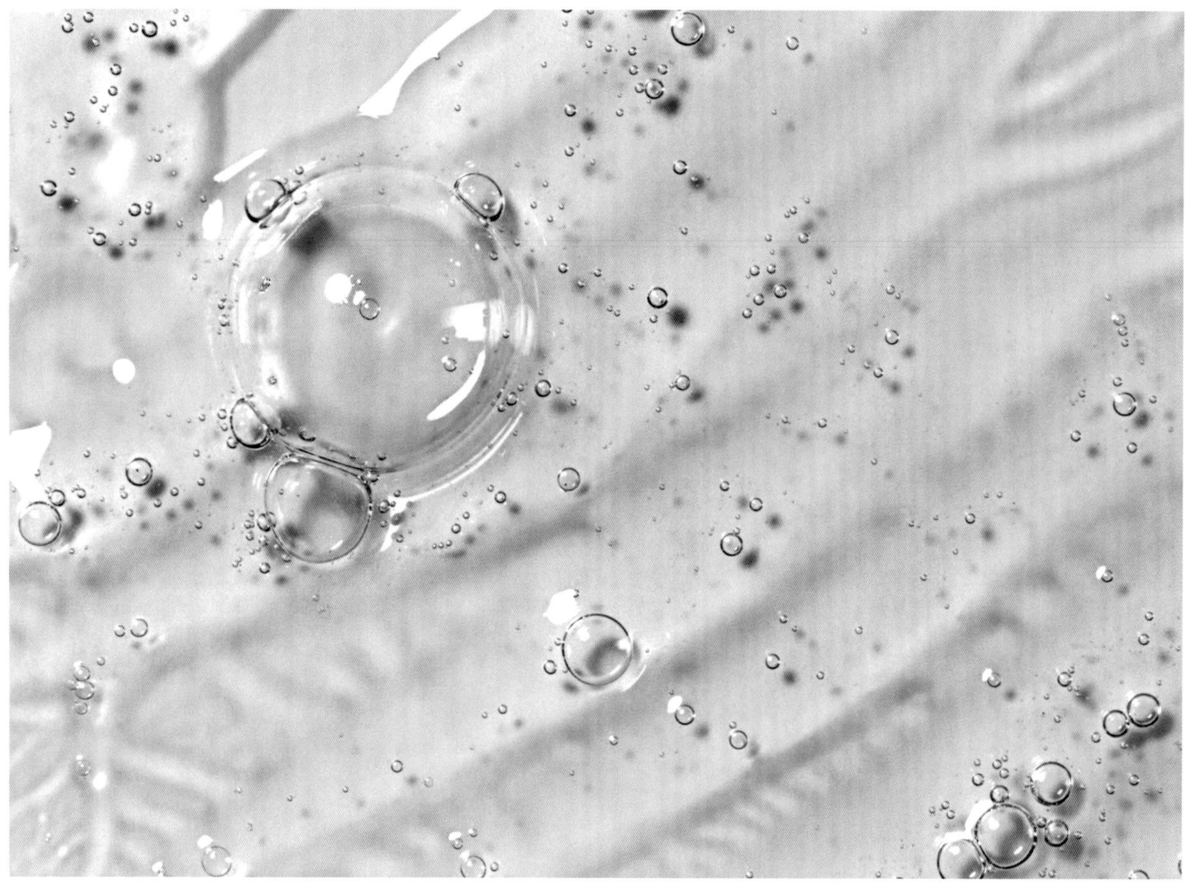

What it is

N-acetylglucosamine (NAG) is a derivative of glucose and a naturally occurring amino sugar found in the structure of glycoproteins and glycosaminoglycans in the skin. Chemically, it consists of a glucose molecule with an acetyl group attached, making it more stable and effective for cosmetic applications. Its molecular structure allows it to interact with the skin's surface, supporting hydration, exfoliation, and the reduction of uneven skin tone.

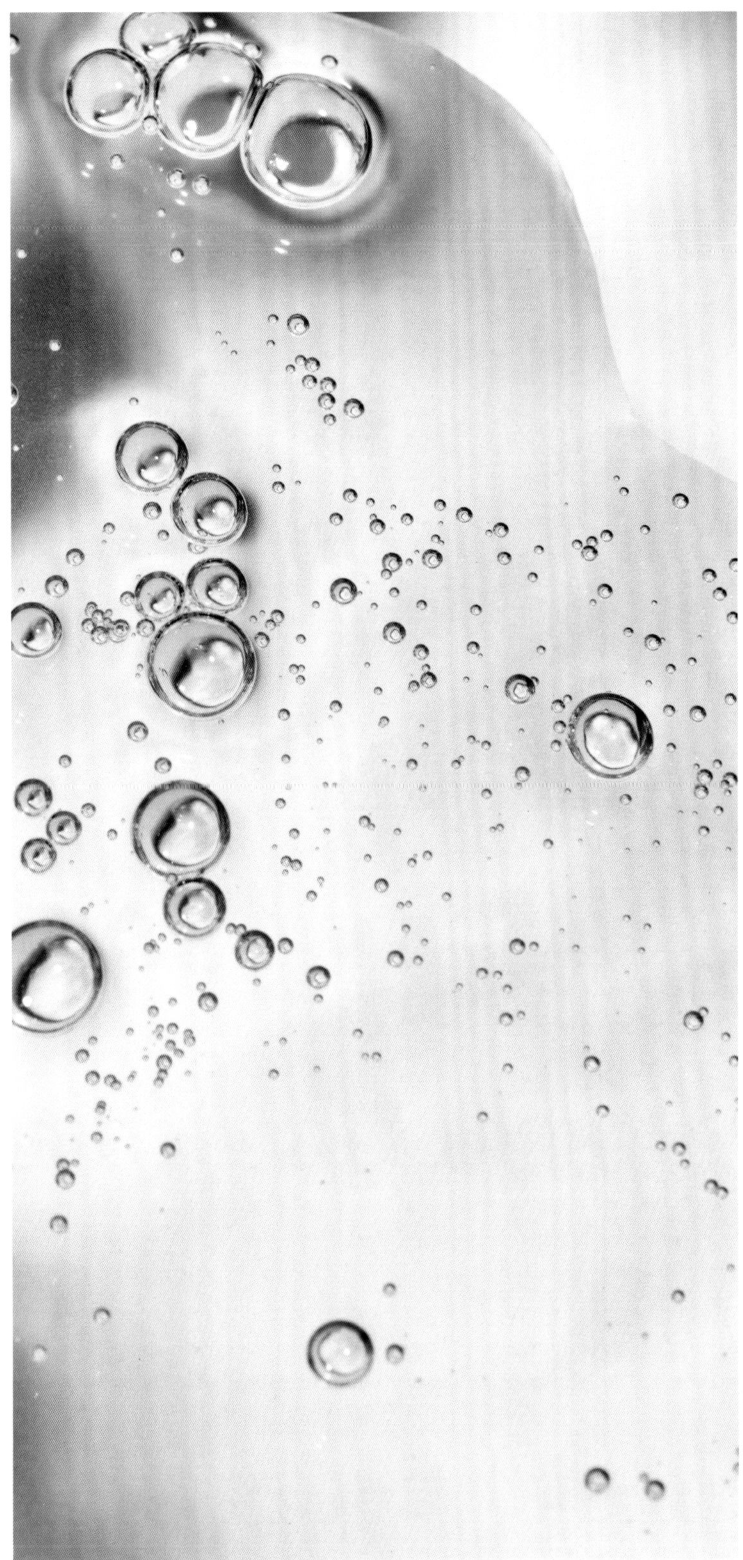

What it does

NAG supports skin health by enhancing hydration, maintaining structural integrity, and stimulating natural hyaluronic acid production. This makes NAG an effective ingredient in skincare formulations targeting hydration, anti-aging, and skin barrier repair. It is also used for its gentle exfoliating properties, improving skin tone and texture by inhibiting melanin production through suppression of tyrosinase activity. This mechanism makes it a valuable ingredient in products helping improve the look of radiance and reduce the appearance of dark spots.

Mechanism of action

In cosmetics, N-acetyl glucosamine (NAG) leverages its structural similarity to glucose and its role as a precursor to hyaluronic acid by supporting the skin's natural mechanisms of promoting hydration and improving the look of texture. NAG enhances hyaluronic acid production, a critical molecule for skin hydration and plumpness, by supplying essential building blocks for its synthesis. This action helps to maintain the skin barrier, reduce water loss, and maintain overall skin health.

Additionally, NAG interacts with melanin synthesis pathways to reduce the appearance of dark spots and uneven skin tone. In in vitro studies, NAG has been demonstrated to reduce the activity of tyrosinase, a key enzyme in melanin production, leading to improvements in uneven pigmentation. Its gentle exfoliating properties also encourage the shedding of dead skin cells, further improving radiance over time. These combined actions make NAG an effective ingredient for hydration, anti-aging, and improving the look of uneven skin tone.

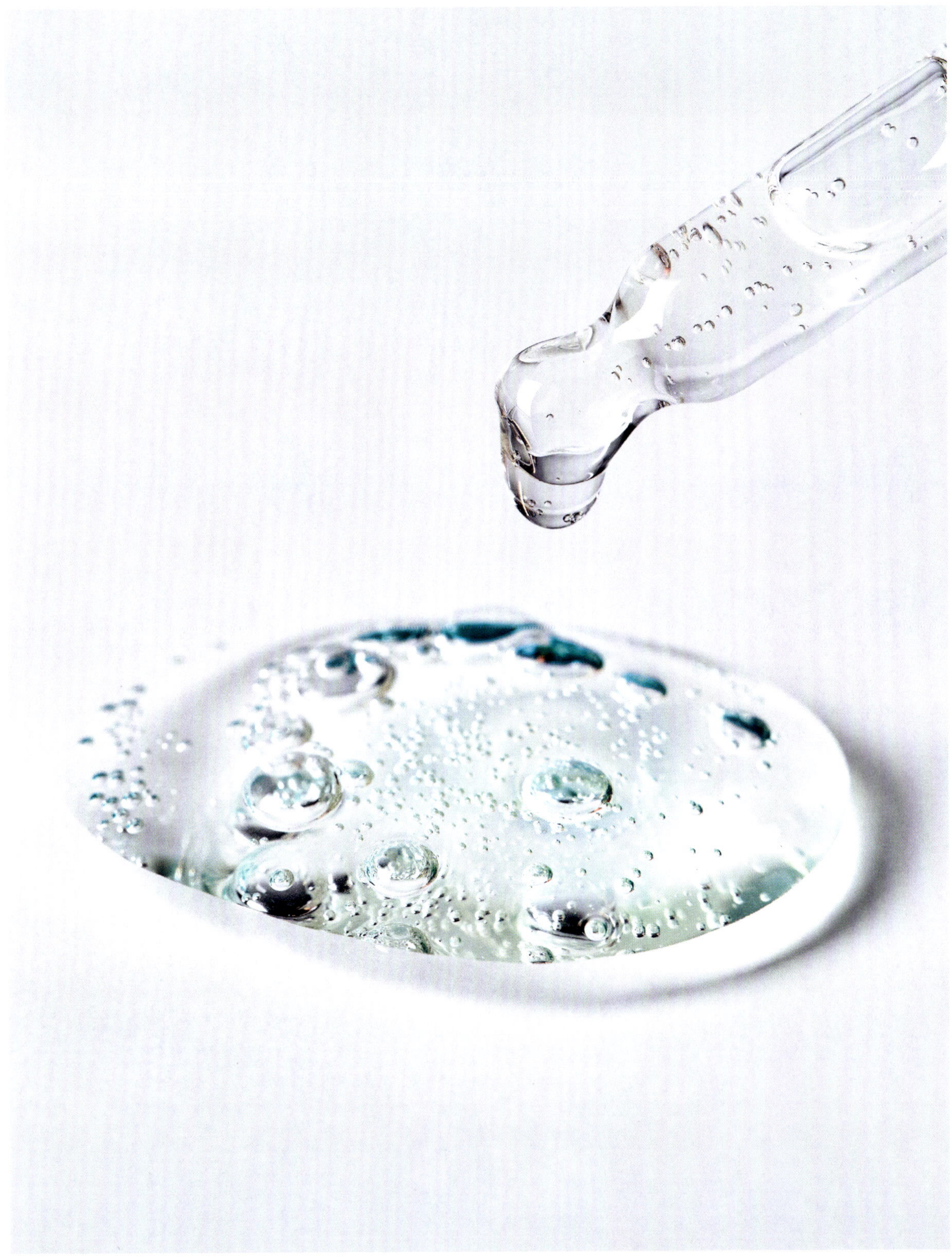

001	**INCI Names:**	Niacinamide
002	**Common/ Other Names**	Nicotinamide, vitamin B3
003	**Classification**	Skin-conditioning agent

Niacinamide

004	**Primary Function**	Multi-functional active
005	**Phonetic Spelling**	Nye-uh-SIN-uh-mide
006	**First Discovered**	Conrad Arnold Elvehjem, 1937
007	**Clinical Concentration(s)**	2–10%

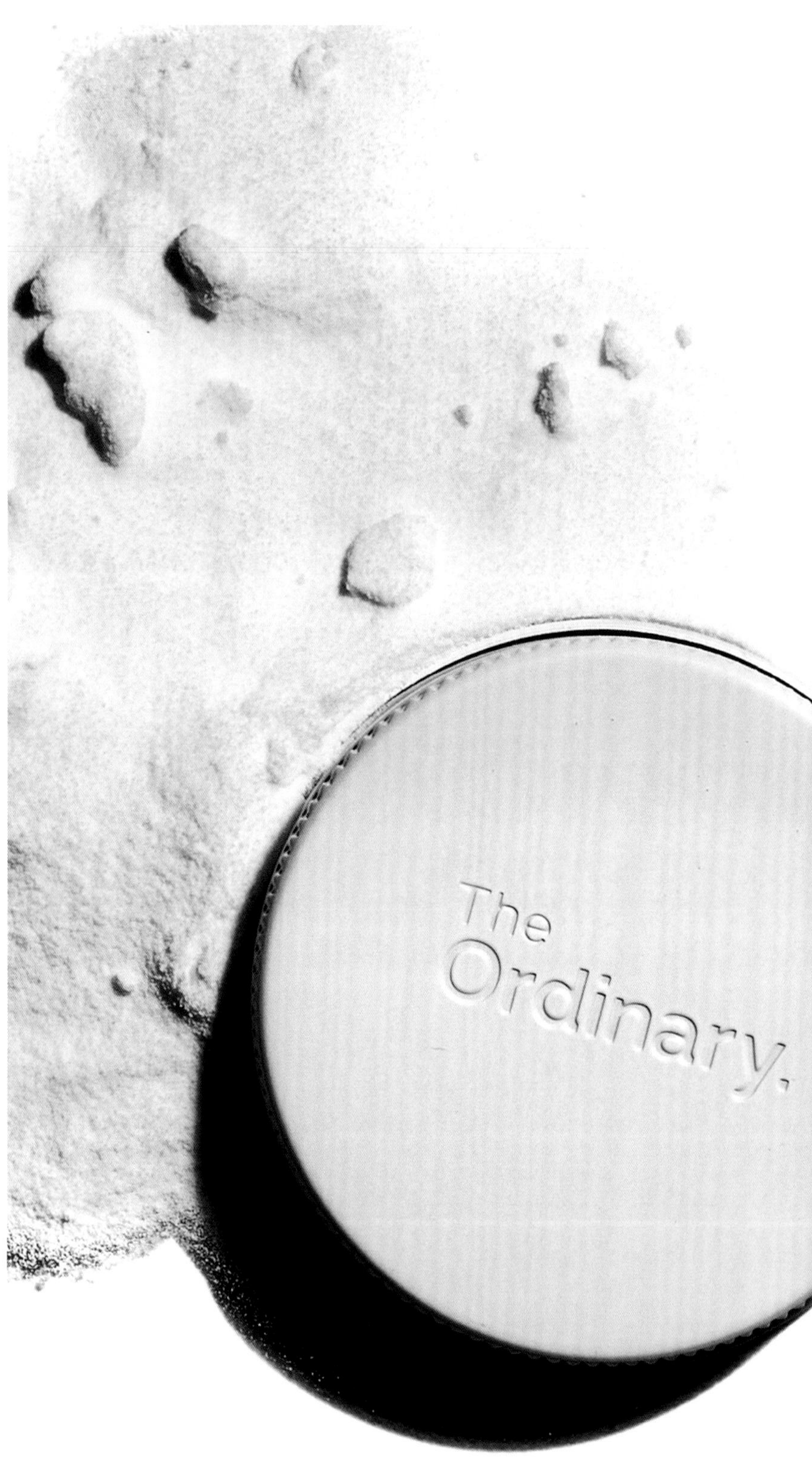

What it is

Niacinamide, also known as nicotinamide, nicotinic acid amide, or 3-pyridinecarboxamide, is a water-soluble form of vitamin B3. It can be found in its varying forms within a range of foods, including meat, dairy, legumes, nuts, grains, and fortified foods like bread and cereal. Most cosmetic forms of niacinamide come from synthetic origin.

What it's used for

Niacinamide is an active ingredient that is used to target a wide range of cosmetic concerns. It is used to improve the look of radiance and target uneven tone, as well as support the skin barrier for improved skin hydration. It is also used to reduce excess oil and pore visibility as well as improve the look of signs of congestion.

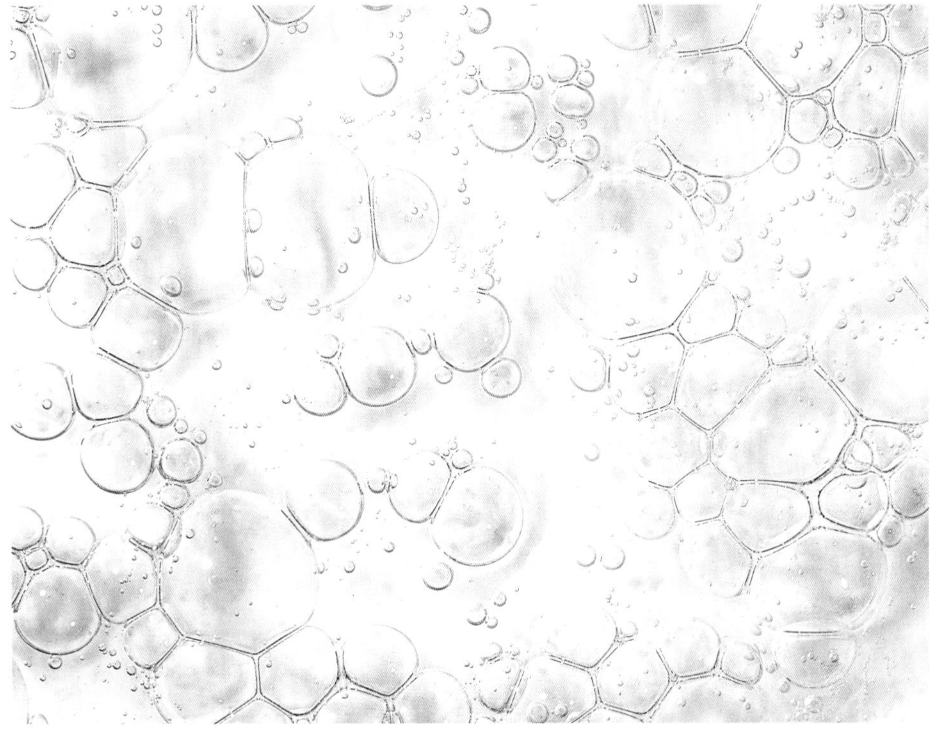

Mechanism of action

Sebum regulation and blemishes

Niacinamide is a helpful ingredient for balancing oil production. Niacinamide helps to regulate the amount of sebum the skin produces (the natural oil that can sometimes lead to a shiny or greasy feeling), thereby improving signs of congestion and boosting radiance. By balancing excess sebum production, niacinamide helps your skin stay hydrated without becoming too oily and helps support blemish-prone skin.

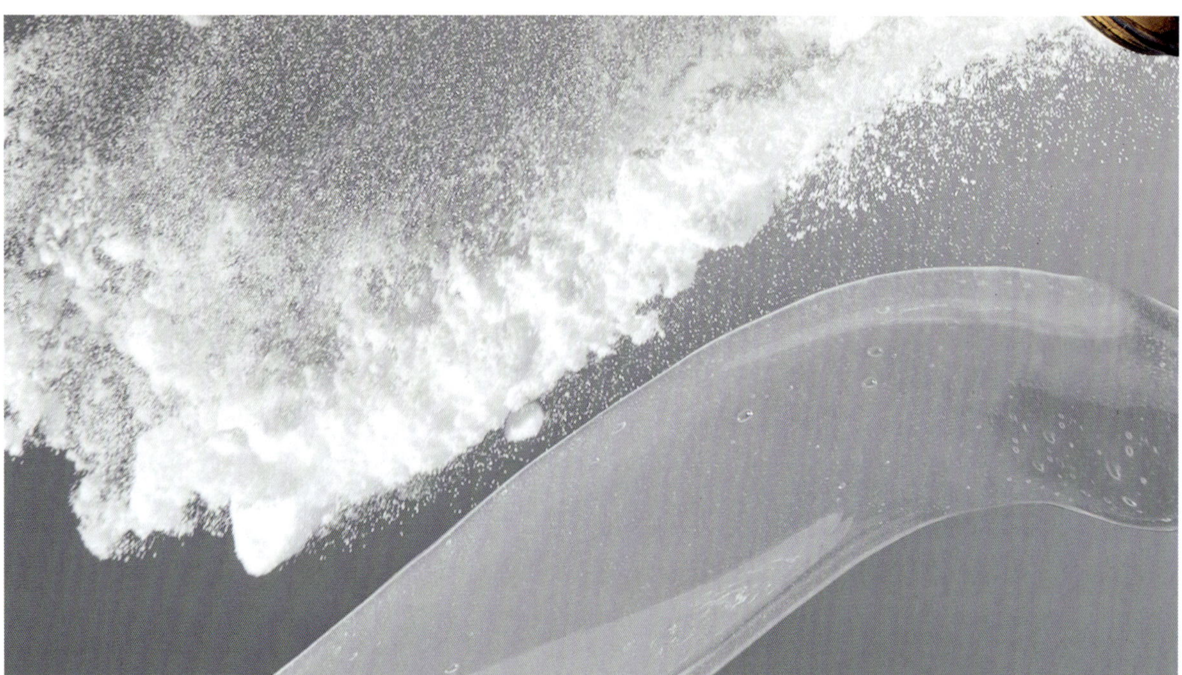

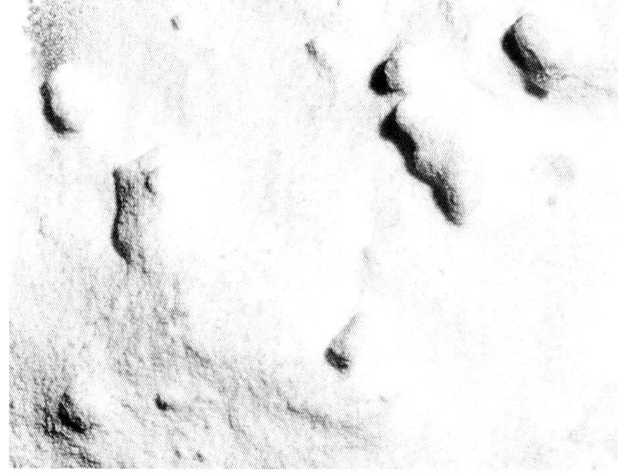

Signs of aging

Research on human participants has shown that using products with 4–5% niacinamide can improve the appearance of fine lines and wrinkles, with noticeable results after about 8 weeks. This anti-aging effect is likely due to niacinamide's impact on important proteins like collagen and elastin. These proteins are key for keeping skin smooth, firm, and elastic. Studies have shown that niacinamide can boost collagen production, even in older skin cells, which helps explain its ability to support more youthful-looking skin.

Barrier support and hydration

Niacinamide goes beyond just supporting collagen—it also helps with the production of other key proteins that keep skin healthy. It plays a role in making keratin, involucrin, and filaggrin, all of which are important for maintaining a strong skin barrier. Keratin helps form the structure of the skin's outer layer, while involucrin helps with skin stability, and filaggrin helps the skin hold on to moisture. Research has also shown that niacinamide boosts the production of essential skin lipids like ceramides. These lipids keep the skin hydrated and act as a shield, protecting it from moisture loss and environmental stressors.

Radiance and texture

Niacinamide promotes a more even skin tone and enhances radiance by supporting the skin's natural renewal process. Studies show that niacinamide helps reduce the appearance of uneven skin tone by inhibiting the transfer of pigment into the visible upper layers of the skin. When uneven pigmentation has developed in the skin, this action helps to minimize visible pigmentation differences and create a more uniform complexion. Human studies have shown that topical application of niacinamide, in concentrations of 2–5%, effectively targets areas of uneven skin tone. By supporting skin renewal, niacinamide contributes to smoother, more radiant skin.

Niacinamide has been shown to support skin renewal, thereby promoting radiance and improving overall texture. People using products with niacinamide often notice smoother, more radiant skin thanks to its ability to boost skin cell turnover and enhance natural exfoliation. It helps strengthen the skin barrier and promotes healthier, more mature skin cells on the surface, resulting in a thicker stratum corneum layer. This leads to better light reflection, which contributes to a more even texture and a radiant, glowing complexion.

Panthenol

001	**INCI Names:**	Panthenol, pantothenic acid
002	**Common/ Other Names**	Provitamin B5, pantothenate, vitamin B5
003	**Classification**	Humectant
004	**Primary Function**	Hydration
005	**Phonetic Spelling**	PAN-then-awl
006	**First Discovered**	Roger John Williams, 1933
007	**Clinical Concentration(s)**	1–5%

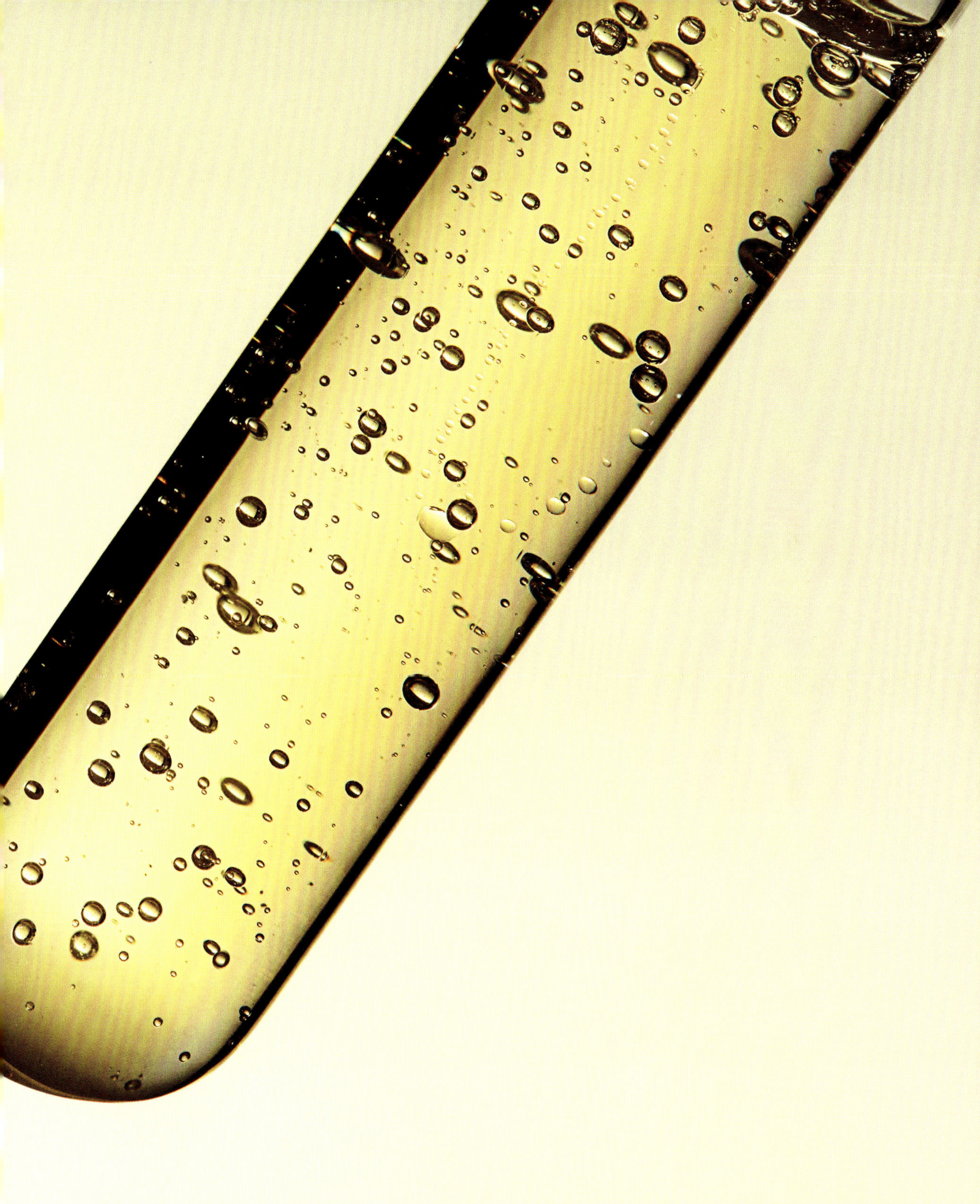

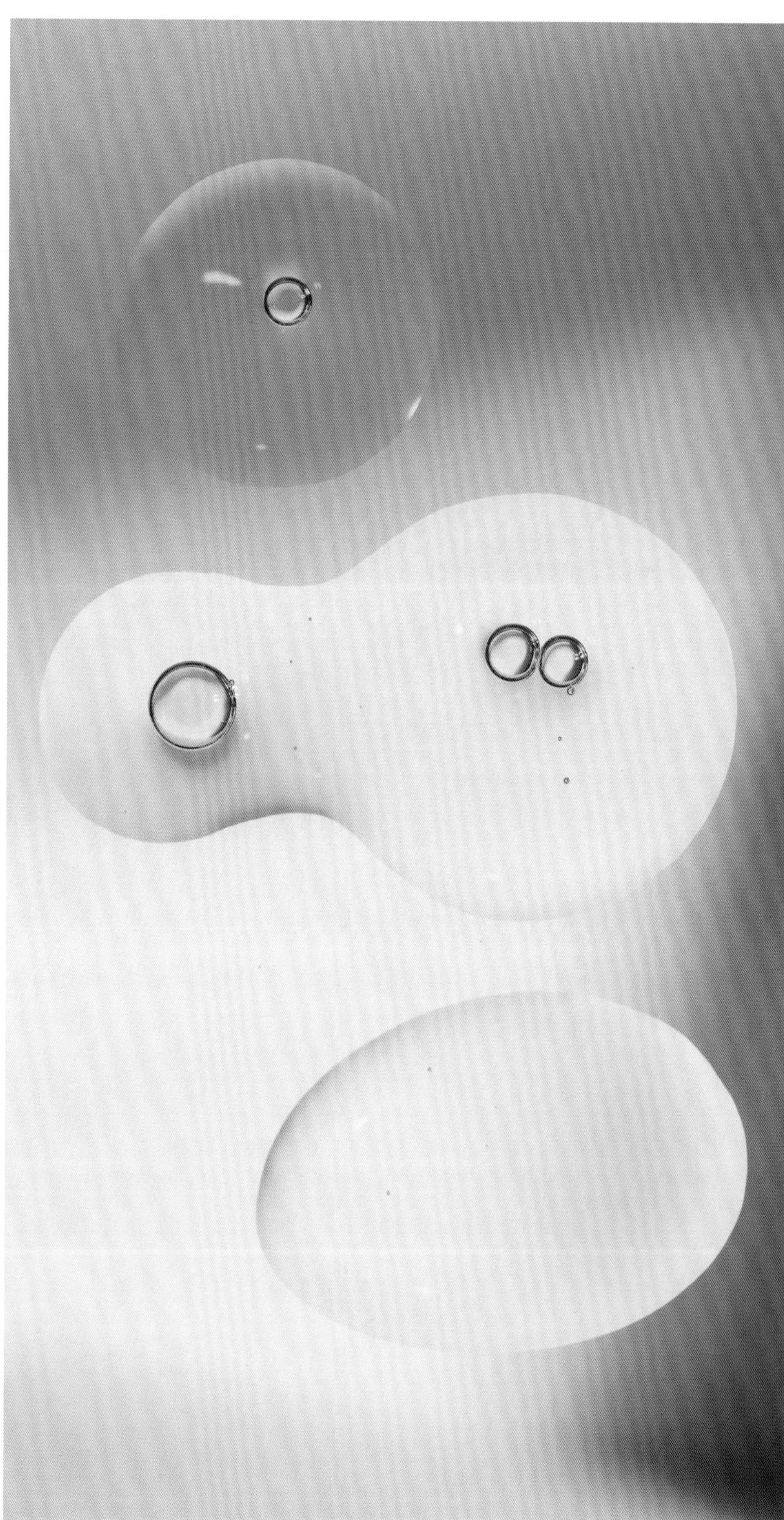

What it is

Panthenol, also known as provitamin B5, is a water-soluble B vitamin that is found in a wide range of foods, including meat, vegetables, and grains, as well as produced by a number of microorganisms. It is an important molecule involved in many processes within the body, and is used in cosmetics for its benefits in supporting skin hydration. Pantothenic acid was first isolated from sheep liver in 1939, and the subsequent synthetic production began in 1940, facilitating its widespread use in various industries including cosmetics.

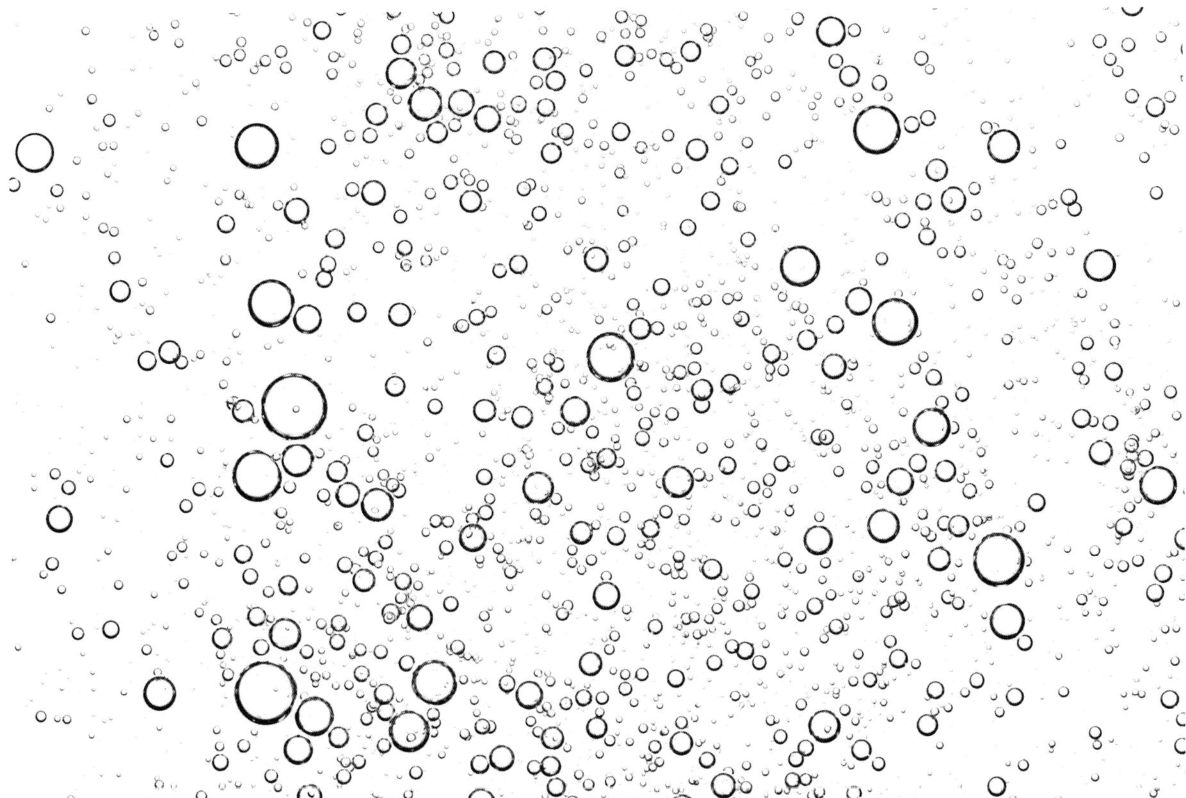

What it's used for

Panthenol, a derivative of vitamin B5, is widely used in cosmetics for its versatile and beneficial properties. As a humectant, panthenol attracts water from the environment and helps the skin retain moisture, leaving it feeling soft and supple. This ability to bind water contributes to improved skin texture and a more hydrated, plump appearance. Panthenol's water-binding nature makes it an ideal choice for moisturizers, serums, and other hydrating products designed to address dryness. Additionally, panthenol's emollient properties help support the appearance of a healthy skin barrier. This barrier consists of the natural oils and lipids that shield the skin from moisture loss while protecting it from potential external irritants.

Mechanism of action

Inside the skin, panthenol is converted into pantothenic acid, which is a key component of coenzyme A. Coenzyme A is required in the early stages of the production of key lipids such as fatty acids, cholesterol, and ceramides. These are key components that contribute to the skin barrier function, helping the skin to retain moisture by trapping and holding water within the skin. A healthy skin barrier ensures a strong protective effect, reducing the permeability of the skin barrier to stop unwanted external molecules penetrating the skin and potentially leading to redness or irritation. Due to these functions, panthenol is an essential molecule in supporting the skin barrier. In vivo research shows that panthenol-containing formulas help to reduce TEWL (transepidermal water loss) and boost skin hydration.

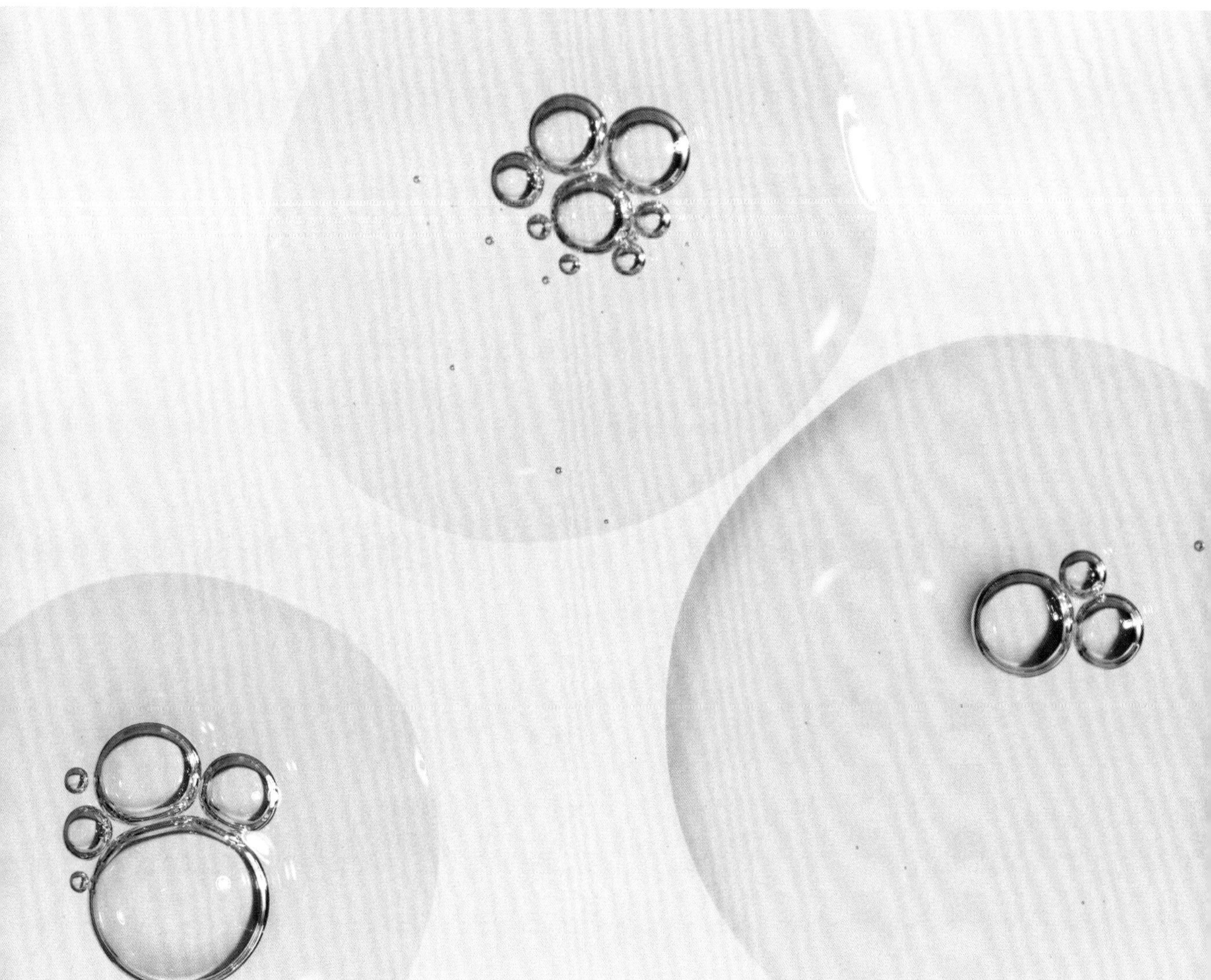

Resveratrol

001	**INCI Names:**	Resveratrol
002	**Common/ Other Names**	Resveratrol
003	**Classification**	Antioxidant
004	**Primary Function**	Antioxidant and brightening
005	**Phonetic Spelling**	rez-VEHR-uh-trawl
006	**First Discovered**	Michio Takaoka, 1939
007	**Clinical Concentration(s)**	0.1–1%

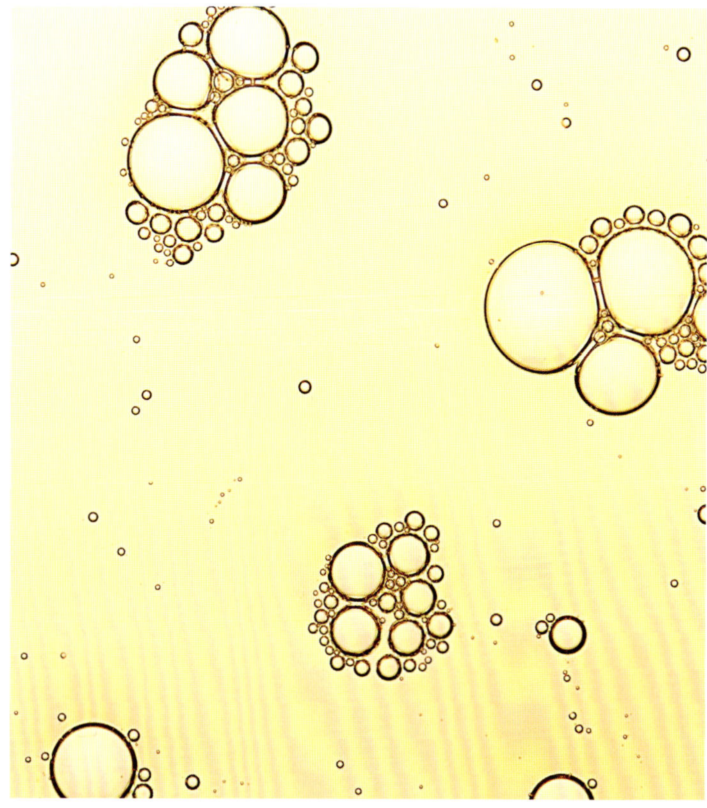

What it is

Resveratrol is a natural polyphenolic compound primarily found in the skins of red grapes, berries, and peanuts. Chemically, it belongs to a class of compounds called stilbenes. Its structure consists of two aromatic rings connected by a double bond, with hydroxyl groups attached at various positions.

What it's used for

In skincare, resveratrol is known for its powerful antioxidant properties, which help protect the skin from the effects of environmental stressors such as pollution and UV exposure. By neutralizing free radicals, resveratrol helps prevent the appearance of visible signs of aging, like fine lines, wrinkles, and uneven skin tone. It also plays a role in helping to soothe sensitive or irritated skin. Additionally, resveratrol's ability to support the skin's natural collagen and elasticity helps maintain a firmer, smoother appearance, contributing to a more youthful-looking complexion.

Beyond its antioxidant and soothing properties, resveratrol also supports the skin barrier, enhancing the skin's ability to retain moisture and defend against external aggressors. This makes it an ideal ingredient for promoting healthy, balanced skin. Whether used alone or in combination with other active ingredients, resveratrol is a versatile addition to skincare routines focused on hydration, protection, and rejuvenation.

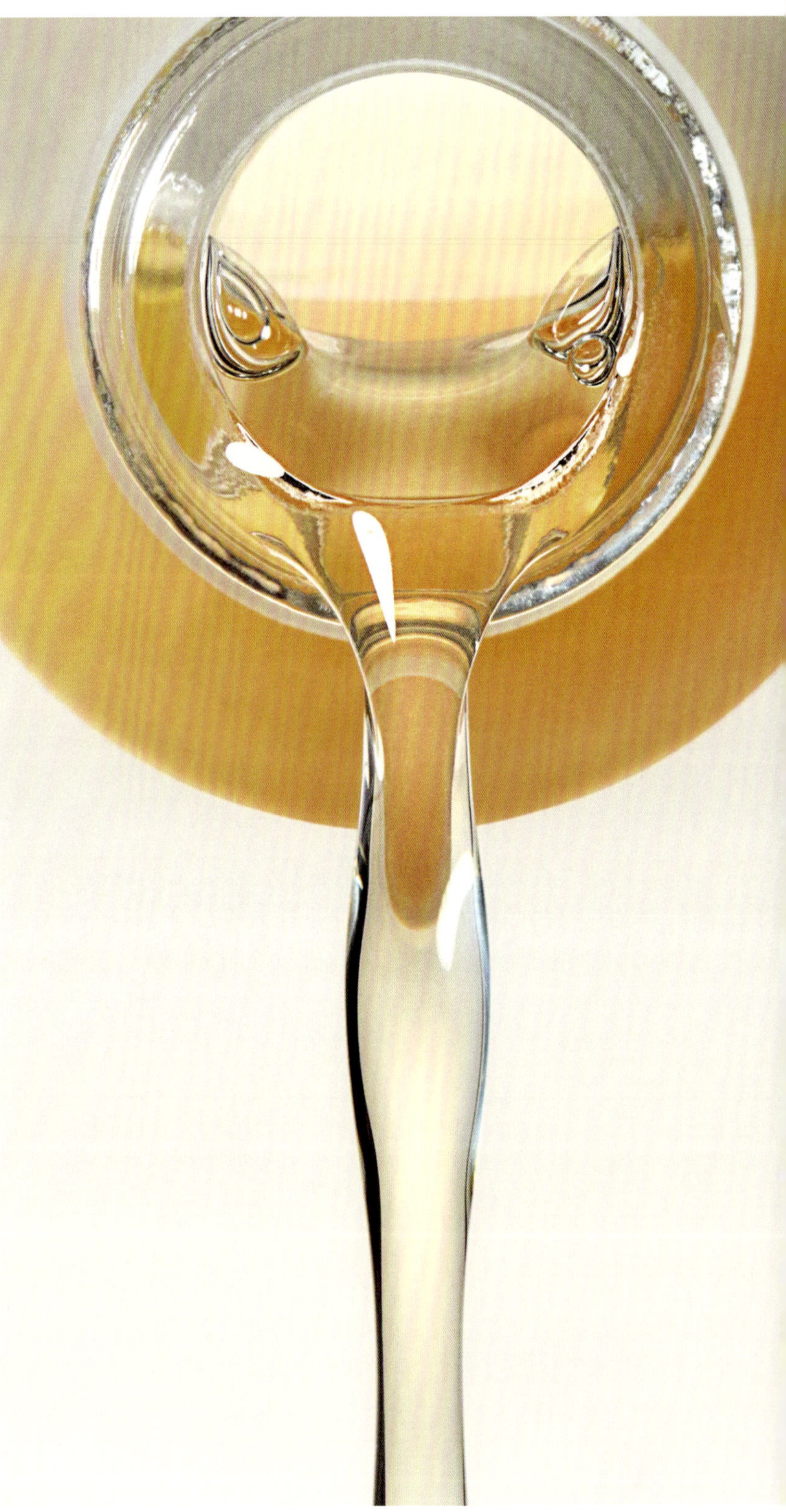

Mechanism of action

The chemical structure of resveratrol allows it to exhibit strong antioxidant activity by scavenging free radicals and modulating the activity of enzymes related to redness and skin aging.

Resveratrol also exerts a photoprotective effect and as a result can reduce the appearance of signs of photoaging, like wrinkles and uneven skin tone. It achieves this by counteracting the impact of repeated UV exposure on the collagen content of the skin. Studies also show that resveratrol-based formulations can stimulate the collagen-producing cells present in the skin's surface, leading to increased collagen III production. These properties make resveratrol a valuable ingredient in anti-aging and protective skincare formulations.

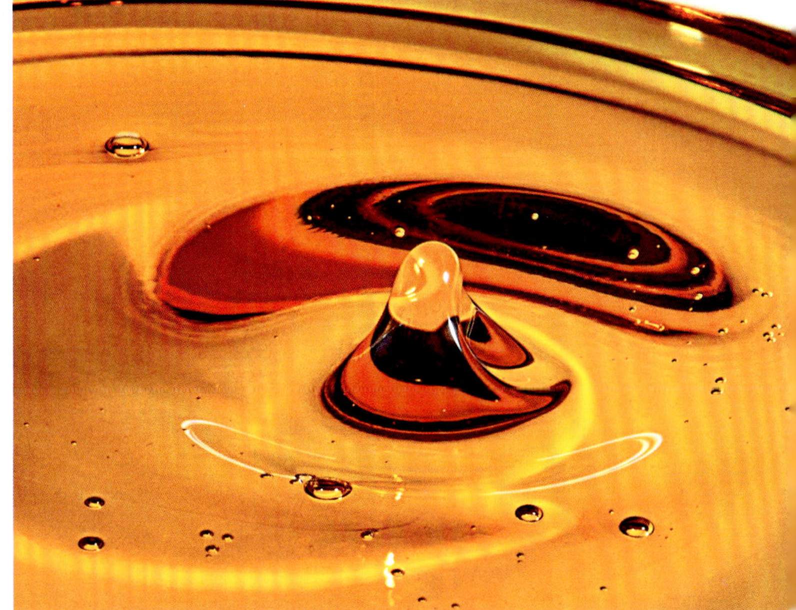

Retinoids

001	**INCI Names:**	Retinol, retinoic aldehyde, retinal, retinoic acid
002	**Common/ Other Names**	Vitamin A derivatives
003	**Classification**	Vitamin A derivative
004	**Primary Function**	Textural irregularities, signs of aging, uneven skin tone
005	**Phonetic Spelling**	Reh-TIN-oid
006	**First Discovered**	Elmer McCollum and Marguerite Davis, 1913
007	**Clinical Concentration(s)**	0.01–3%

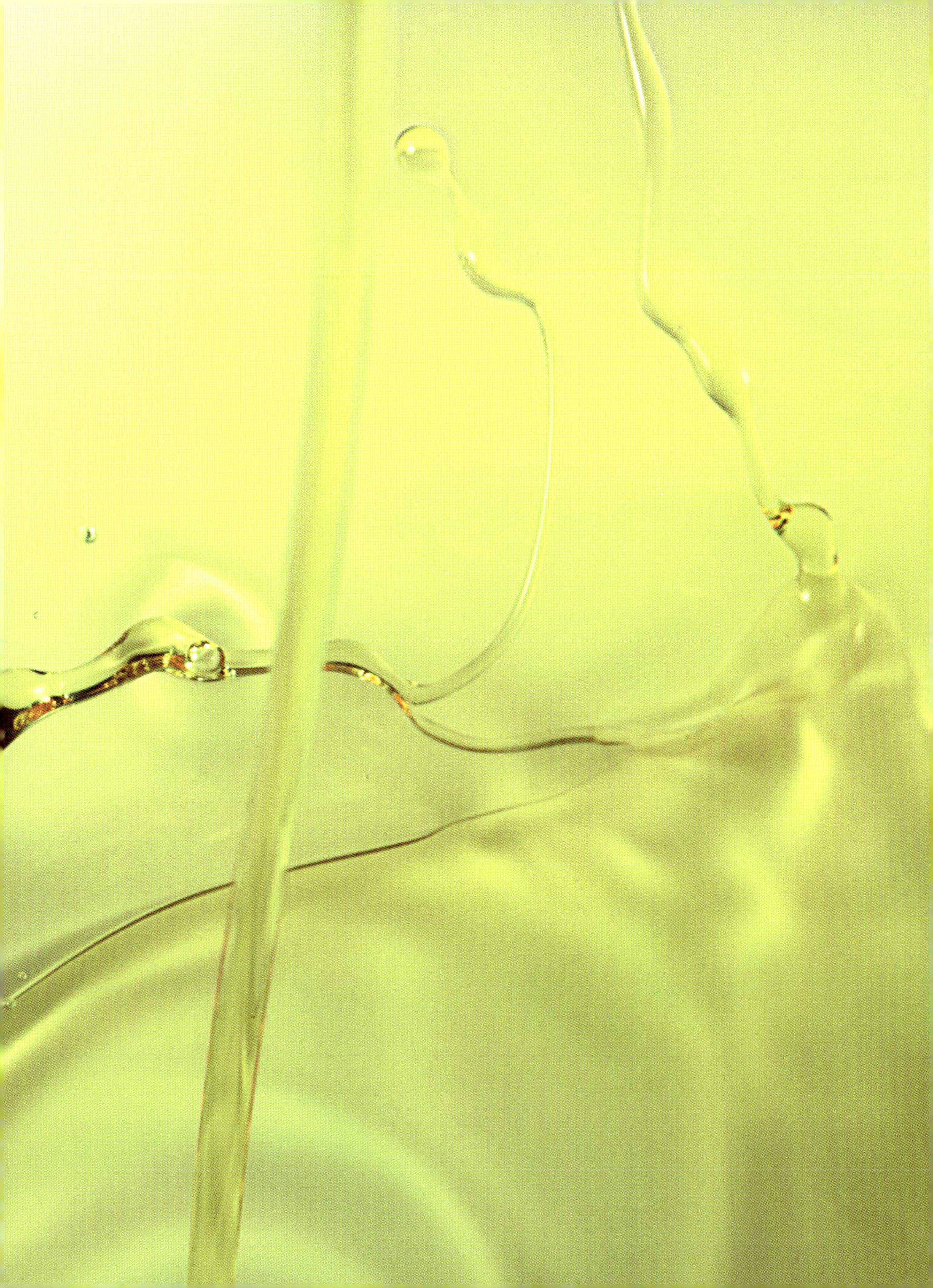

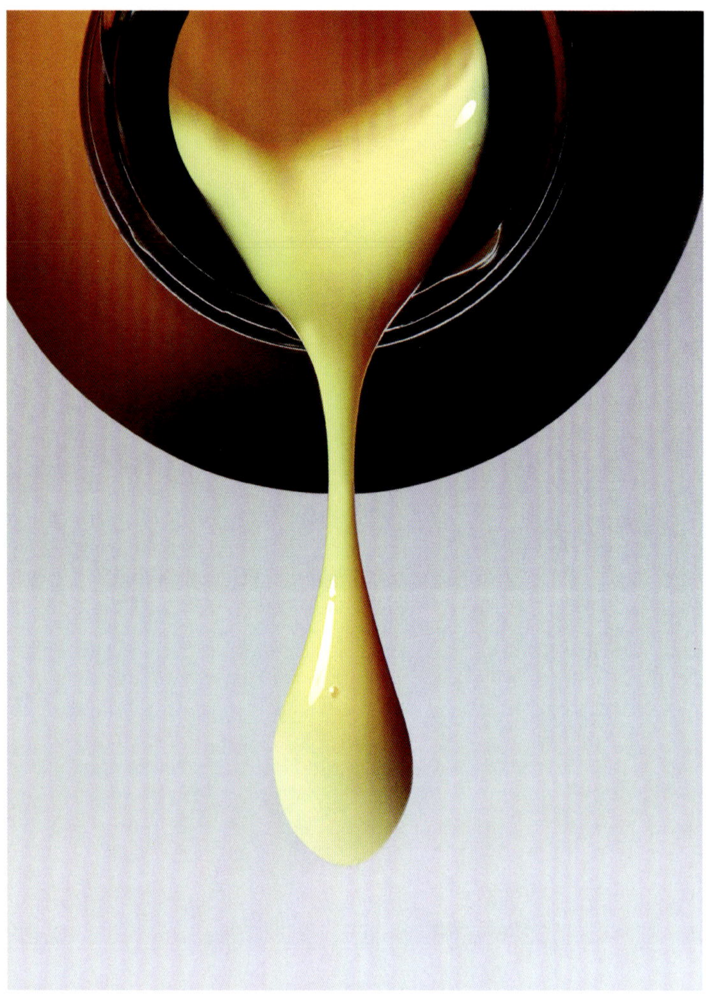

What it is

Retinoids are a class of compounds that are either derived from vitamin A, or have structural and/or functional similarities to vitamin A. Initially used for their ability to improve night blindness, retinoids have since been extensively studied for dermatologic applications. In general, they are categorized into four main classes based on their molecular structure and properties:

1. Non-aromatics: includes retinol, retinaldehyle, tretinoin, isotretinoin and alitretinoin.

2. Mono-aromatics: includes etretinate and acitretin.

3. Poly-aromatics: includes adapalene and tazarotene.

4. Pyranones: includes seletinoid G.

What it's used for

Retinoids are used in both cosmetic and medicinal products to address an array of skin conditions. For cosmetic use, retinoids are used at concentrations of up to 1% to address signs of aging, uneven skin tone, and textural irregularities. They may also be used at concentrations higher than 1% to treat medical skin conditions, such as acne vulgaris, and pigmentation disorders like post-inflammatory hyperpigmentation.

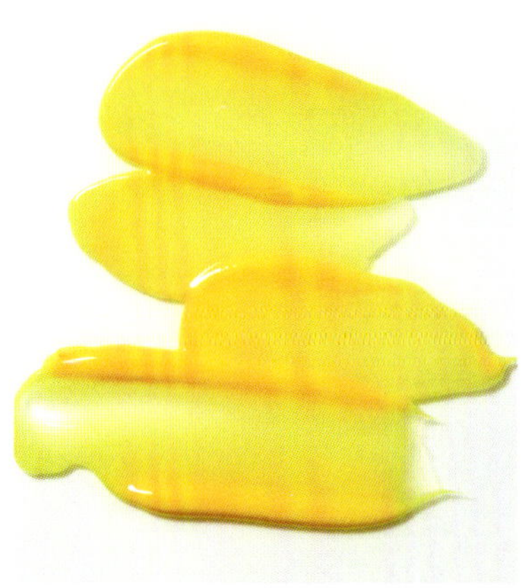

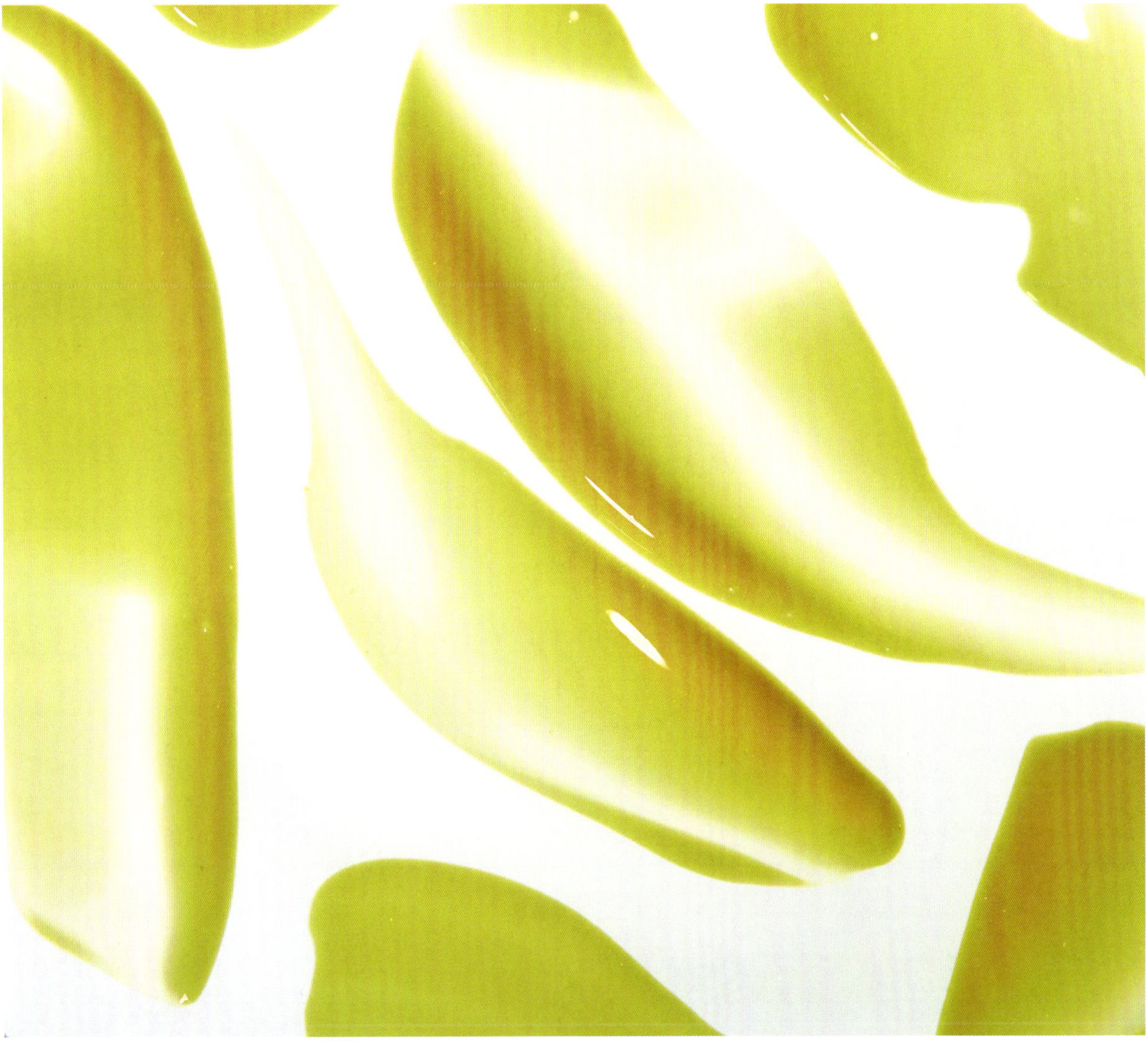

Mechanism of action

Retinoids become biologically active when they are converted into retinoic acid within the skin. Upon conversion, they bind directly to retinoic acid receptors (RARs), forming complexes that activate the functions of retinoic acid.

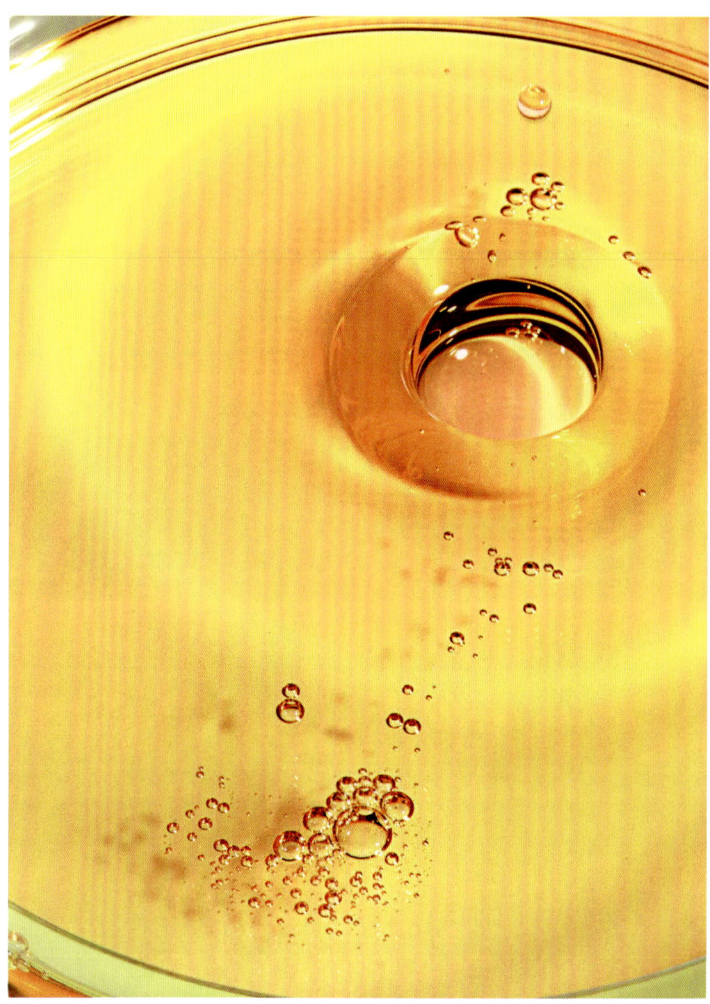

Uneven skin tone

Retinoids are also used to help address the appearance of uneven skin tone because of their ability to impact the distribution of visible pigment within the skin. Over time, factors such as natural aging, repeated sun exposure, or disruptions to the skin's surface can affect melanocyte activity, leading to the appearance of uneven pigmentation and dark spots. Retinoids work to refine the look of skin tone by influencing melanocyte function in several ways. They help distribute melanin more evenly within the skin, reduce the transfer of melanin to surface cells, and minimize overactive melanocyte behavior. These actions contribute to a visibly smoother, more balanced complexion.

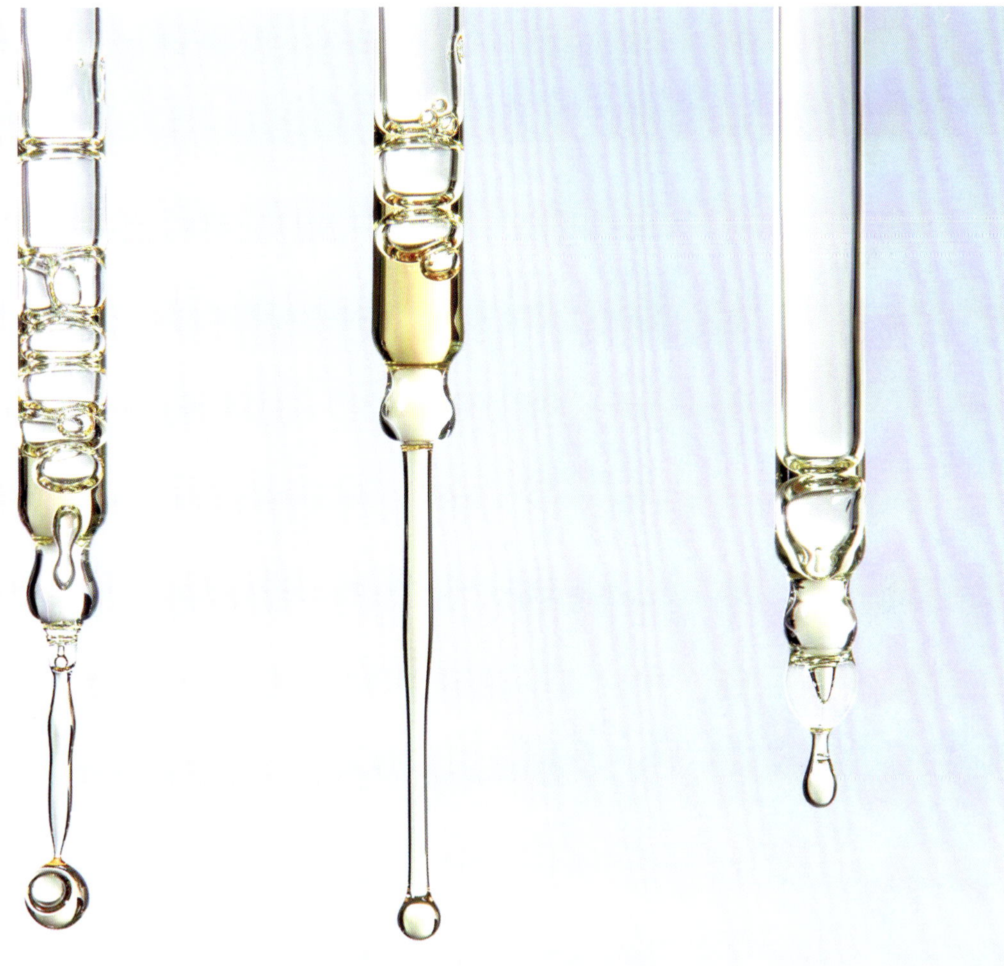

Anti-aging

Retinoic acid is the active form of vitamin A and plays a pivotal role in delivering the cosmetic benefits associated with retinoids. Topically applied retinoids, such as retinol or retinaldehyde, undergo a conversion process within the epidermis to become retinoic acid. This multi-step conversion begins with retinol being oxidized to retinaldehyde, which is then further oxidized to retinoic acid. Once formed, retinoic acid interacts with skin cells in the epidermis, promoting natural cell turnover and enhancing the skin's surface texture. This mechanism helps to visibly reduce the appearance of fine lines, wrinkles, and uneven skin tone, leaving the skin looking refreshed and smooth. By supporting skin renewal at the epidermal level, retinoids are a cornerstone of many skincare routines focused on achieving a more youthful and radiant complexion.

001 **INCI Names:** Rosa canina seed oil

002 **Common/ Other Names** Rosehip, dog rose

003 **Classification** Emollient, plant-derived oil

Rose Hip Seed Oil

004 **Primary Function** Moisturization

005 **Phonetic Spelling** ROWZ-hip SEED OYL

006 **First Discovered** Unknown (thought to be used in ancient Egyptian, Mayan, and Native American cultures)

007 **Clinical Concentration(s)** 1–100%

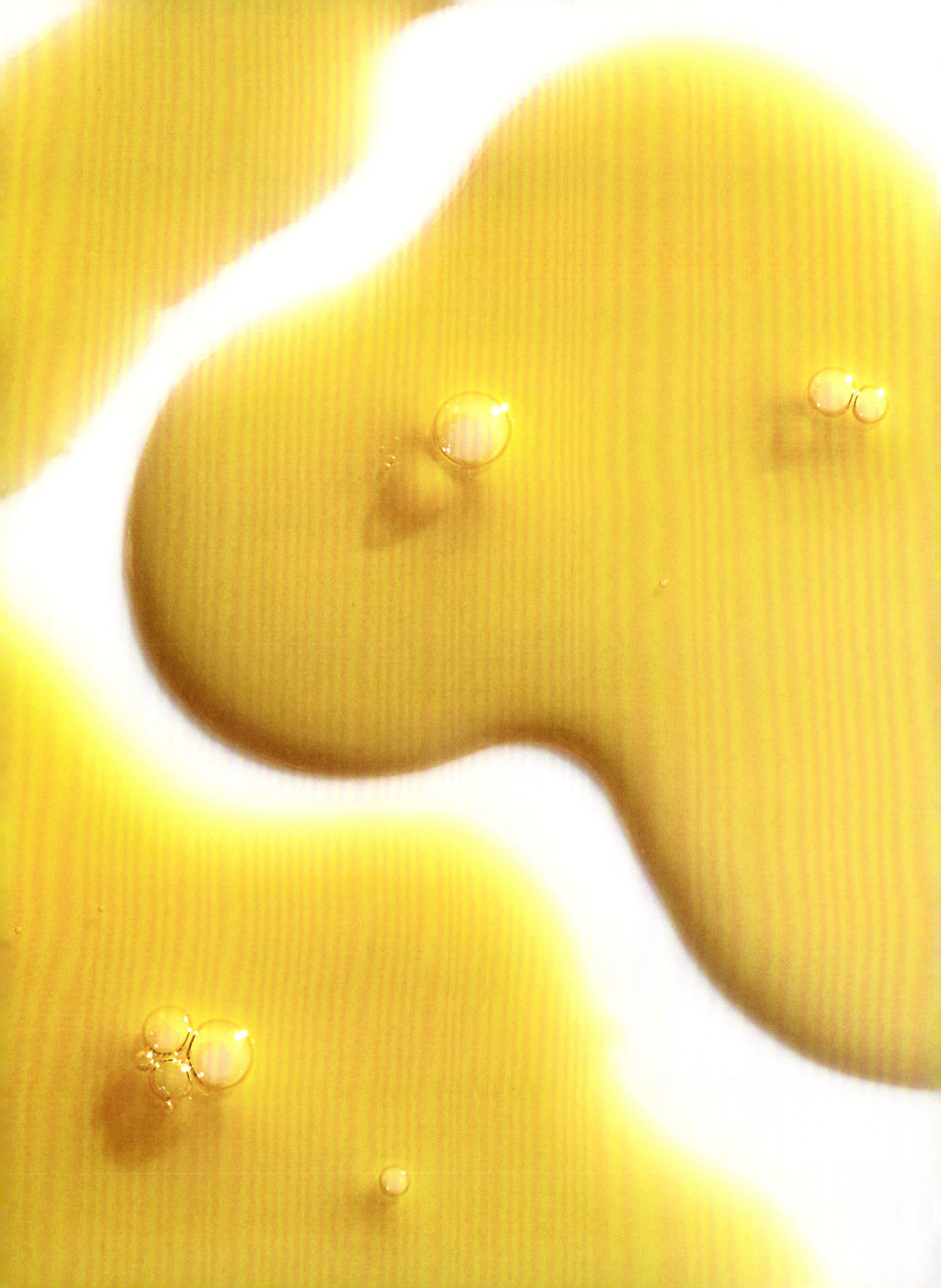

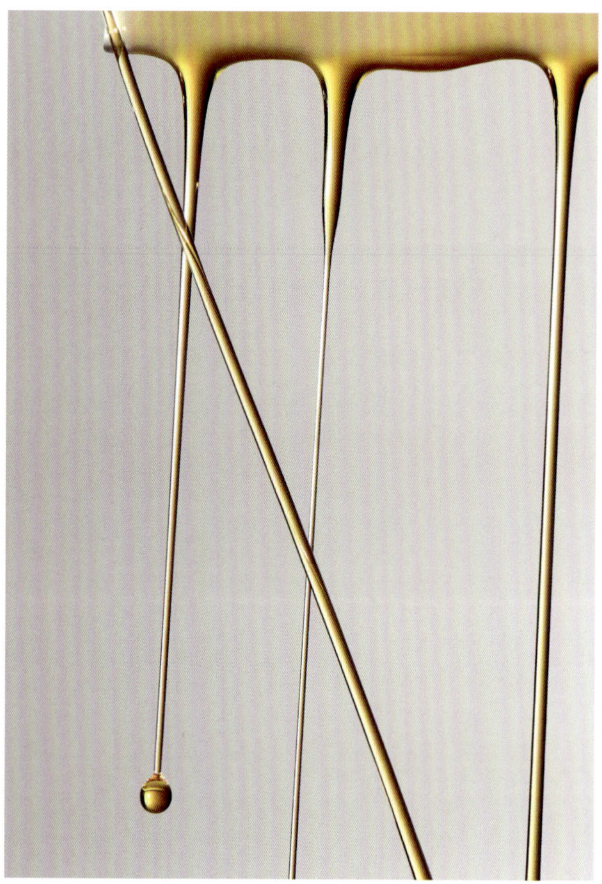

What it is

Rose hip is the common name given to a number of rose species of which the fruit and seeds are used for cosmetic purposes. The two most common of these are *Rosa canina* and *Rosa rubiginosa*; however for the purposes of this discussion we will be focusing on *Rosa canina*. The seed oil consists of a number of lipid components, including fatty acids and sterols, which topically provide moisturization through helping to reinforce the lipid barrier. Rose hip seed oil also contains a variety of other components, including antioxidants and phenolic compounds, which result in an oil with greater antioxidant properties than other common seed oils. It is important to note, however, that while the composition has been documented in literature, this can vary due to the geographical origin of the plant stock, the extraction methods, and several other factors.

What it's used for

Rosehip seed oil is valued in skincare for its emollient properties, largely due to its high content of essential fatty acids. These fatty acids help to support the skin's natural lipid barrier, improving moisture retention and reducing transepidermal water loss (TEWL). By reinforcing the skin's barrier function, rosehip seed oil helps the skin feel smoother and more hydrated. The oil's sterol content also aids in the production of ceramides, which are essential for maintaining the skin's protective barrier.

In addition to its hydrating benefits, rosehip seed oil contains a variety of antioxidants, including vitamin E (tocopherol), carotenoids such as lycopene and beta-carotene (a precursor of vitamin A), and potentially retinoic acid, the active form of vitamin A. These antioxidants help protect the skin from environmental stressors and contribute to improving the appearance of uneven skin tone and signs of aging.

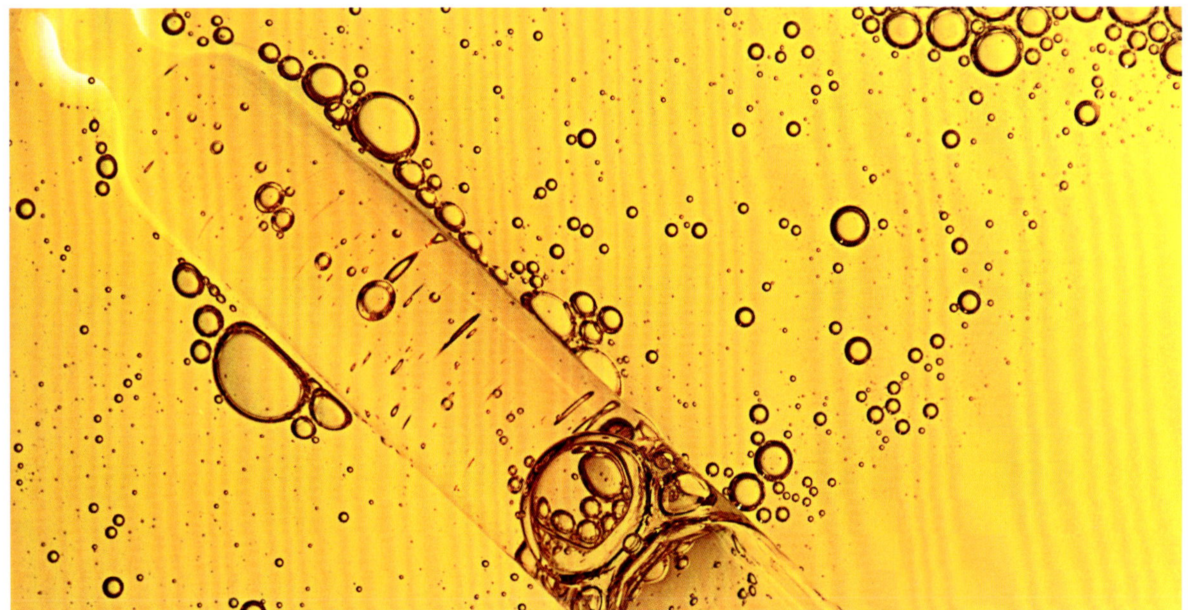

Mechanism of action

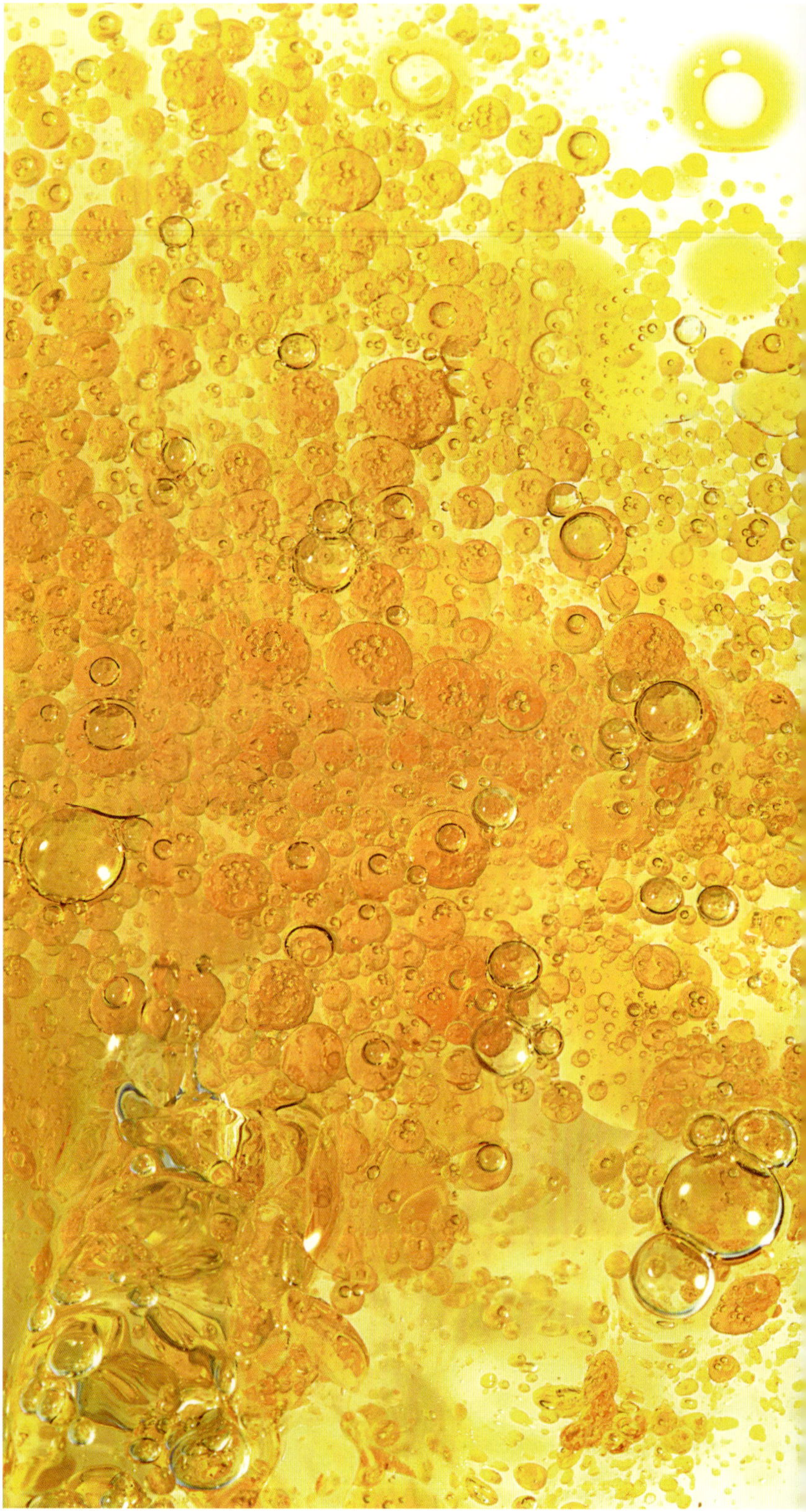

Rose hip seed oil is renowned for its emollient properties, primarily due to its rich content of essential fatty acids, including linoleic acid and oleic acid. These fatty acids play a key role in enhancing the skin's natural lipid barrier, which helps the skin retain moisture by reducing transepidermal water loss (TEWL). By reinforcing this protective barrier, rose hip seed oil helps the skin stay hydrated and feel smoother. The fatty acids also help to soften the skin, making it more supple and less prone to dryness or irritation, which is particularly beneficial for those with dry or sensitive skin.

In addition to its fatty acids, rose hip seed oil contains sterols, which are lipids that support the production of ceramides, another key component of the skin's barrier. Ceramides are crucial for maintaining the skin's hydration and preventing moisture loss. By promoting ceramide synthesis, rose hip seed oil further supports the skin's ability to retain moisture, contributing to healthier and more resilient skin.

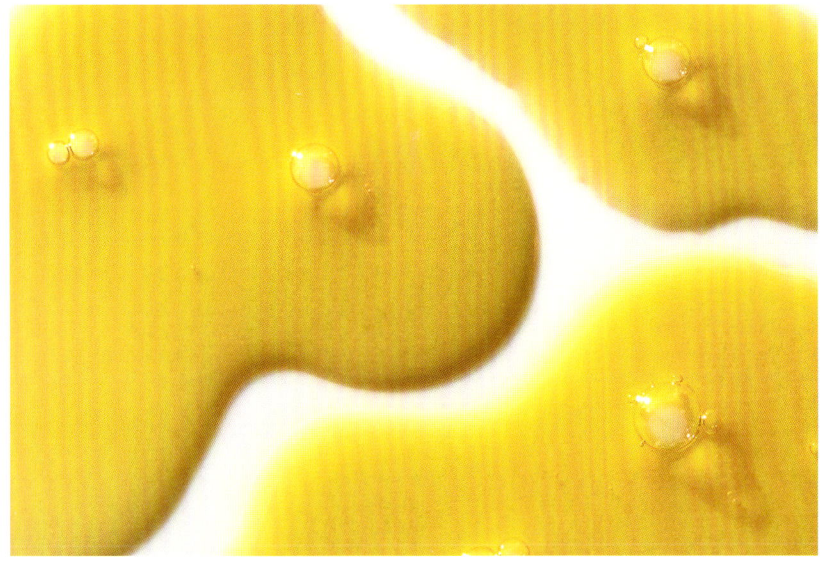

The oil's emollient properties are further enhanced by its rich array of antioxidants, such as vitamin E (tocopherol) and carotenoids like lycopene and beta-carotene. These antioxidants help protect the skin from oxidative stress caused by free radicals, which can lead to the premature appearance of signs of aging and skin damage. As an emollient, rose hip seed oil not only nourishes and hydrates the skin but also helps to soothe the feel of irritation, reduce the appearance of redness, and promote an even skin tone.

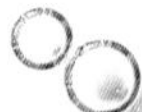
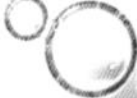

001	**INCI Names:**	Salicylic acid
002	**Common/ Other Names**	Salicylic acid
003	**Classification**	Exfoliant, decongesting active

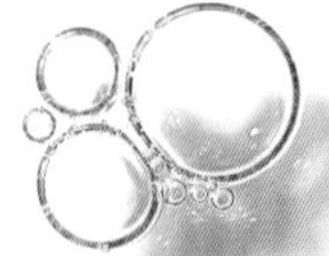

Salicylic Acid

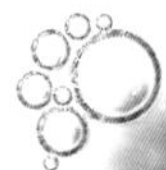

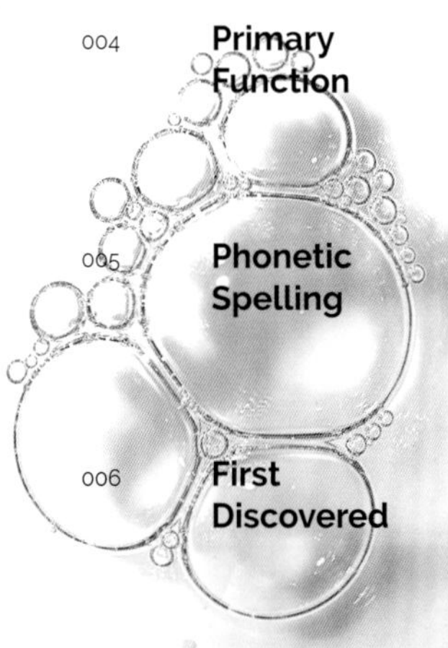

004	**Primary Function**	Decongestion, exfoliation
005	**Phonetic Spelling**	SAL-ih-SIL-ik AS-id
006	**First Discovered**	Charles Frédéric Gerhardt, 1838
007	**Clinical Concentration(s)**	0.5–2%

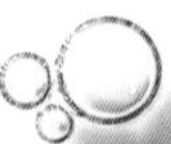

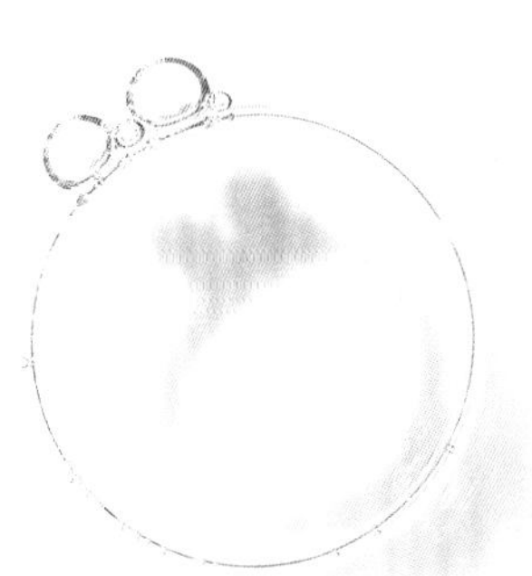
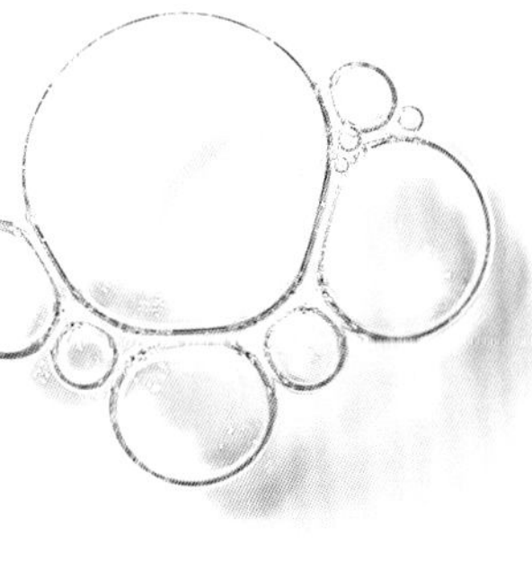
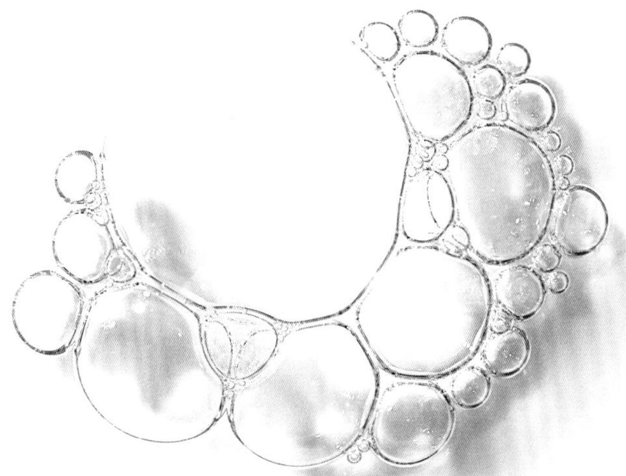
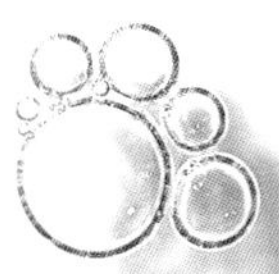

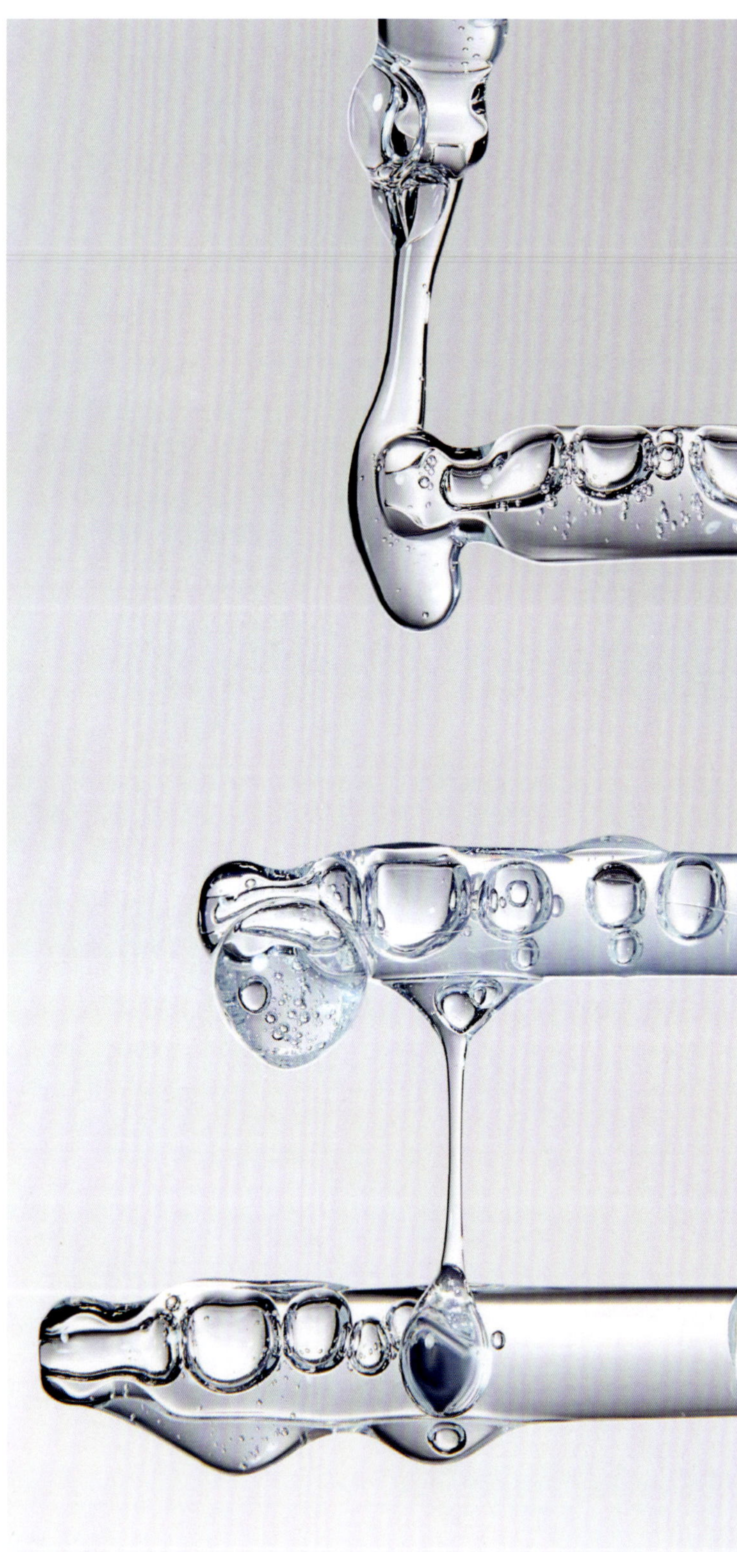

What it is

Salicylic acid is a beta hydroxy acid (BHA) and an organic compound with the chemical formula $C_7H_6O_3$. It is derived from natural sources such as willow bark but can also be synthetically produced. Chemically, it consists of a benzene ring with hydroxyl (-OH) and carboxylic acid (-COOH) groups, giving it both lipophilic and acidic properties. This unique structure allows it to interact with oil and sebum on the skin's surface, making it particularly suitable for addressing oily or blemish-prone skin. Salicylic acid is a widely used ingredient in skincare formulations for its ability to gently refine the appearance of skin texture and improve clarity.

What it's used for

Salicylic acid's lipophilic nature allows it to penetrate into the pores, where it can dissolve excess sebum (oil) and other impurities that contribute to blemishes. By promoting exfoliation, salicylic acid can help unclog pores and prevents the buildup of debris, excess oil, and bacteria that may contribute to blemish formation. This makes it highly effective in treating blemish-prone skin.

Salicylic acid is commonly found in a variety of skincare products, including cleansers, toners, serums, spot treatments, and medicinal acne creams. The concentration of salicylic acid in these products typically ranges from 0.5% to 2%, depending on the formulation and intended use. Lower concentrations are often used in daily skincare routines for gentle exfoliation and maintenance, while higher concentrations are generally reserved for more targeted treatments and blemish-lesion management.

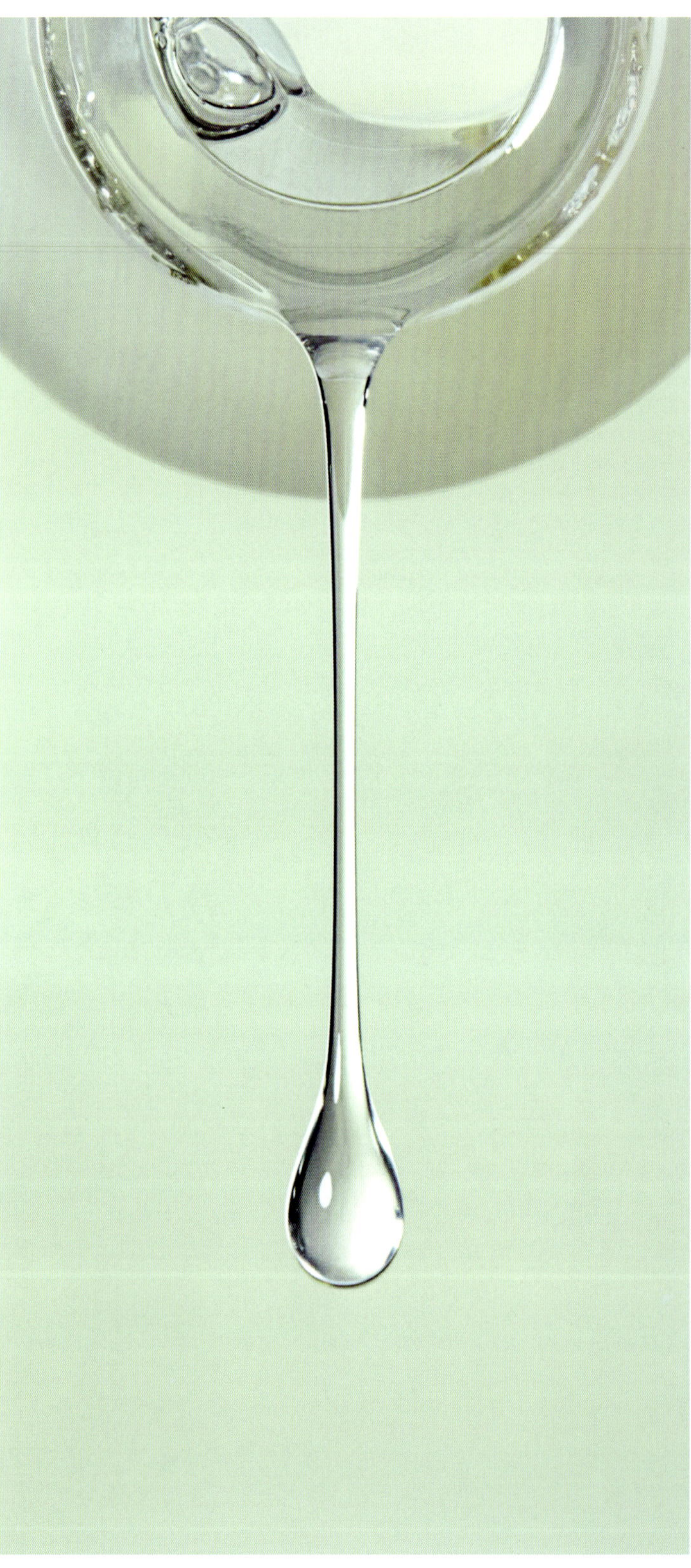

Mechanism of action

Salicylic acid is highly effective for targeting blemish-prone skin due to its unique ability to interact with oil and sebum on the skin's surface. As a beta hydroxy acid (BHA), it is oil-soluble, which allows it to penetrate into the pores more effectively than water-soluble acids. Once inside the pores, salicylic acid helps to break down the buildup of dead skin cells, oil, and debris that can clog pores and contribute to the appearance of blemishes. By addressing these blockages, salicylic acid helps to keep the pores clear, reducing the likelihood of future breakouts.

In addition to its exfoliating properties, salicylic acid has a keratolytic effect, meaning it works to soften and loosen the bonds between dead skin cells on the outermost layer of the skin. This gentle exfoliation smooths the skin's texture, reduces the appearance of unevenness, and helps to prevent further congestion. By promoting a clearer, more refined skin surface, salicylic acid contributes to an overall healthier-looking complexion.

Squalane

001	**INCI Names:**	Squalane
002	**Common/ Other Names**	Squalane
003	**Classification**	Emollient
004	**Primary Function**	Hydration, moisturization
005	**Phonetic Spelling**	SKWAY-lane
006	**First Discovered**	Mitsumaru Tsujimoto, 1906 (squalene from shark liver oil) F.J. Moore, 1931 (identified the squalene precursor, from plant oils) Hydrogenation of squalene to squalane, 1910 to 1930s
007	**Clinical Concentration(s)**	0.5–97%

What it is

Squalane is a stable, saturated derivative of squalene, a naturally occurring oily substance. Although squalane and squalene sound very similar and both have benefits for the skin, they differ in their origin and composition. Squalene is a compound produced by human skin cells and it is also found minimally in certain plants. Historically, squalene was commercially obtained from fish oils, specifically shark liver oil. On the other hand, squalane is a more stable version of squalene that is sustainably sourced from sugar cane and other plant sources.

Although it looks and feels like an oil, pure squalane is oil-free. As a hydrocarbon, squalane's molecular structure is slightly different from typical plant-based or mineral oils. Hydrocarbons are exclusively composed of carbon and hydrogen atoms, whereas oils (typically plant-derived oils) are liquids that contain a variety of organic molecules such as wax esters, fatty acids, antioxidants, and vitamins, alongside hydrocarbons. While many oils are indeed hydrocarbons (such as mineral oils derived from petroleum), not all oils are pure hydrocarbons.

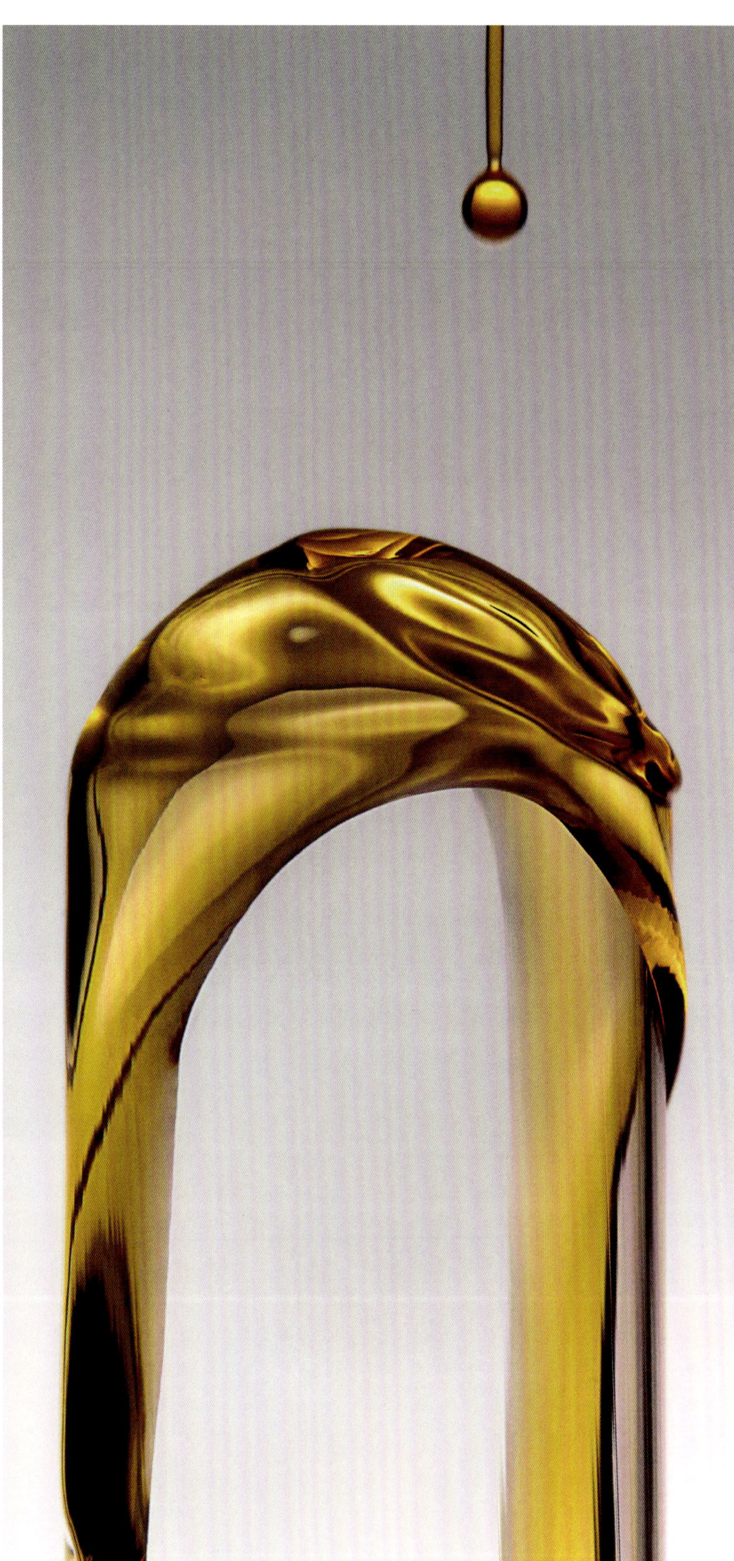

What it's used for

Squalane is valued for its emollient properties, meaning it helps to soften and smooth the skin, but it has a lighter texture compared to many traditional oils. When included in products such as moisturizers, squalane helps increase hydration for healthier-looking skin. As a non-comedogenic substance, squalane does not clog pores and is typically suitable for all skin types, including oily or acne-prone skin.

Mechanism of action

Human sebum functions to lubricate and protect the skin, maintaining moisture and preventing dryness; it contains approximately 13% squalene as one of its major constituents. With age, the amount of squalene produced in the skin declines, which can leave the skin feeling drier. Because squalane resembles this natural emollient found in skin, it moisturizes the skin and contributes to a softer feel and healthier appearance. Research indicates that squalane's moisturizing effect is likely due to its ability to retain moisture in the stratum corneum.

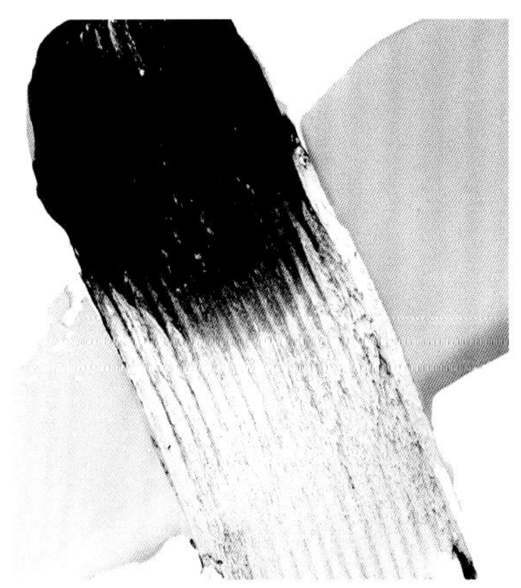

Sulfur

001	**INCI Names:**	Sulfur
002	**Common/ Other Names**	Sulfur
003	**Classification**	Exfoliant
004	**Primary Function**	Exfoliation
005	**Phonetic Spelling**	SUHL-fuhr
006	**First Discovered**	Antoine Lavoisier, 1777
007	**Clinical Concentration(s)**	2–10%

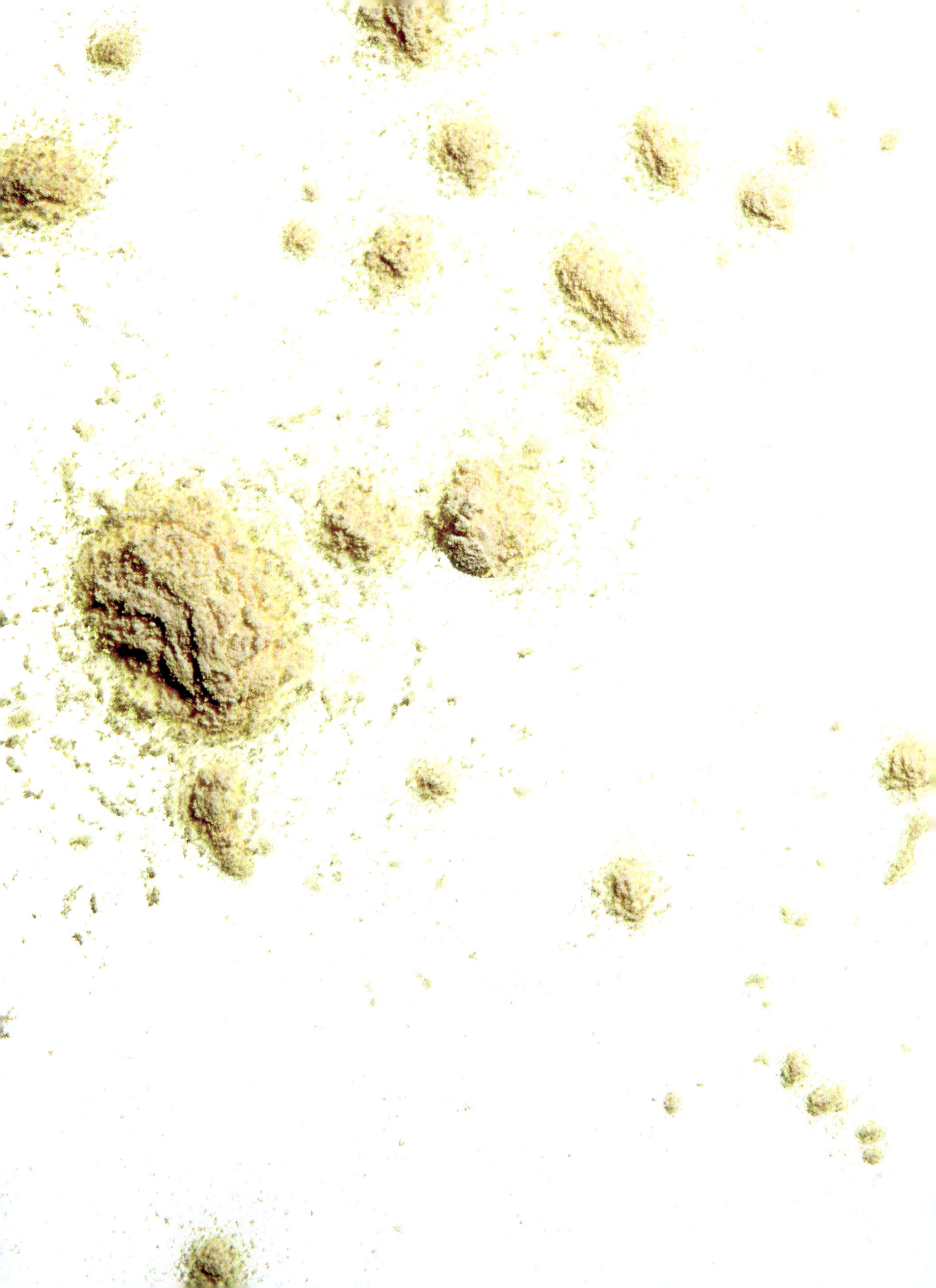

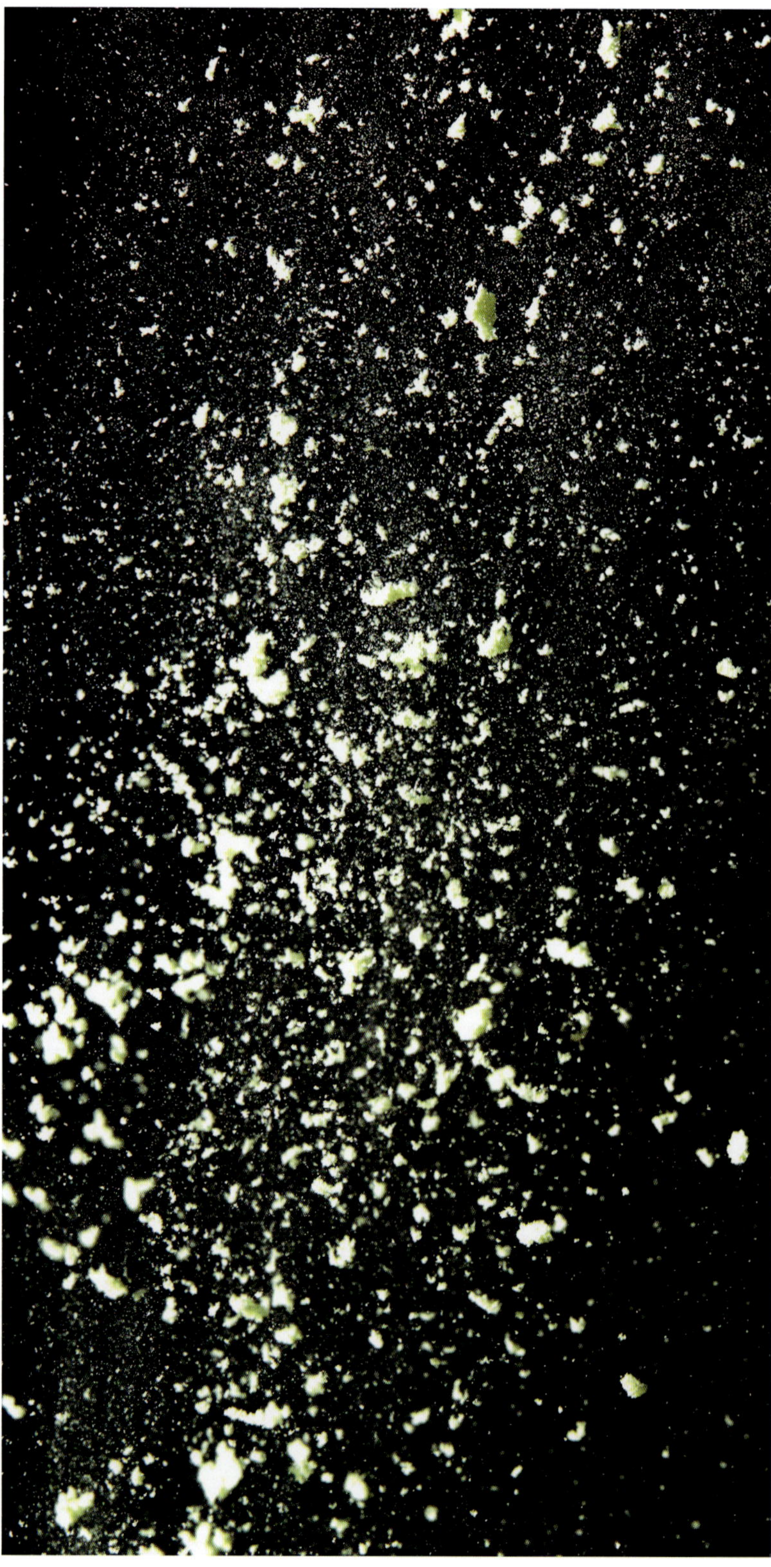

What it is

Sulfur is a naturally occurring mineral that has long been used in cosmetics due to its beneficial properties for the skin. Historically, sulfur has been utilized for centuries in various cultures for its skin-healing benefits. Ancient Egyptians, for instance, used sulfur in their skincare regimens, and it has continued to be a staple in traditional medicine. In modern cosmetics, sulfur is commonly found in spot treatments, masks, and cleansers for its purifying effects.

Sulfur's cosmetic applications were solidified in the 19th and 20th centuries, with the advent of modern skincare products. The compound is often used in combination with other ingredients like salicylic acid to improve the appearance of blemish-prone skin, and it remains a popular choice in formulations aimed at clarifying and smoothing the skin's texture.

What it's used for

Sulfur has been well researched in cosmetics for its ability to gently exfoliate the skin, helping to remove dead skin cells and unclog pores, which is particularly useful for helping mitigate blemish-prone skin. Its exfoliating properties make it effective in controlling oily skin and helping to clear up blemishes.

Due to its ability to help regulate sebum on the skin, sulfur is an effective ingredient for managing both oily blemish-prone skin and the symptoms of dandruff, which has made it a common feature in shampoos and topical treatments. Sulfur's unique ability to treat a variety of skin issues while promoting a healthier, clearer complexion continues to make it an invaluable ingredient in the beauty industry.

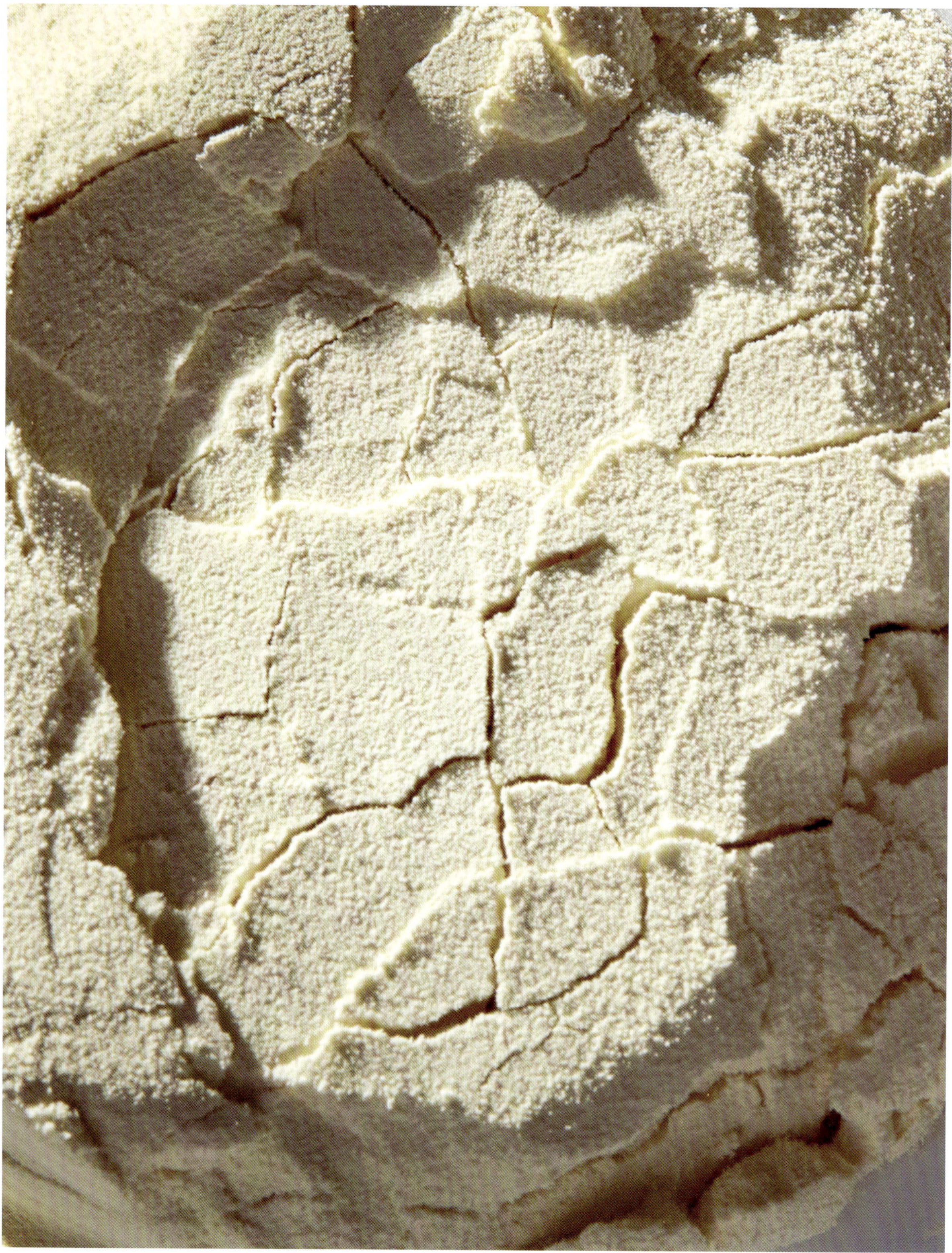

Mechanism of action

As a keratolytic agent, sulfur is reduced to hydrogen sulfide, thereby breaking down keratin in the skin. This helps to exfoliate by breaking down the bonds between dead skin cells, which aids in clearing clogged pores. This action reduces the buildup of sebum and dead cells on the skin and in pores, which can contribute to blemish formation. Its exfoliating effect also improves the look of skin texture and reduces the appearance of post-blemish lesions.

Sulfur also acts as an absorbent, drawing excess oil from the skin's surface. This helps to control shine that is typically associated with oily skin. By decreasing sebum production, sulfur prevents the accumulation of oil that can lead to pore blockage.

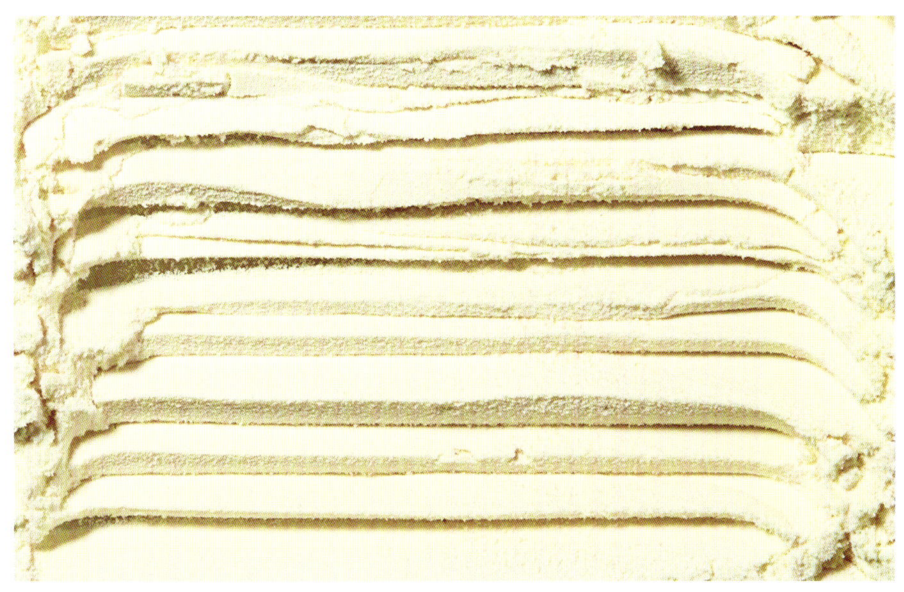

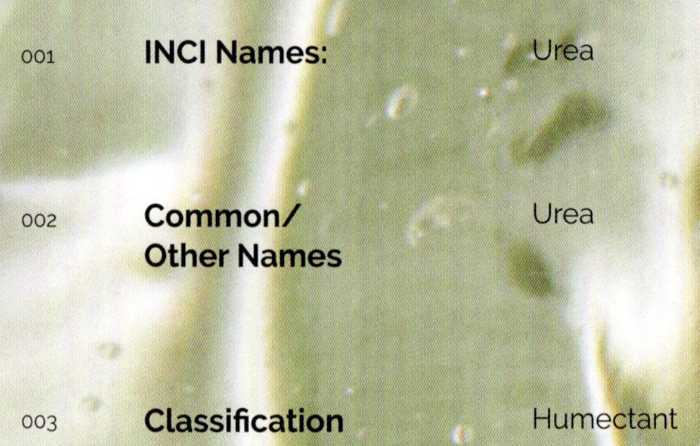

Urea

001	**INCI Names:**	Urea
002	**Common/ Other Names**	Urea
003	**Classification**	Humectant
004	**Primary Function**	Humectant
005	**Phonetic Spelling**	yoo-REE-uh
006	**First Discovered**	Friedrich Wöhler, 1828
007	**Clinical Concentration(s)**	2–30%

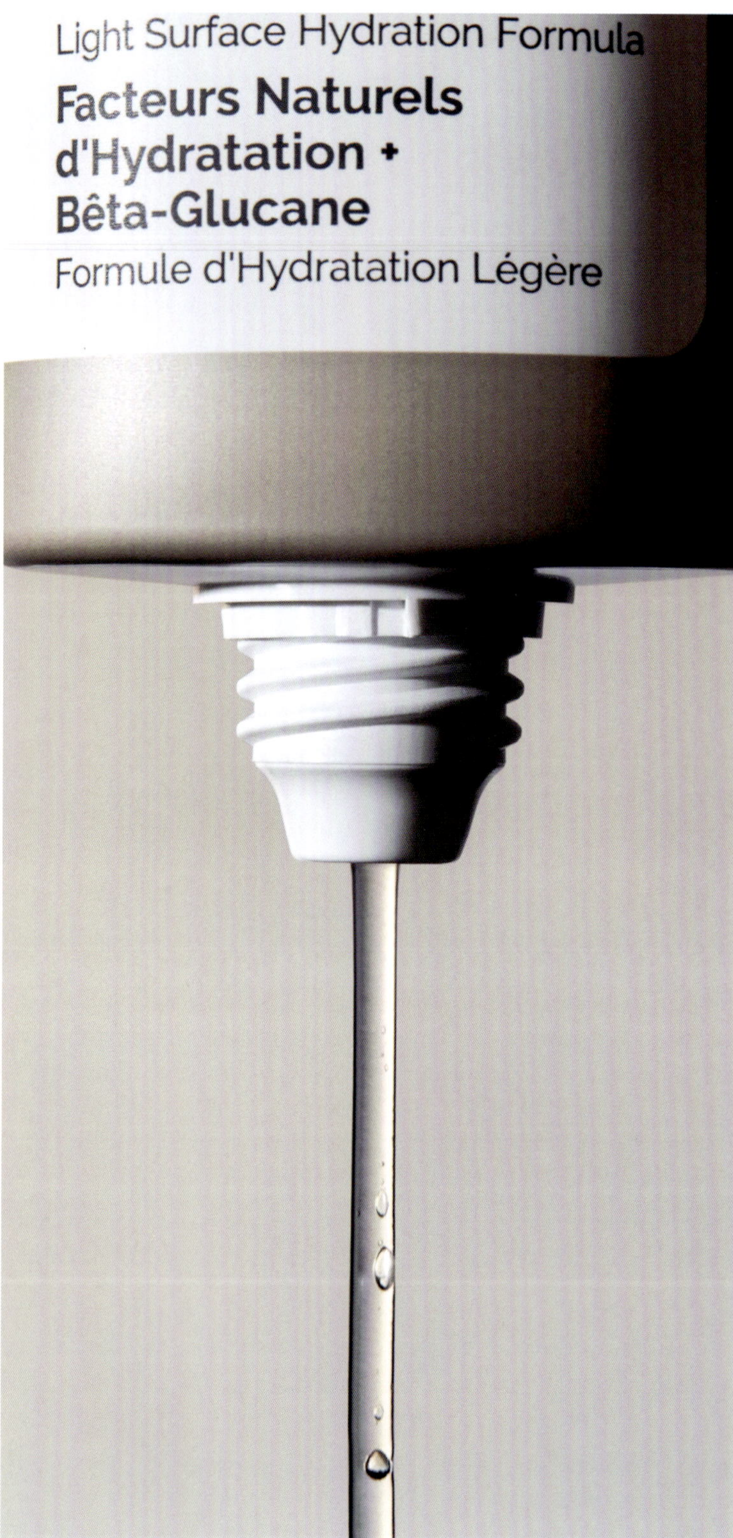

What it is

Urea is a low-molecular-weight organic molecule consisting of a carbonyl group linked to two amine groups. Naturally produced in the liver as a byproduct of protein metabolism, urea is an essential component of the body's waste elimination process, being excreted primarily through urine. In the context of skincare, urea plays a significant role as a hydrating agent.

Because of its ability to absorb and retain water, urea is present in the epidermis as a key component of the Natural Moisturizing Factors (NMF), which is vital for maintaining the skin's hydration, elasticity, and overall barrier function. Proper levels of urea in the skin help to maintain the integrity of the stratum corneum (the outermost layer of the skin).

What it's used for

Urea is a multifaceted ingredient in skincare, known for its powerful hydrating and exfoliating properties. Urea helps decrease transepidermal water loss (TEWL), boosts water retention, and enhances the stratum corneum's ability to withstand osmotic stress. Additionally, urea can function as a natural humectant, maintaining moisture levels in low-humidity environments.

In addition to its moisturizing properties, urea is also a potent keratolytic agent. In higher concentrations, urea helps to break down the connections between dead skin cells on the surface of the skin, promoting their exfoliation and improving the look of skin texture. Furthermore, urea has been shown to enhance the skin's barrier function by increasing the expression of ceramides, which are essential lipids that protect the skin from environmental stressors and pathogens.

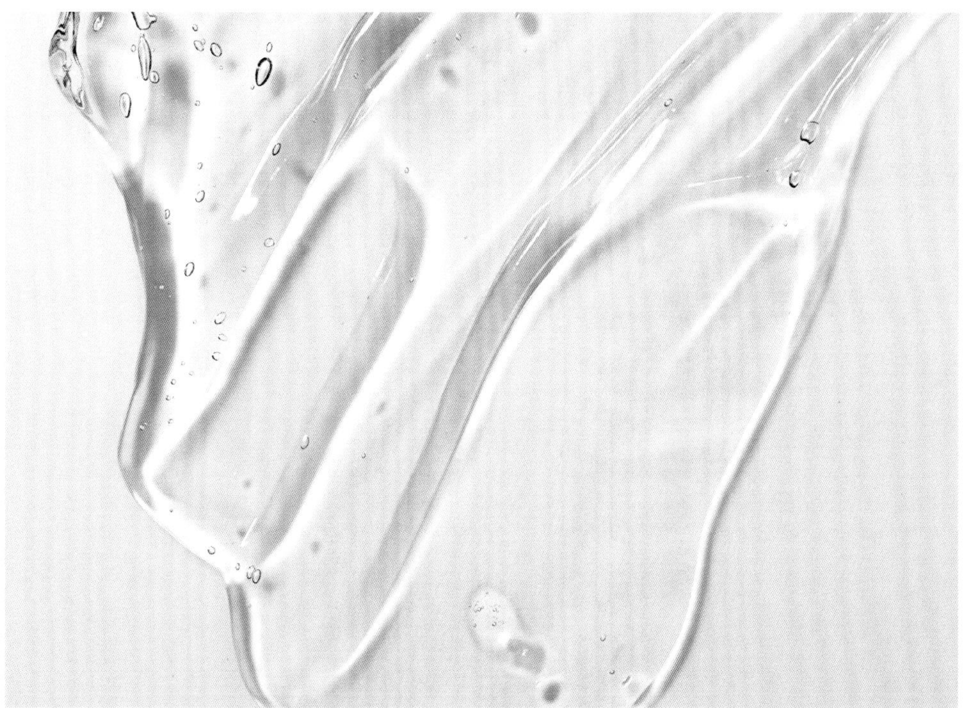

Mechanism of action

The mechanism of action of urea in skincare involves multiple effects that enhance skin health.

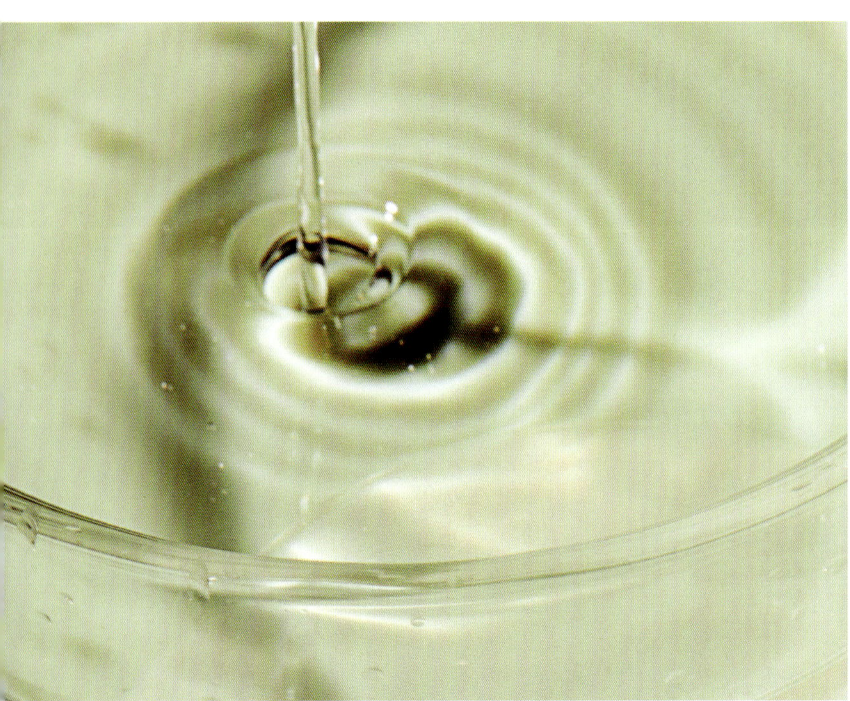

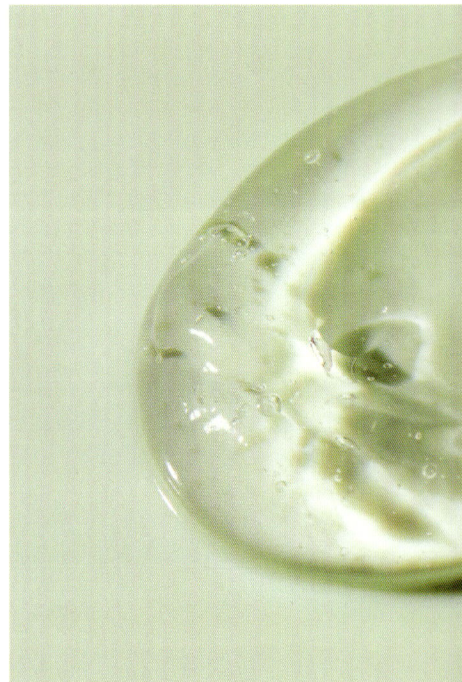

Moisturization

Urea is a hygroscopic molecule, meaning it can absorb and retain moisture from the environment, which helps to keep the skin soft and supple. Urea's ability to attract and hold water in the stratum corneum (the outermost layer of the skin) is vital for maintaining a healthy skin barrier, reducing transepidermal water loss (TEWL), and preventing dryness.

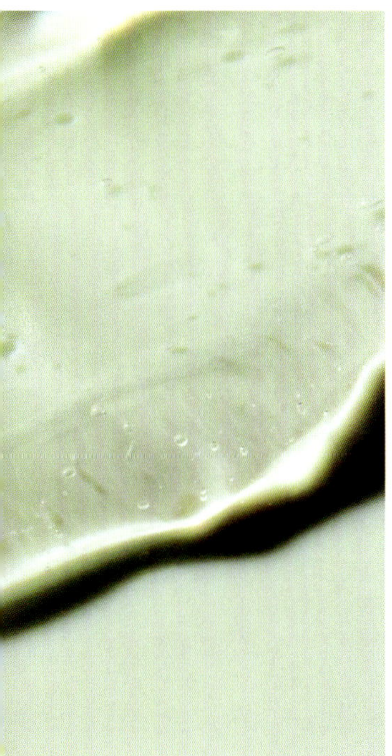

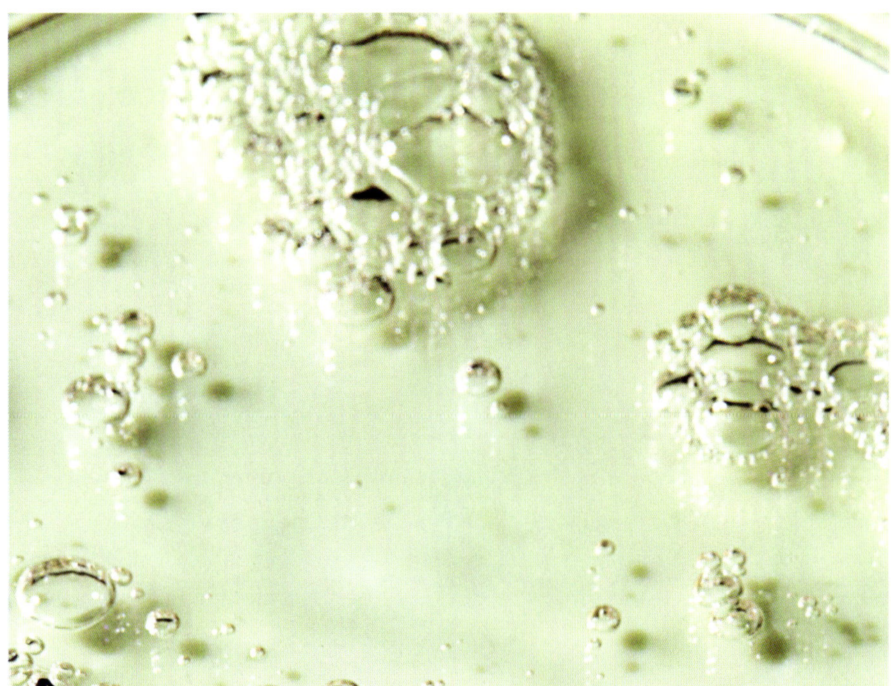

Keratolytic action

As an exfoliating agent, urea works by breaking down the protein structures (keratin) in the outermost layer of the skin, which loosens and dissolves dead skin cells. This action helps to smooth the skin's surface, reduce rough patches, and improve overall texture. Urea's ability to exfoliate is concentration-dependent, with higher concentrations (typically 10% or more) showing more pronounced keratolytic effects.

Vitamin C

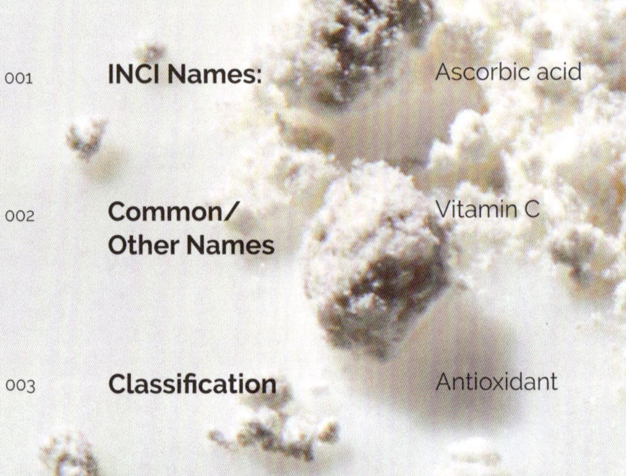

001 **INCI Names:** Ascorbic acid

002 **Common/ Other Names** Vitamin C

003 **Classification** Antioxidant

004 **Primary Function** Brightening and antioxidant support

005 **Phonetic Spelling** VY-tuh-min see

006 **First Discovered** Albert Szent-Györgyi, 1912

007 **Clinical Concentration(s)** 5–20%

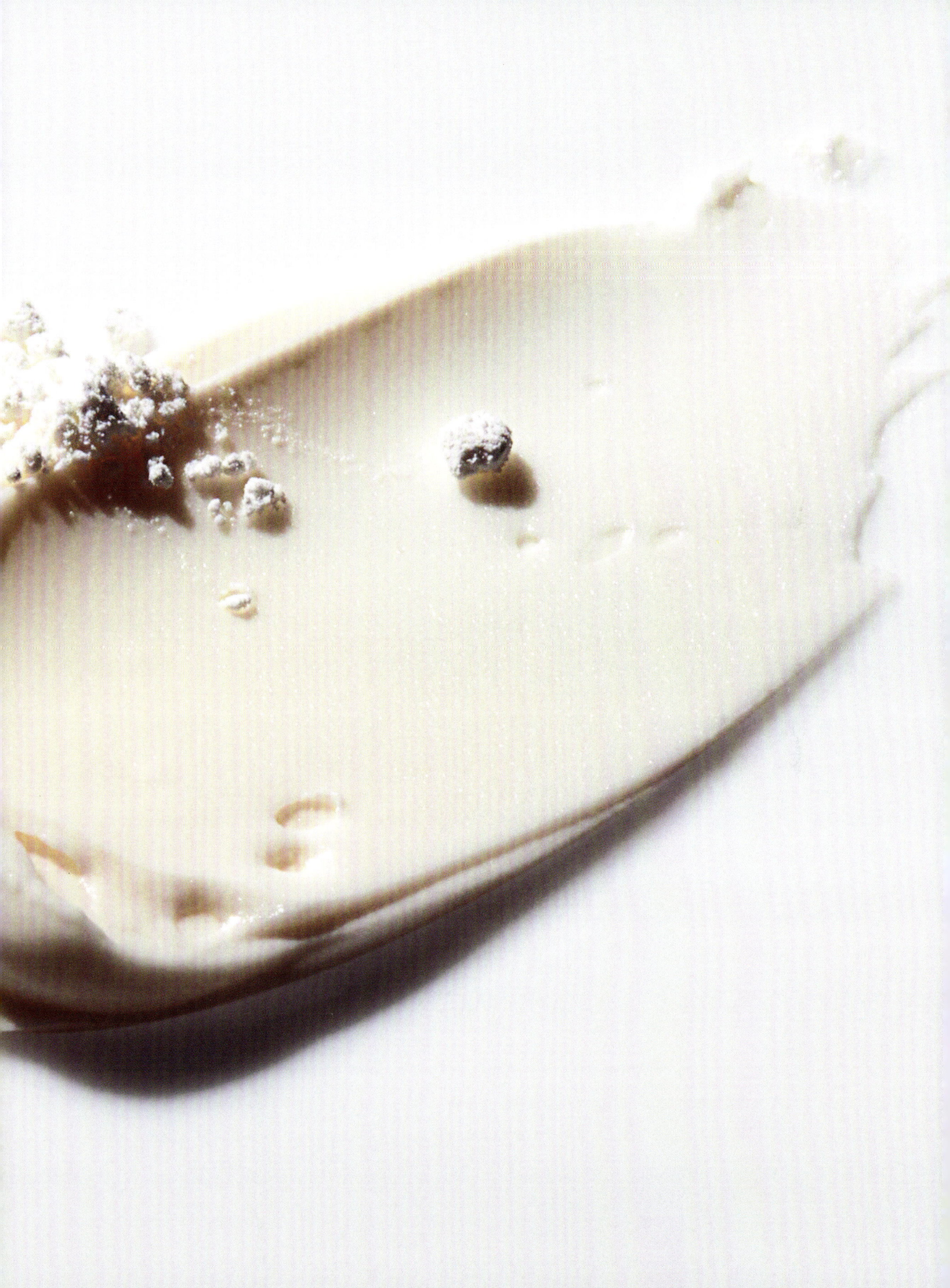

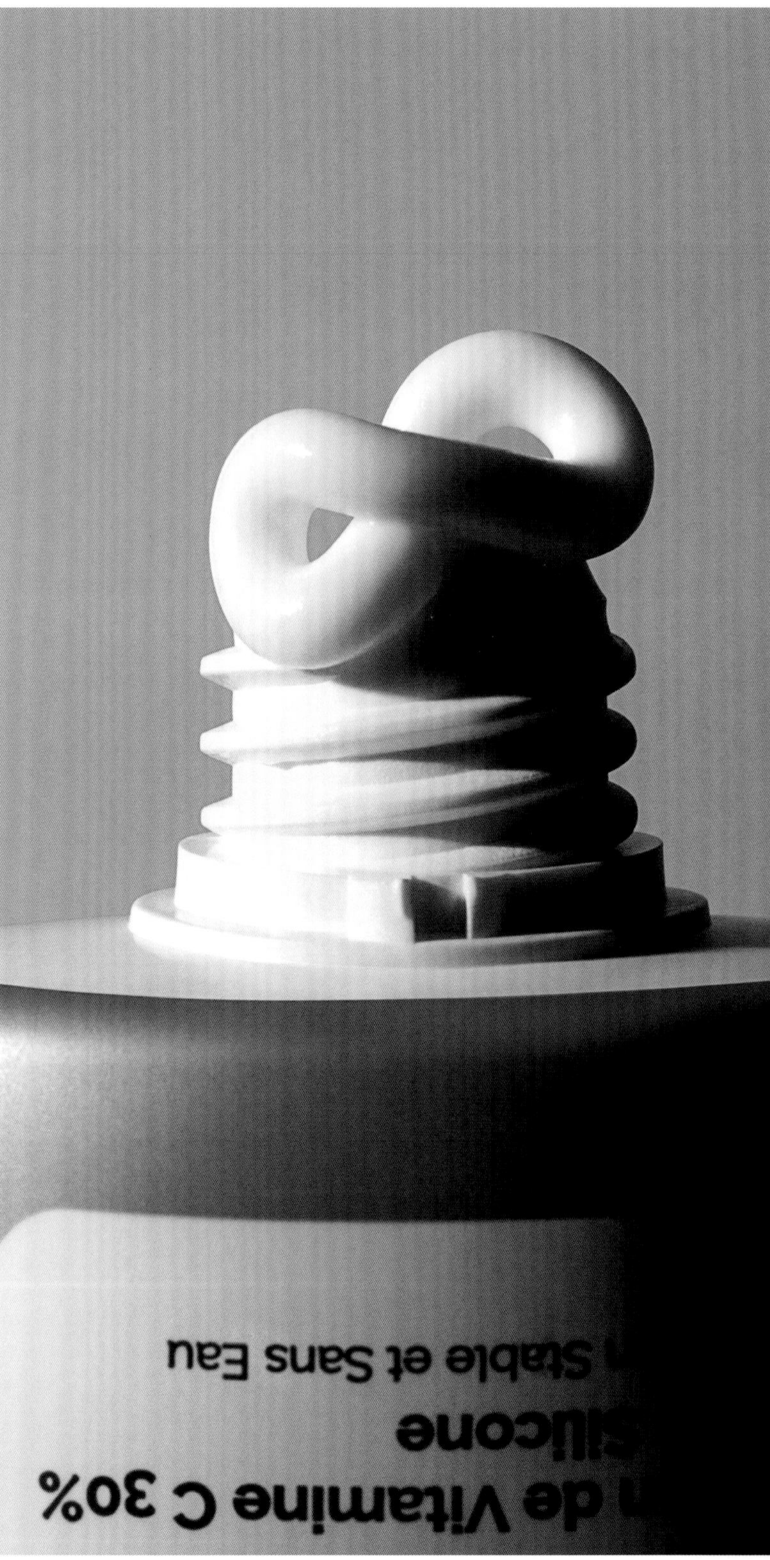

What it is

Vitamin C, also known as ascorbic acid, is a water-soluble antioxidant that plays a crucial role in skincare by neutralizing free radicals, which can damage the skin and accelerate the appearance of aging. Chemically, it is a small molecule composed of carbon, hydrogen, and oxygen, with a unique structure that enables it to easily donate electrons to reactive molecules, effectively neutralizing them. This antioxidant activity helps to protect the skin from oxidative stress caused by environmental factors such as UV exposure and pollution.

In skincare formulations, ascorbic acid is often used in its pure form or in stabilized derivatives like ascorbyl glucoside, which are designed to be more stable and less prone to oxidation. Pure ascorbic acid can often be unstable in formulas, so other forms are often used to enhance its stability and effectiveness in skincare products.

What it's used for

Vitamin C is a potent antioxidant that is widely used in skincare for its ability to improve the look of skin radiance. This powerful ingredient helps to visibly improve the appearance of dull, tired skin by promoting a more radiant and even skin tone. It works by neutralizing free radicals, which can contribute to the look of premature skin aging and environmental damage. As a result, vitamin C helps to refresh the skin, giving it a more youthful, glowing appearance.

In addition to its brightening effects, vitamin C supports the skin's natural protection against environmental stressors and helps to maintain a smooth, refreshed complexion. It is often included in formulations aimed at evening out skin tone and enhancing overall skin clarity. Regular use of vitamin C can leave the skin looking visibly more vibrant, radiant, and revitalized.

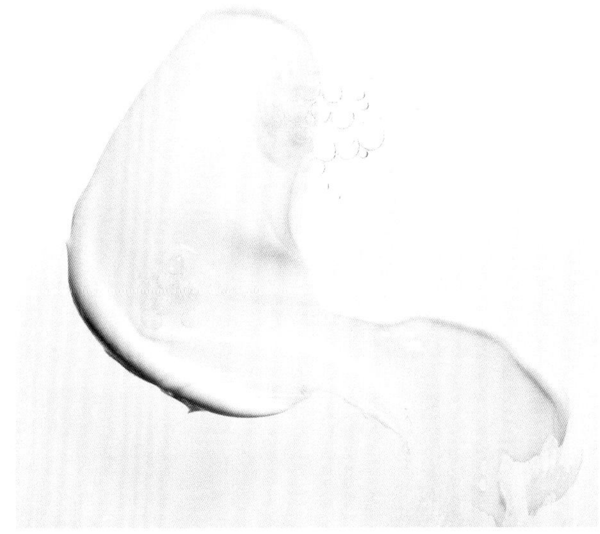

Mechanism of action

Vitamin C operates through several key mechanisms in skincare, providing a multitude of benefits that enhance skin health and appearance.

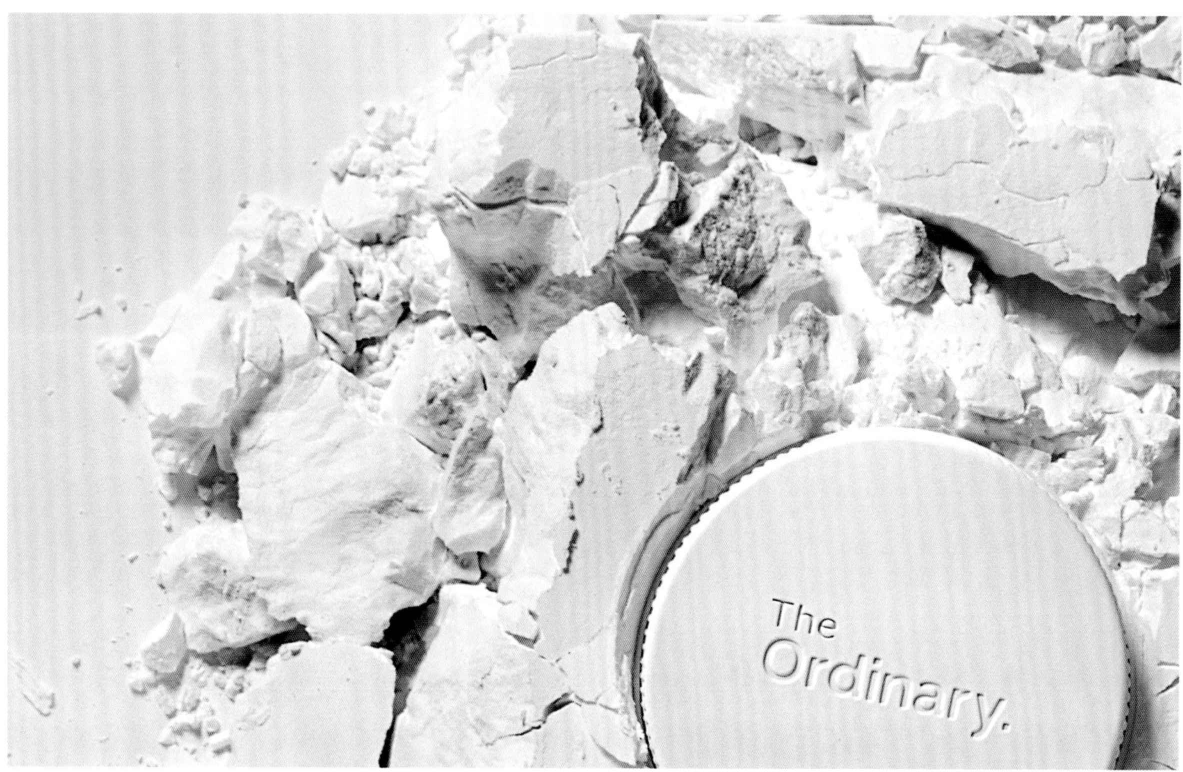

Antioxidant activity

As an antioxidant, vitamin C neutralizes free radicals—unstable molecules generated by UV exposure, pollution, and other environmental stressors. These free radicals have unpaired electrons, making them highly reactive and capable of causing damage that can then lead to signs of premature aging. Vitamin C donates electrons to these free radicals, stabilizing them and preventing them from reacting with and damaging important cellular components such as proteins and lipids. This protective action helps to prevent the appearance of premature aging of the skin, characterized by fine lines, wrinkles, and loss of elasticity.

Additionally, vitamin C's antioxidant capacity helps to regenerate other antioxidants within the skin, such as vitamin E. When vitamin E neutralizes free radicals, it becomes oxidized and inactive. Vitamin C can regenerate oxidized vitamin E back to its active form, thereby maintaining the antioxidant network in the skin. This synergistic effect enhances the overall protective mechanism against oxidative stress, contributing to a healthier, more resilient skin barrier and a brighter, more youthful complexion.

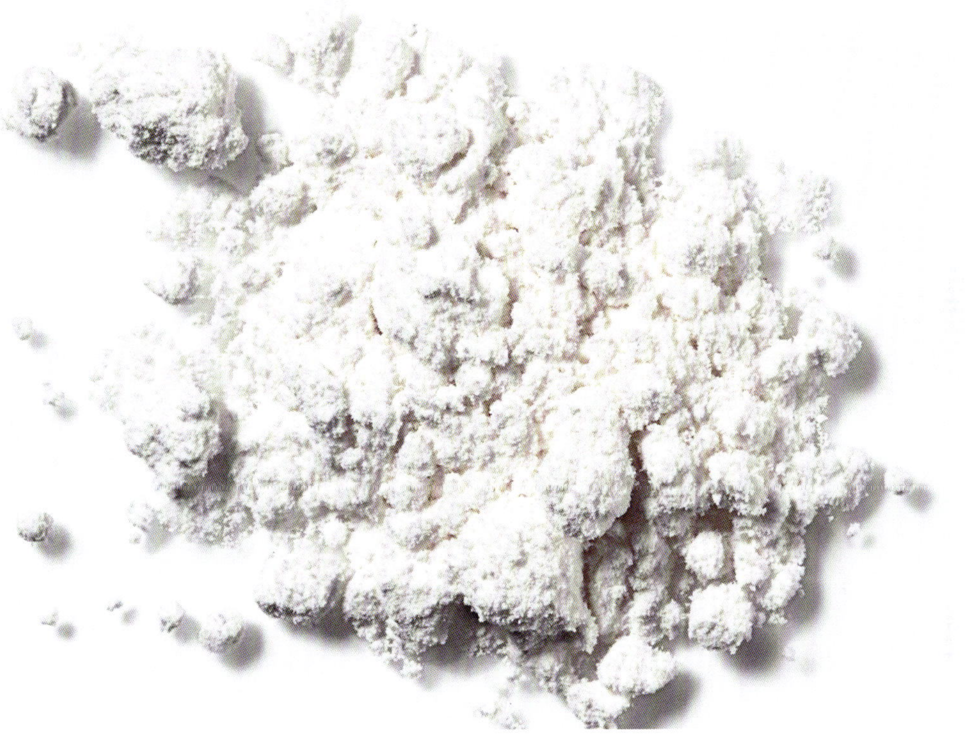

Uneven skin tone

In addition to its antioxidant properties, vitamin C is also known for its ability to improve the look of uneven skin tone. It helps to even out skin tone by inhibiting the production of melanin, the pigment responsible for dark spots and discoloration. As a result, skin appears refreshed and rejuvenated, with a healthier and more youthful glow.

Vitamin E

001	**INCI Names:**	Tocopherol
002	**Common/ Other Names**	Vitamin E
003	**Classification**	Antioxidant
004	**Primary Function**	Antioxidant support
005	**Phonetic Spelling**	VIT-uh-min Ee
006	**First Discovered**	Herbert McLean Evans and K. S. Bishop, 1922
007	**Clinical Concentration(s)**	0.5–5%

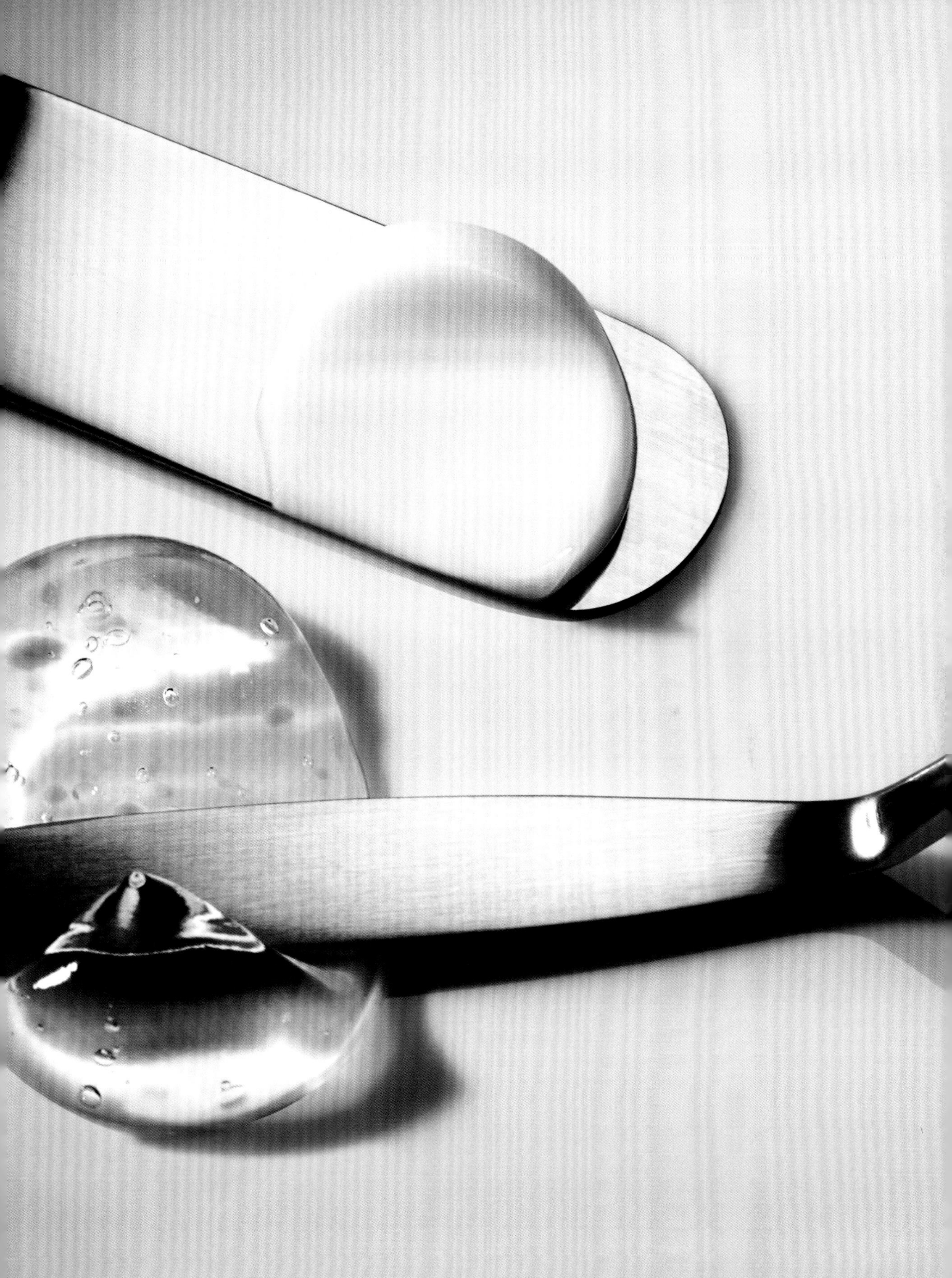

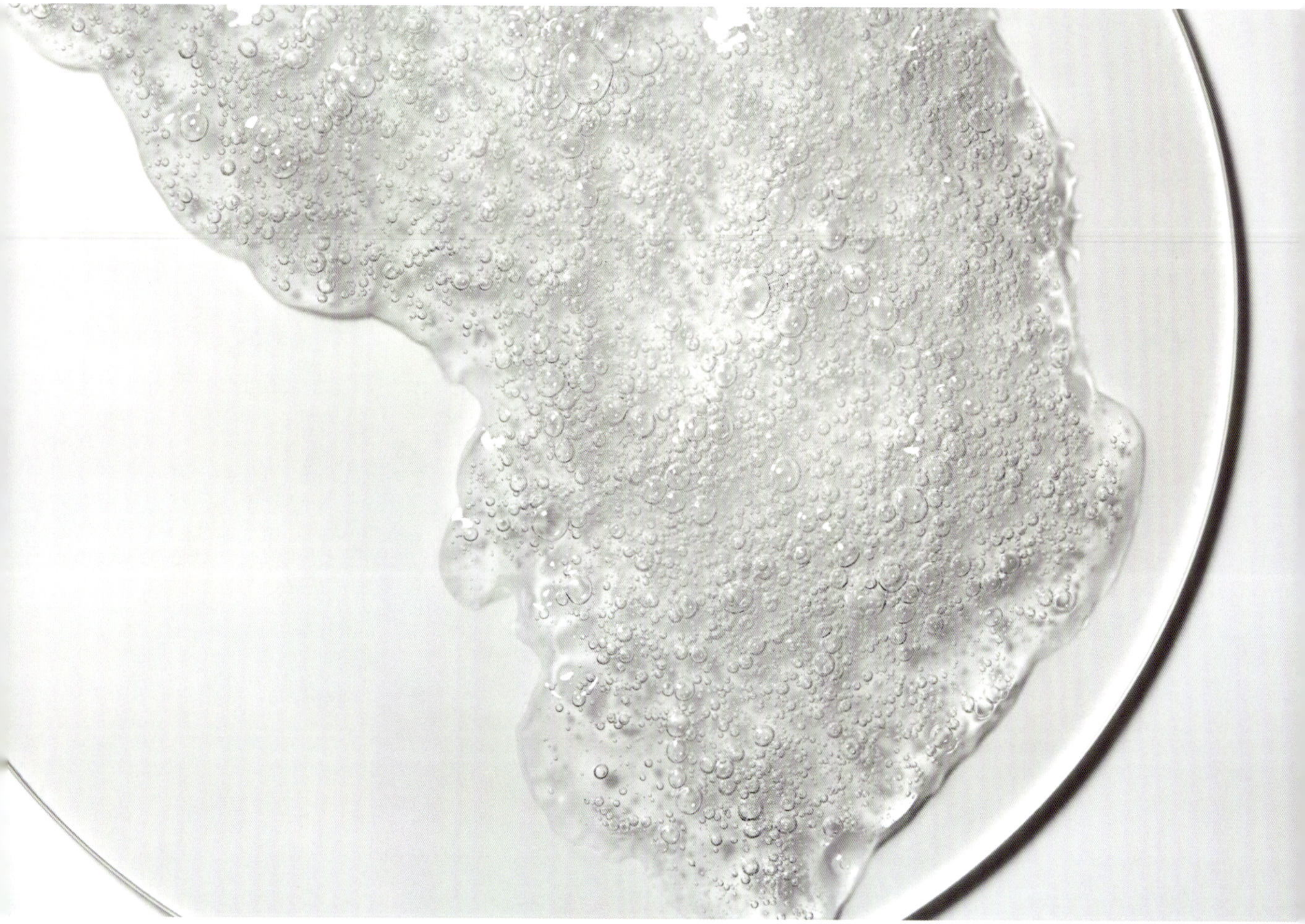

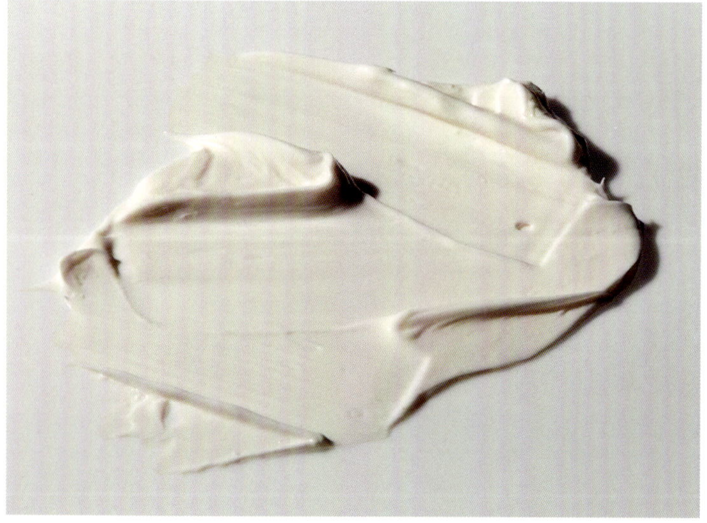

What it is

Vitamin E refers to a group of fat-soluble compounds, primarily composed of tocopherols and tocotrienols, that function as antioxidants. Chemically, these molecules share a similar structure: a chromanol ring attached to a hydrophobic isoprenoid side chain. This structure enables vitamin E to play a key role in protecting lipids from oxidative damage caused by free radicals.

The slight differences in chemical structures between tocopherols and tocotrienols influence their antioxidant potency and bioavailability. These characteristics make vitamin E a versatile and essential nutrient in skincare formulations.

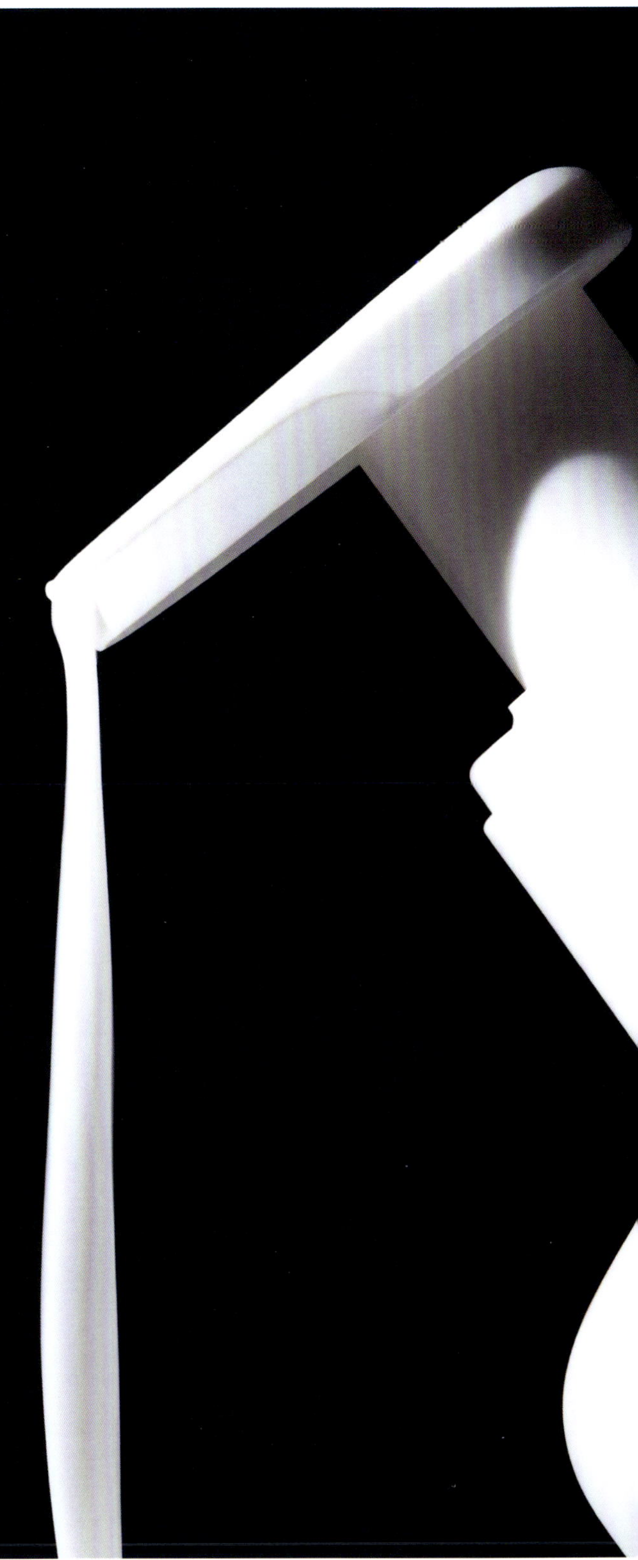

What it's used for

In skincare, vitamin E serves several important functions that contribute to maintaining healthy, youthful-looking skin. Primarily, it acts as a powerful antioxidant, protecting the skin from oxidative stress caused by free radicals. UV radiation from the sun generates free radicals that can damage skin cells, and vitamin E neutralizes these, so it is used to combat signs of aging that can be caused by UV exposure, as well as fine lines and wrinkles. Vitamin E also plays a key role in moisturizing the skin. It enhances the skin's natural barrier, which helps to lock in moisture and prevent dryness.

The largest body of scientific evidence for the role of topical vitamin E is it's role in protecting against signs of photoaging due to its potent antioxidant properties. UV radiation from the sun generates free radicals that can damage skin cells, leading to the appearance of premature signs of aging. Vitamin E helps neutralize these free radicals, reducing oxidative stress and minimizing the potential damage and visible signs of aging that can be caused by UV exposure.

Mechanism of action

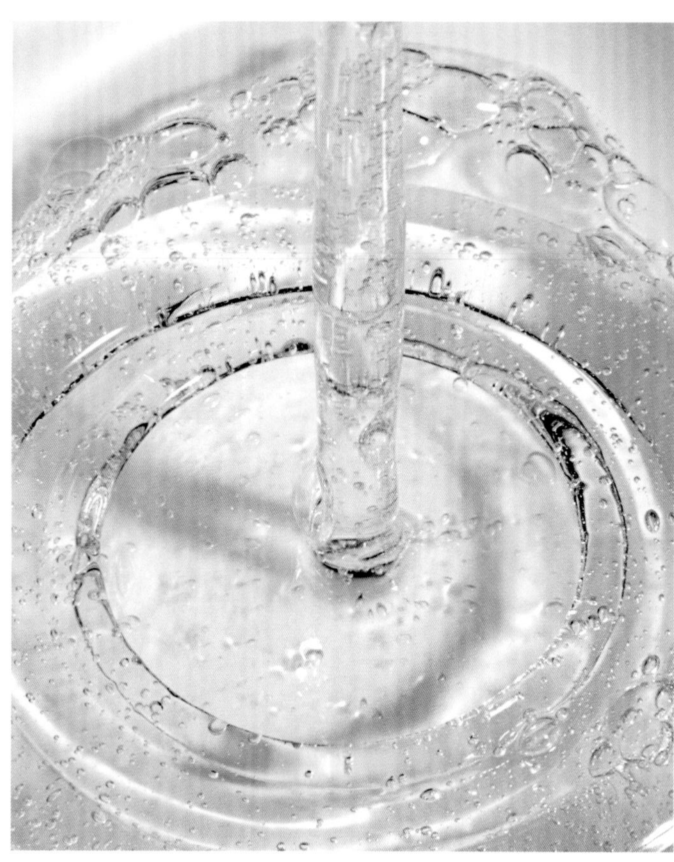

Antioxidant protection

Vitamin E is a prominent fat-soluble antioxidant renowned for its ability to counteract pro-oxidant activity caused by reactive oxygen species (ROS). This helps prevent the degradation of components like lipids and proteins. It neutralizes free radicals produced by both internal and external sources, such as UV radiation, drugs, and environmental pollutants, thereby mitigating their harmful effects. The antioxidant properties of vitamin E are closely associated with its capacity to prevent lipid peroxidation in unsaturated fatty acids. Vitamin E effectively inhibits the oxidation of lipids, helping protect from external damage.

Skin barrier and moisturization

Vitamin E enhances the skin's natural barrier function by stabilizing lipids. This integration into the lipid bilayer helps to prevent moisture loss and improve overall hydration. Additionally, by reinforcing the skin barrier, vitamin E can reduce dryness and irritation, making it beneficial for maintaining smooth and healthy skin.

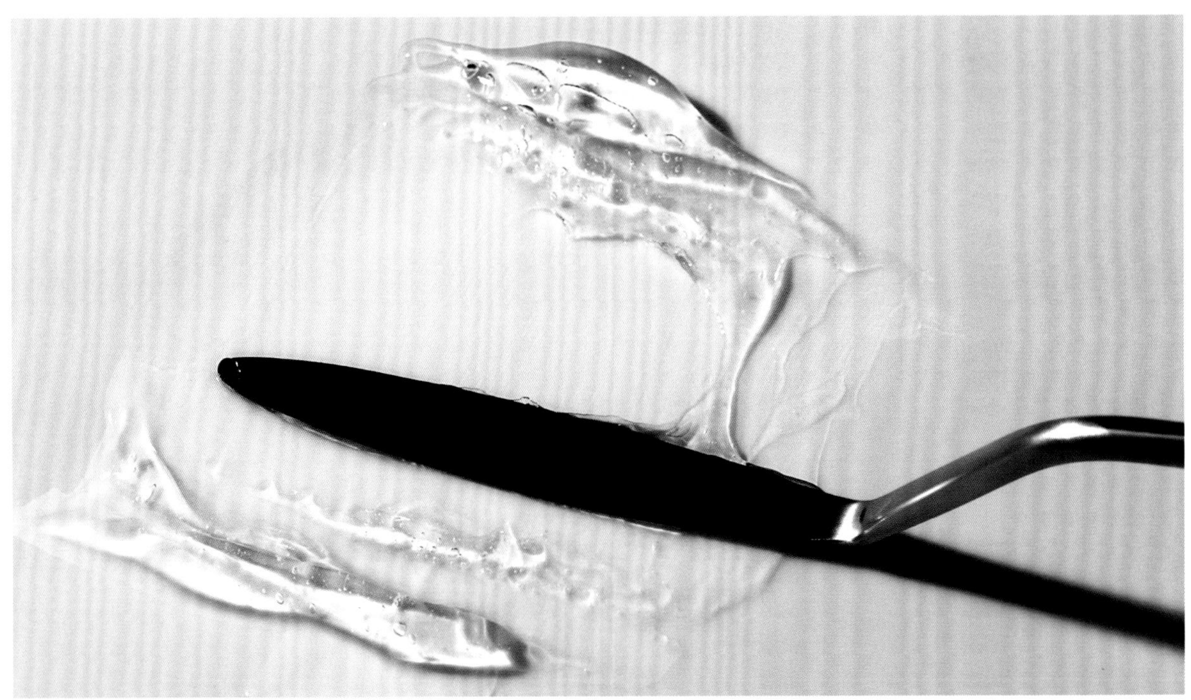

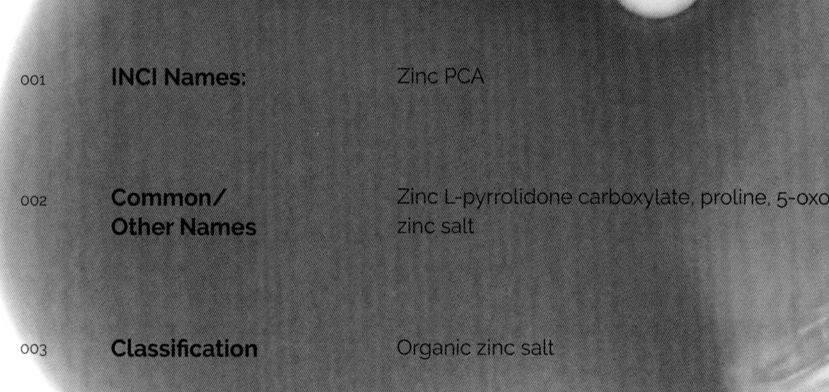

001 **INCI Names:** Zinc PCA

002 **Common/ Other Names** Zinc L-pyrrolidone carboxylate, proline, 5-oxo, zinc salt

003 **Classification** Organic zinc salt

Zinc PCA

004 **Primary Function** Acne and blemishes, sebum regulation

005 **Phonetic Spelling** ZINK PEE-ESS-AY

006 **First Discovered** 1980s

007 **Clinical Concentration(s)** 1%

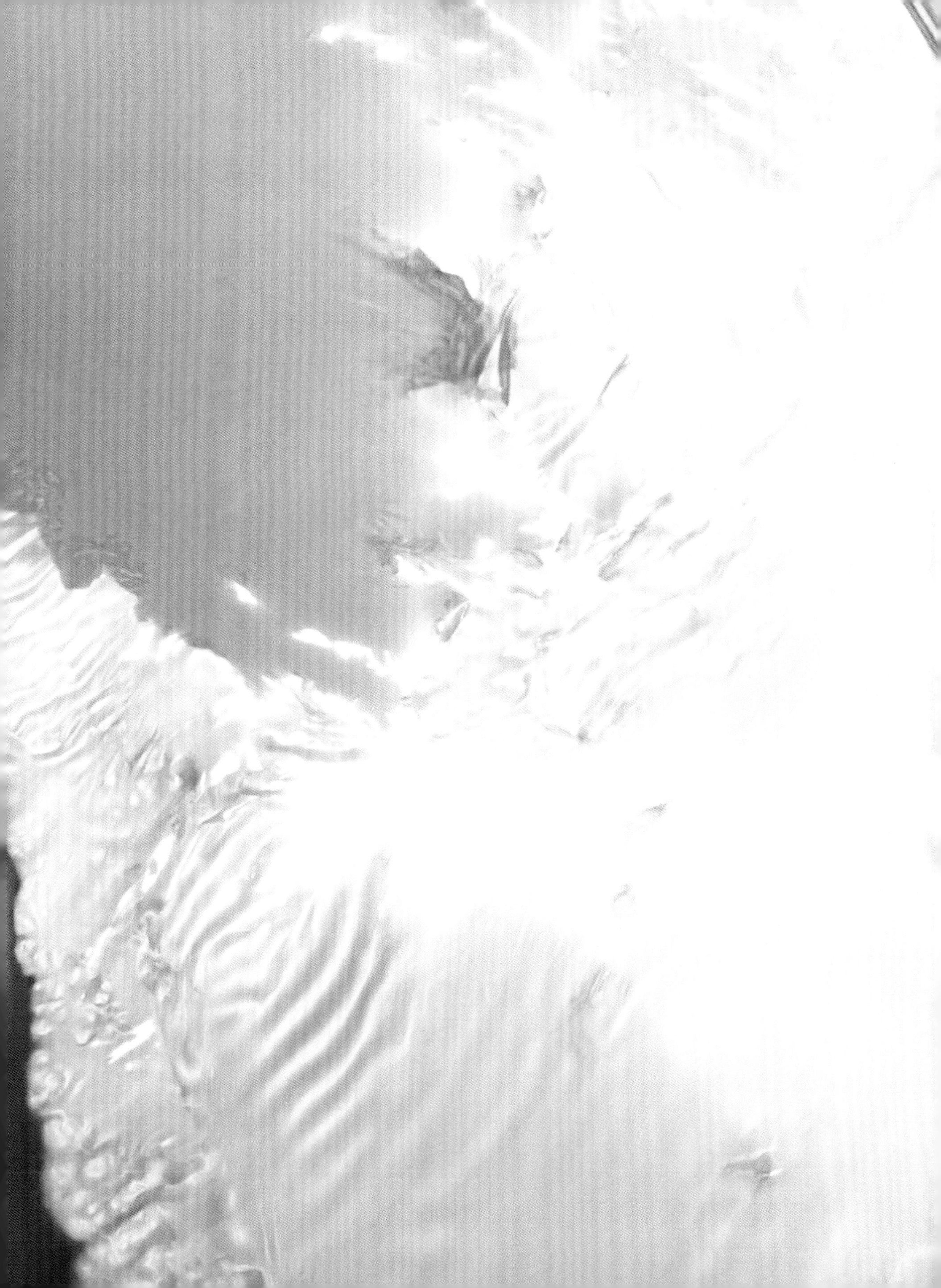

What it is

Zinc PCA, also known as zinc L-pyrrolidone carboxylate, is a water-soluble organic zinc salt composed of zinc, an essential trace element with diverse biological roles, and pyrrolidone carboxylic acid (PCA), a natural moisturizing factor and humectant found in the skin. This combination makes Zinc PCA a valuable ingredient in skincare formulations, as it exhibits a range of beneficial effects.

What it's used for

In skincare, Zinc PCA is commonly found in formulations designed for blemish-prone skin due to its sebum-regulating and soothing properties. It is frequently combined with other ingredients known for targeting the appearance of blemishes, such as niacinamide, sulfur, and salicylic acid. A less common, but promising application for Zinc PCA is its inclusion in products that target signs of aging, specifically those that arise from a loss of structural integrity within the skin over time.

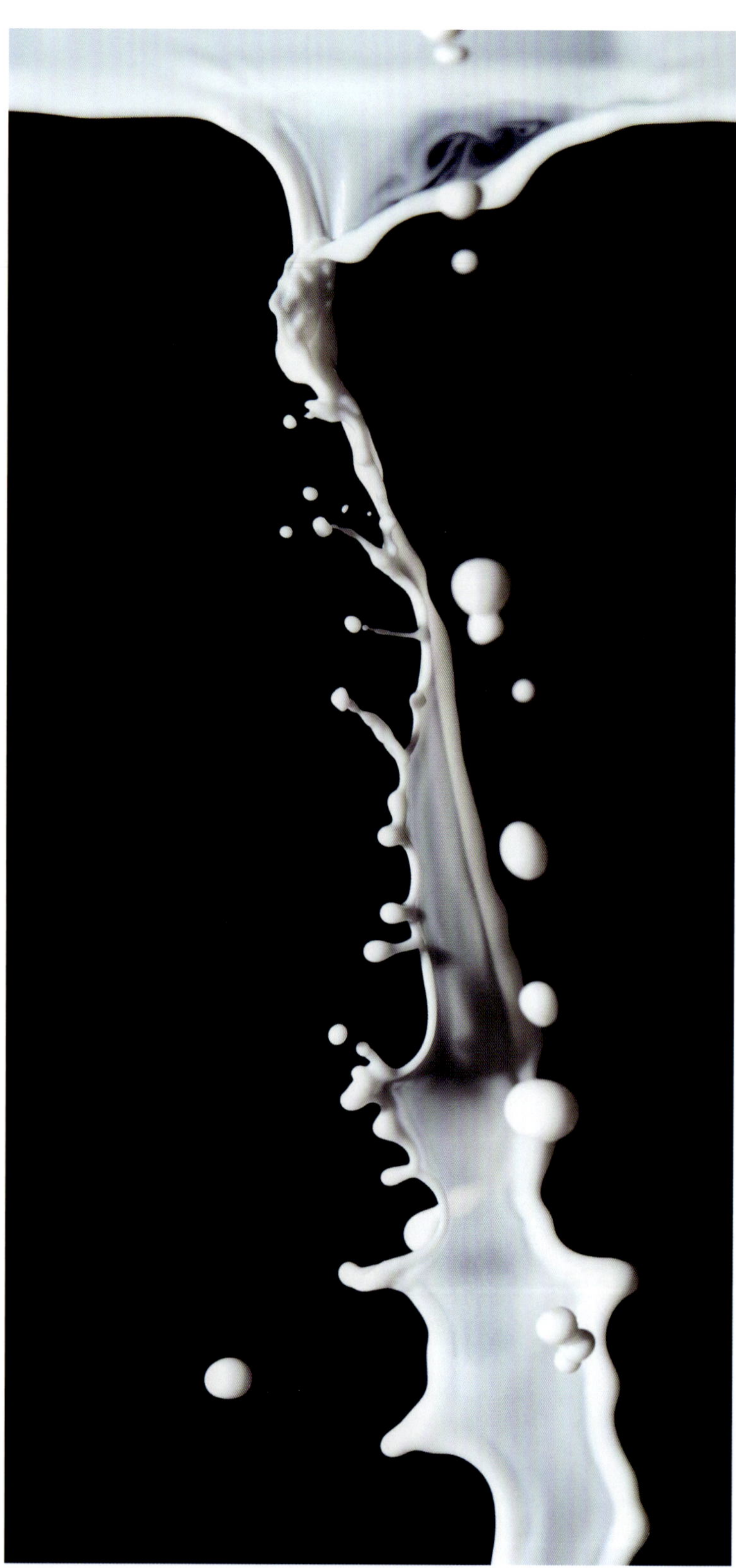

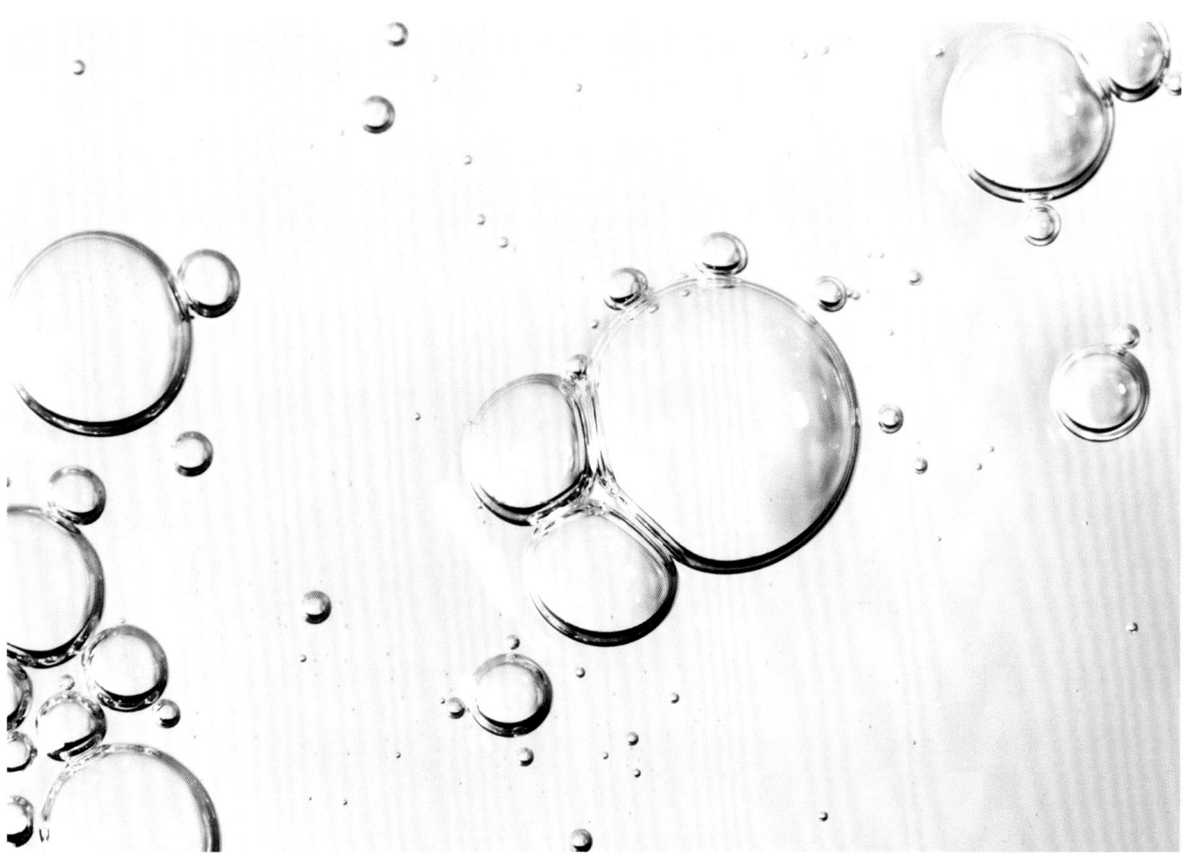

Mechanism of action

Zinc PCA has been shown to reduce the appearance of redness and skin discomfort, which can be experienced by those with blemish-prone skin. While the exact mechanism is not fully elucidated in scientific literature, Zinc PCA is reported to help regulate excess sebum and therefore, reduces the appearance of oily skin. This makes it particularly beneficial for individuals with blemish-prone skin, as excess sebum can contribute to clogged pores and breakouts.

In vitro studies also suggest that Zinc PCA can play a supportive role in maintaining the skin's natural collagen content. As an important structural protein, changes to the skin's natural collagen content can lead to fine lines and wrinkles, as well as loss of elasticity and firmness. Further research is needed to understand the potential of Zinc PCA as a collagen-supporting ingredient.

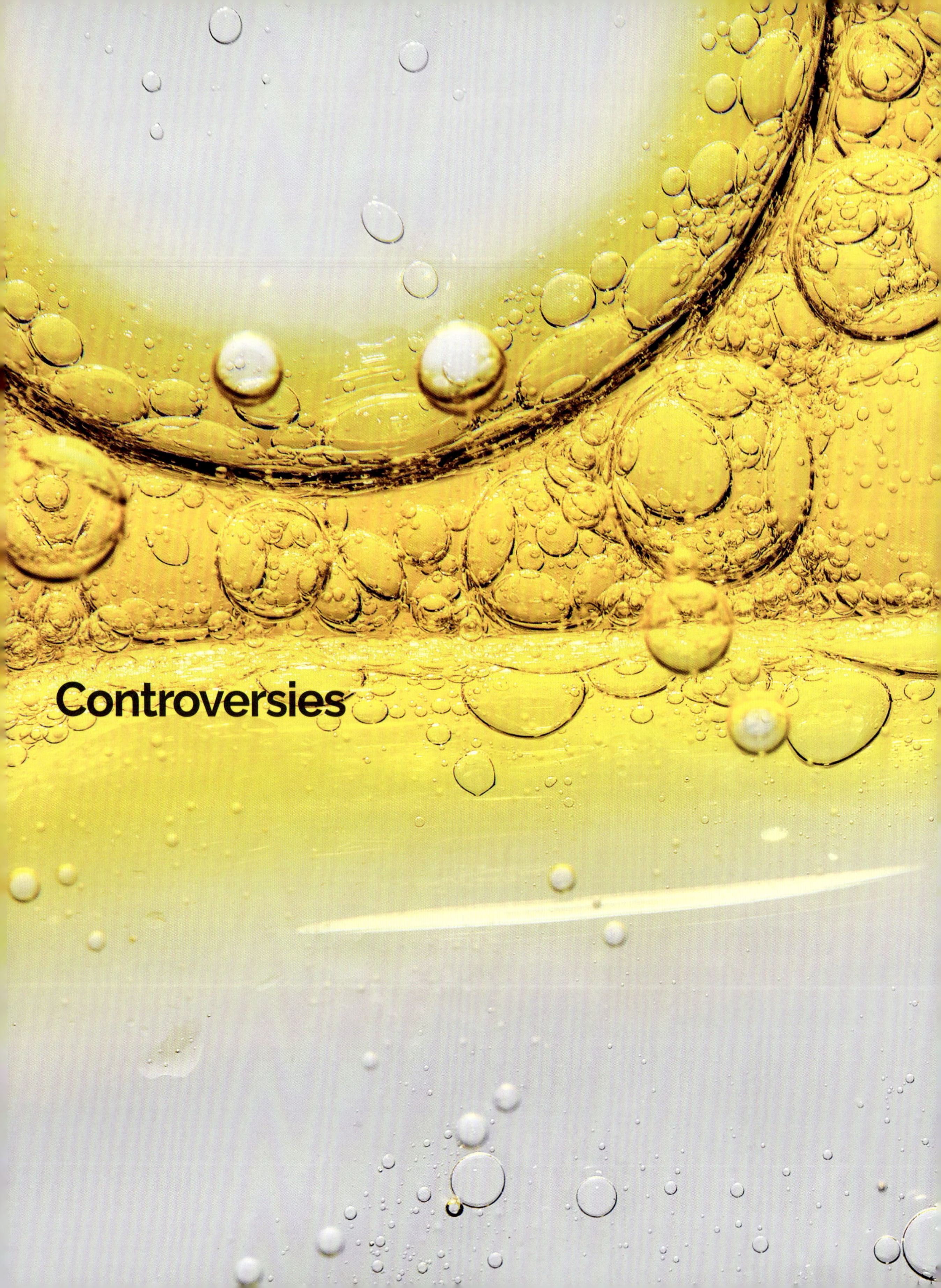

Controversies

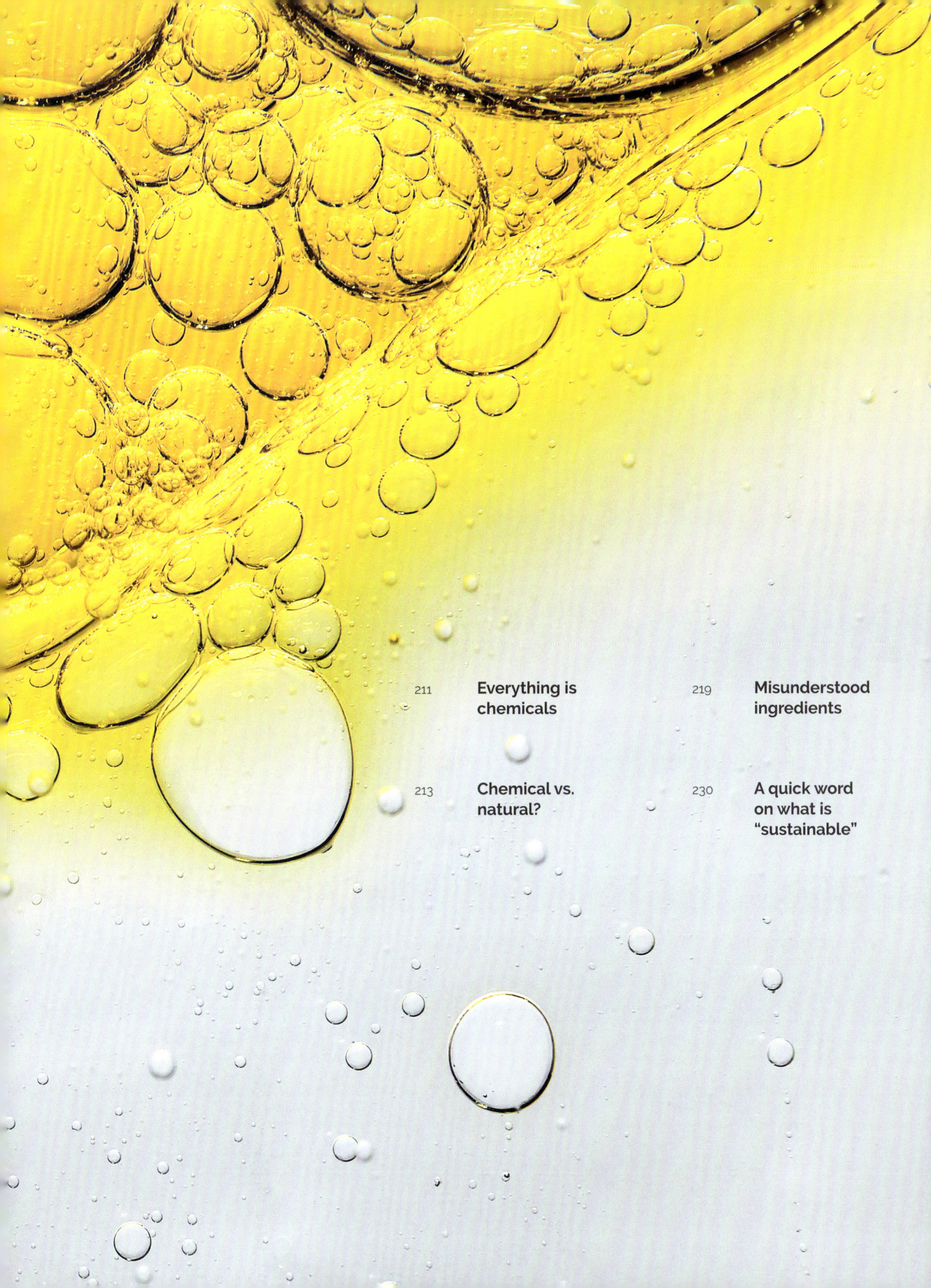

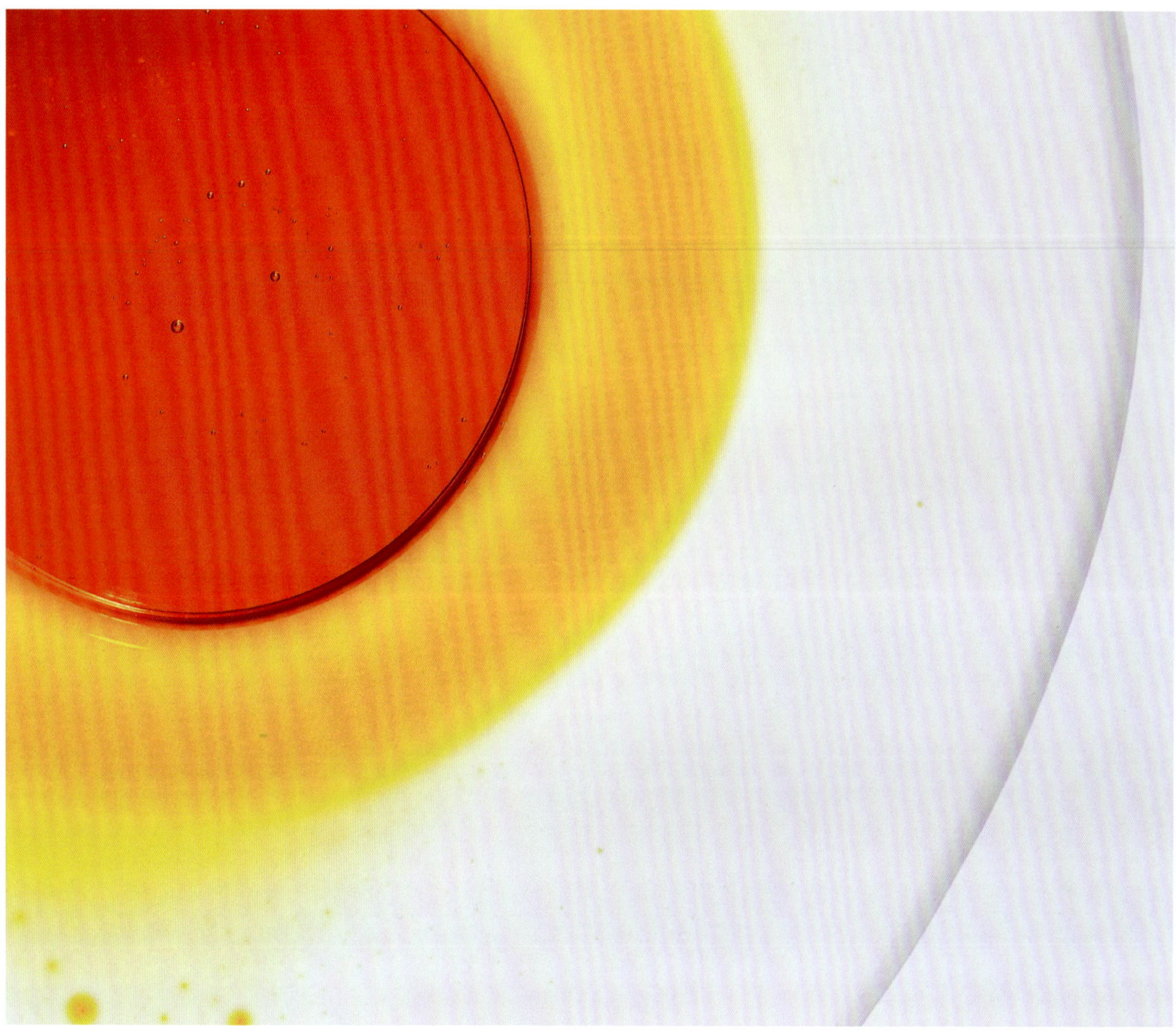

Controversies

Like any industry, the world of skincare has its misconceptions. From buzzwords and convoluted claims to misunderstood ingredients, navigating this space can feel overwhelming. In today's digital age, the rapid proliferation of information online has made things even more complicated—especially when scientific findings can be reduced to catchy one-liners, taken out of context, or misinterpreted entirely.

It's not surprising. While skincare is a part of daily life for many, the science behind it is complex and not always easy to understand. One key concept to keep in mind is that correlation does not equal causation—just because two factors may be related does not mean that one directly causes the other. Drawing conclusions without considering the full scope of a study—its methodology, variables, and limitations—and other studies on the same topic can lead to misinformation.

But because this is an industry rooted in science, and science is about looking at the full picture—not just the data points that confirm our assumptions—taking a deeper look can help cut through the noise and bring clarity.

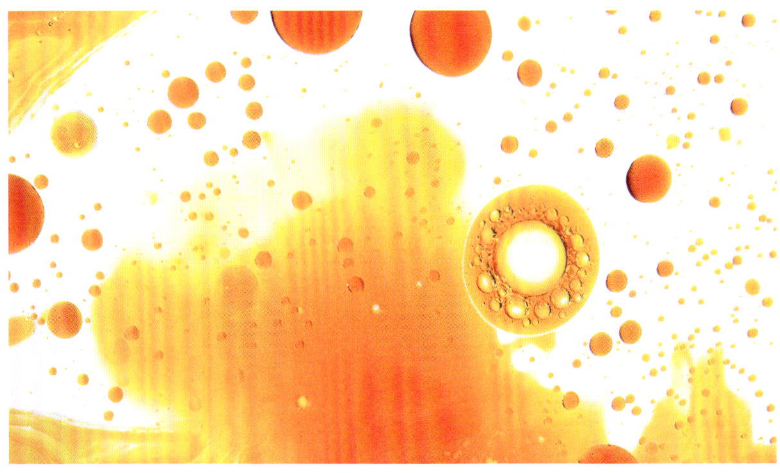

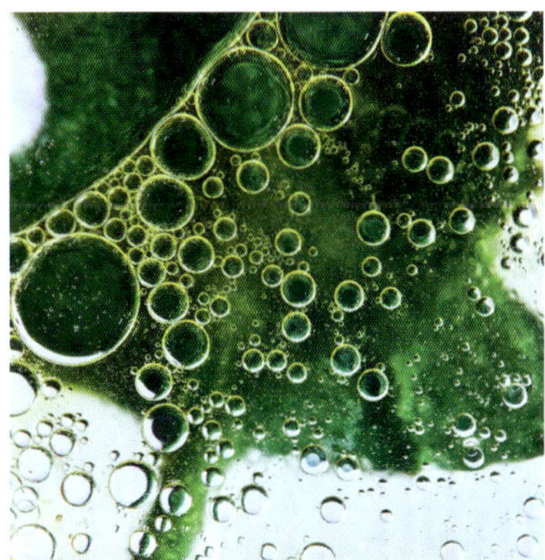

Everything is chemicals

The word "chemical" has taken on a negative connotation—whether in beauty and cosmetics, other consumer goods, or many of the things we interact with in our daily lives. But let's be clear: everything is chemicals. They existed long before humans had the language to describe them. Over time, we developed chemistry as a way to understand and communicate how things are in the world around us. Rather than something to be feared, chemistry is simply the language we use to explain how everything—natural or synthetic—is constructed.

In chemistry, everything in the world can be understood as small building blocks—atoms—that come together to form molecules, which in turn make up matter, the foundation of everything around us. And everything in nature, from the air we breathe to the food we eat, is made of chemicals. For example, one atom of oxygen (O) and two atoms of hydrogen (H) combine to form H_2O—the chemical formula for water. Chemistry calls it H_2O, while everyone else calls it water, but no matter the name, fundamentally, it's still water and it's still a chemical.

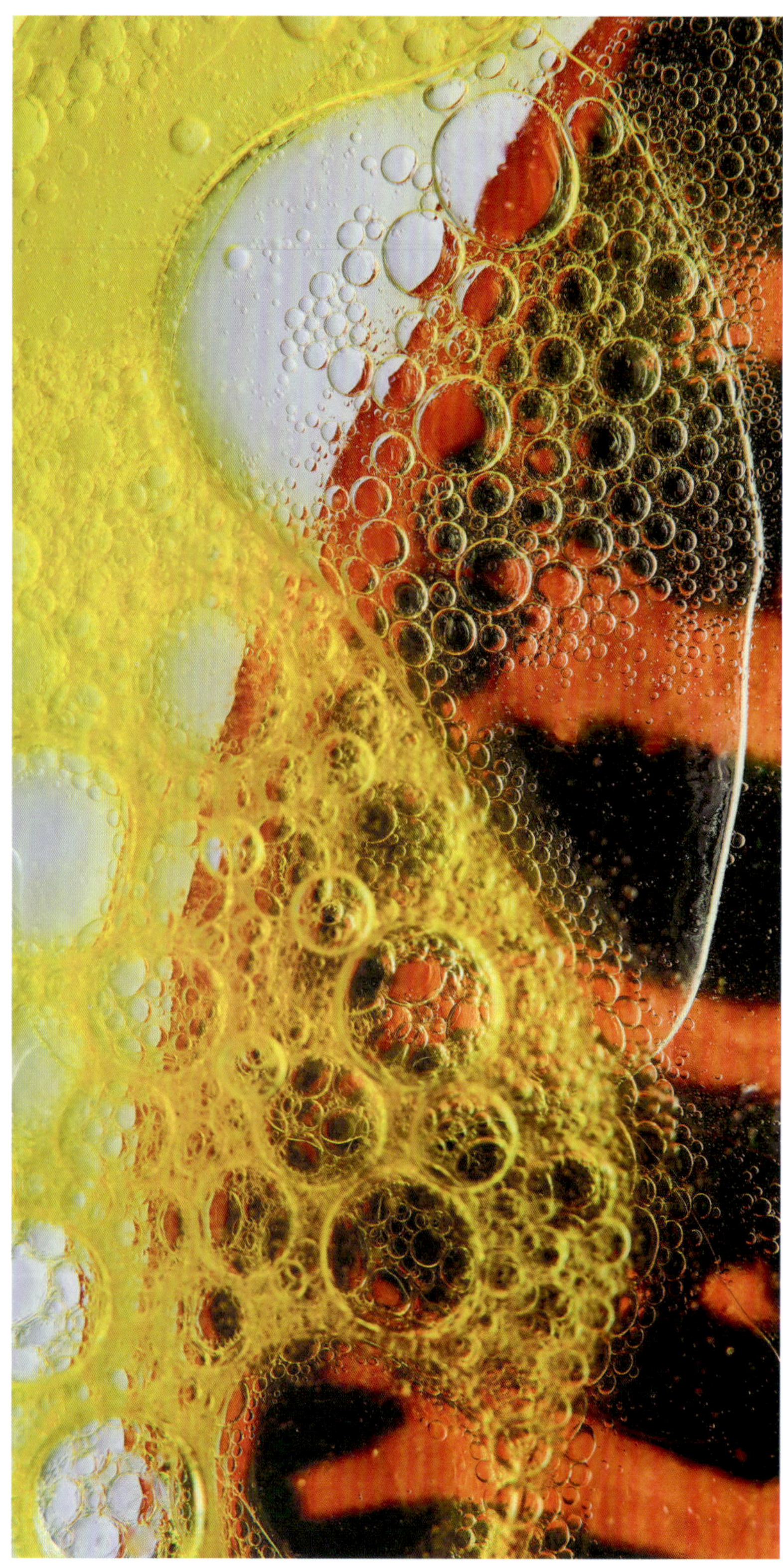

Similarly, humans are made entirely of chemicals, just like everything we see, touch, and taste. For example, you might be sitting on a chair made of $C_6H_{10}O_5$—cellulose, or, as we'd typically call it, wood. Or you might sprinkle NaCl—sodium chloride, better known as salt—onto your dinner. In everyday conversation, we use familiar, colloquial words to describe these things, but we could just as easily use the language of chemistry. It's all the same matter, just different ways of naming it.

The challenge is that the language of chemistry can be like a foreign language. It's entirely normal and understandable to fear the unknown and seemingly incomprehensible, so it's easy to see how chemophobia—the fear of chemicals—has infiltrated the world of cosmetics. Unfortunately, instead of demystifying the science, chemophobia and consumer misconceptions have sometimes been manipulated and amplified by marketing strategies.

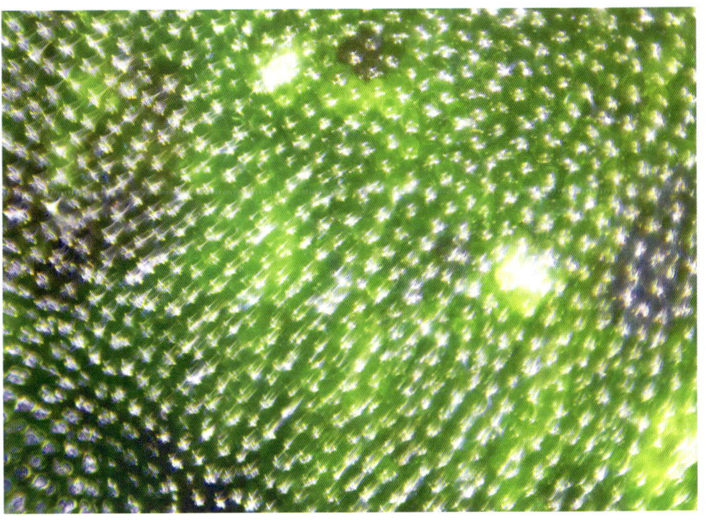

Chemical vs natural?

Chemical is not the opposite of natural. Everything in nature, from the soil to the plants growing in it, is made up of chemicals. The air we breathe, the water we drink, and even the fruits and vegetables we eat are all composed of chemical compounds. When we talk about chemicals in nature, we're simply recognizing that the natural world is built from the same fundamental building blocks as everything else—it's just chemistry at work.

The chemicals that make up the ingredients for the products we all use can be derived from both naturally occurring and synthetic sources, and, while the term "natural" can often be interpreted by consumers to mean a product is safer for skin and the environment, this isn't always the case. Just because an ingredient is natural doesn't mean it's free from risks, as the potential for ingredient contamination is assessed in both natural and synthetic materials. Bacteria and fungi can naturally develop during the growing, harvesting, and processing stages, and, if the product is not properly preserved, they can shorten an ingredient's or a product's shelf life. Additionally, natural ingredients can sometimes contain trace amounts of heavy metals like lead and mercury, which are naturally found in soil, regardless of pollution. If the soil a natural ingredient is grown in is contaminated, or if the equipment used to process the ingredients isn't properly cleaned, the risk of contamination increases.

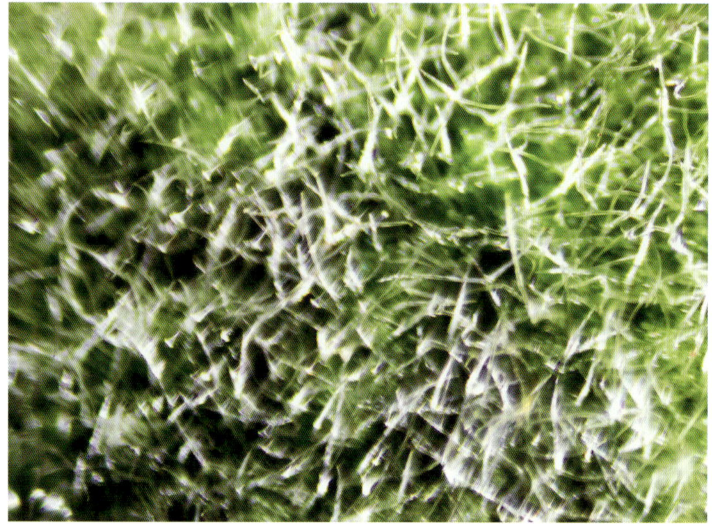

This is why natural doesn't automatically mean safer for skin or for the environment. The impact of an ingredient, whether natural or synthetic, depends on many factors, including how it's sourced, processed, and used. In some cases, natural ingredients may have a greater environmental and human safety impact than synthetic alternatives, while in other, the opposite may be true. There are also instances where both can have a similar impact, but in different ways. Rather than assuming one is always better than the other, it's important to recognize that both natural and synthetic ingredients have unique impacts, and that comparisons should be carefully nuanced.

Chemical vs clean?

You've likely heard the term "clean beauty," but it's understandable if you're not entirely sure what it means. The term is unregulated, which means there is no official definition or standard for what qualifies as "clean." Without a clear, regulated definition, brands can interpret and market the term in their own way, leading to confusion and a lack of consistency for consumers.

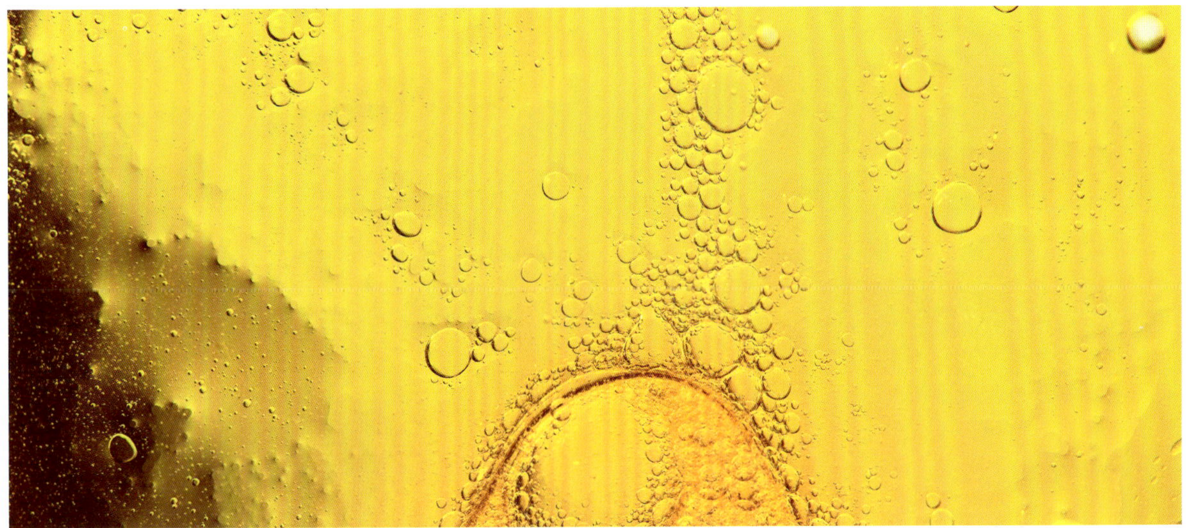

Generally, "clean" beauty brands claim to avoid certain ingredients due to concerns over their potential negative interactions with skin or the environment, though these concerns are sometimes based on speculative information or single-study results. Additionally, some extreme "clean" lists with several hundreds of ingredients can arguably be deemed unfair or deceptive marketing if they include many ingredients not generally used in cosmetics. These extensive clean lists carry an implied claim that other cosmetic companies are formulating with those ingredients. This type of marketing can be misleading to consumers and contributes to misinformation and fear around cosmetics and cosmetic ingredients.

Marketing campaigns are not the only source of misinformation about cosmetics. When information sourced from scientific research is cherry-picked or taken out of context, it can easily lead to misinterpretation of the science, fueling unnecessary misconceptions about the potential risks of certain ingredients. Ingredients may be labeled as harmful and avoided, sometimes based on a single study or isolated piece of evidence, even when the broader body of research indicates they pose little to no significant risk to human health or the environment. In some cases, studies suggesting a risk may be based on extreme conditions, such as very high concentrations, that don't reflect typical real-world exposures or conditions.

However, risk is more nuanced than that. Toxicologists—the experts who study the effects of substances on humans, the environment, and other living organisms—evaluate risk by considering both the hazard (or potential harm) of a substance and the level of exposure. This includes factors such as how much of the substance you're exposed to, how long the exposure lasts, the pathway for exposure, and how likely it is that you'll come into contact with it.

You might also have heard this explained as "the dose makes the poison," which is a key principle of toxicology. Take apple seeds, for example. They contain a chemical called amygdalin, which, if ingested, is converted into cyanide by enzymes in our digestive system, potentially leading to cyanide poisoning. However, you'd need to eat around 200 apple seeds in a limited amount of time to experience this effect. Even if you ate one seed a day for 200 days, you're highly unlikely to get cyanide poisoning, as cyanide doesn't accumulate in the body and our excretory system can easily handle small amounts of it.

When toxicologists assess the safety of cosmetic ingredients, they consider all of these factors, including the body's ability to protect itself through the skin and efficiently dispose of unwanted compounds. The guidelines for the ingredients used in cosmetics are based on these comprehensive risk assessments, along with multiple studies on ingredient safety. This ensures that, as long as you're purchasing from a reputable brand and retailer, the product and its ingredients are safe for use.

From this, we hope you now understand that the absence of certain ingredients doesn't automatically make a product risk-free, just as a "clean" label doesn't necessarily indicate that a product is safer.

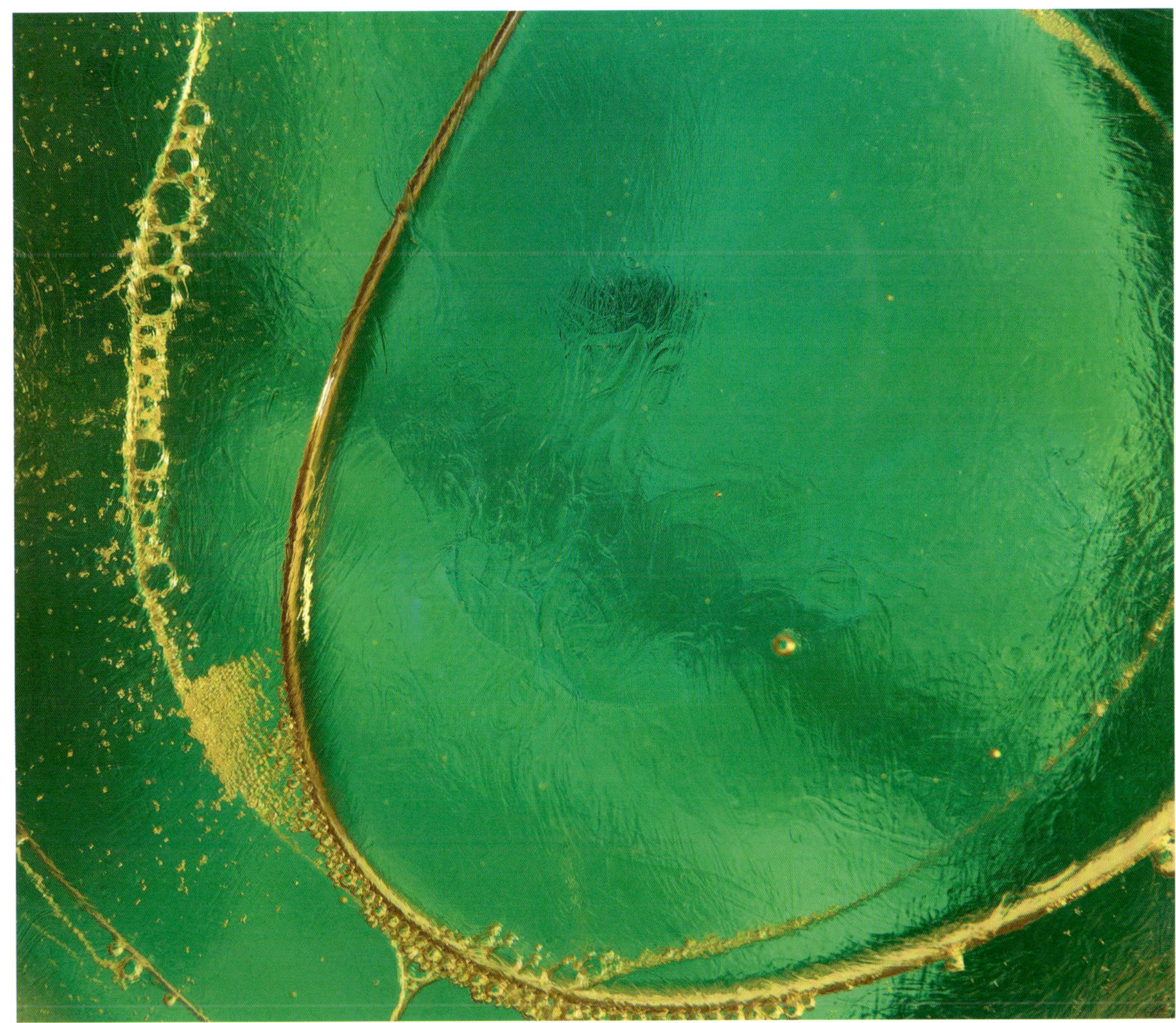

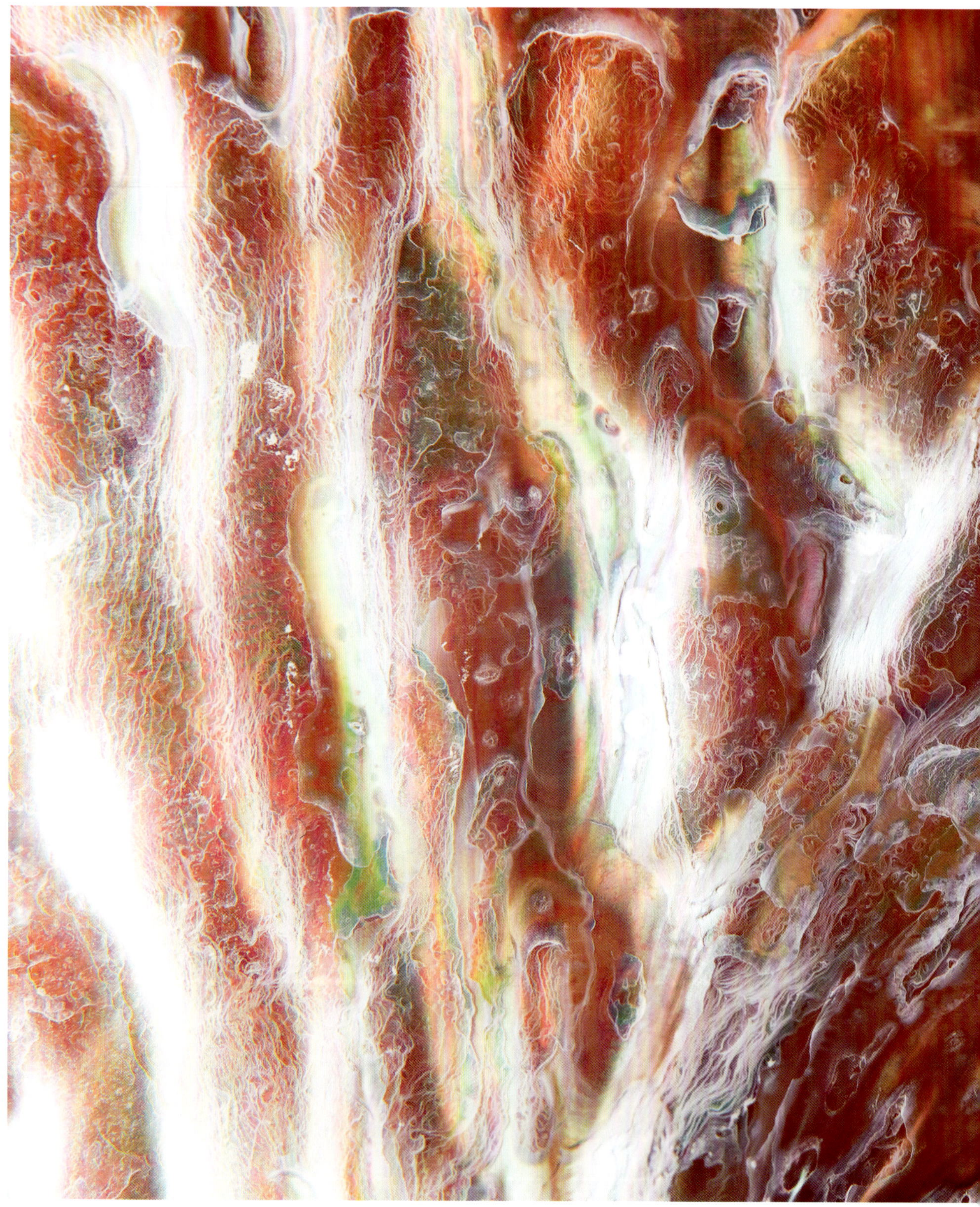

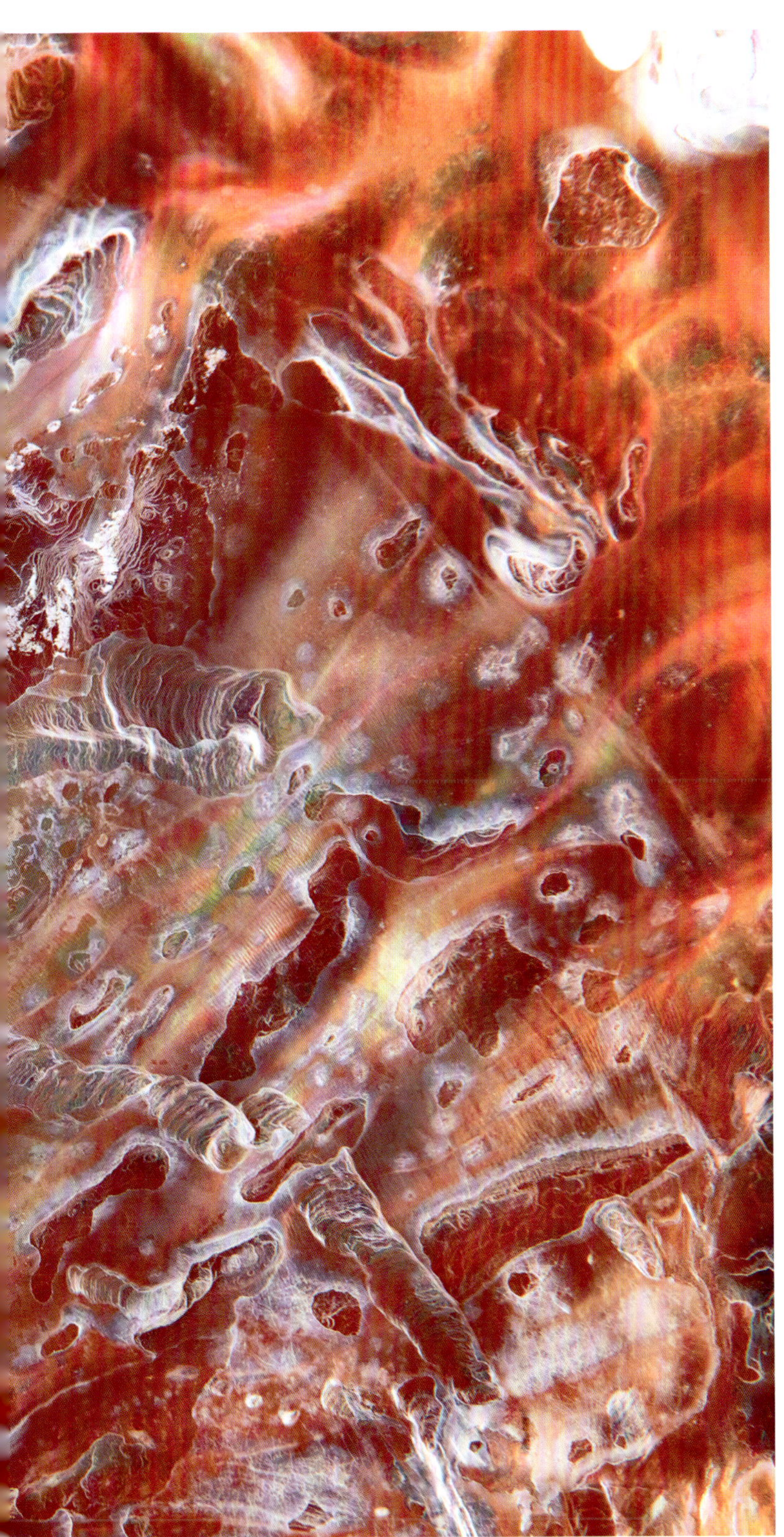

Misunderstood ingredients

In the world of skincare, some ingredients can be misunderstood or misrepresented, leading to confusion about their safety or effectiveness. This is largely due to how data is presented, often with certain studies being selectively highlighted to support specific claims. In this chapter, we'll explore a few ingredients that have been subject to such misunderstandings and discuss how considering the full body of research, and remembering that correlation does not equal causation, are crucial to developing a more accurate understanding.

Aluminum

Aluminum is one of the most common elements on Earth. It's found in our food, water, and even in some cosmetics. Aluminum salts are commonly used in antiperspirants to temporarily block sweat ducts, while aluminum oxide can be found in creams to thicken formulations, enhance color in lipsticks, and provide a gentle scrubbing action in toothpastes. Over the years, various studies have linked aluminum to certain health conditions, but it's important to remember that an association does not equate to causation. Public concerns over aluminum in cosmetics prompted the Scientific Committee on Consumer Safety (SCCS), an independent body of experts from different European Union (EU) countries, to assess the safety of aluminum in cosmetic products.

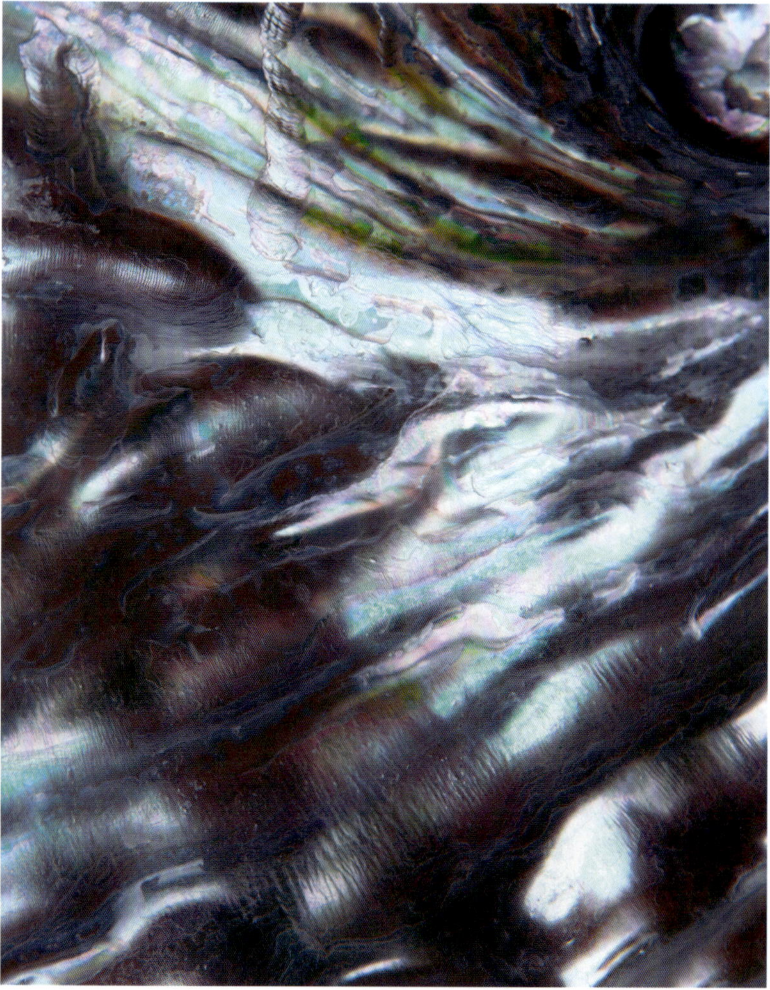

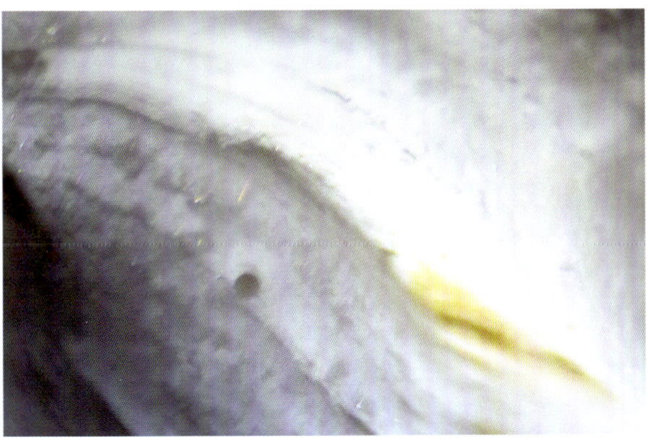

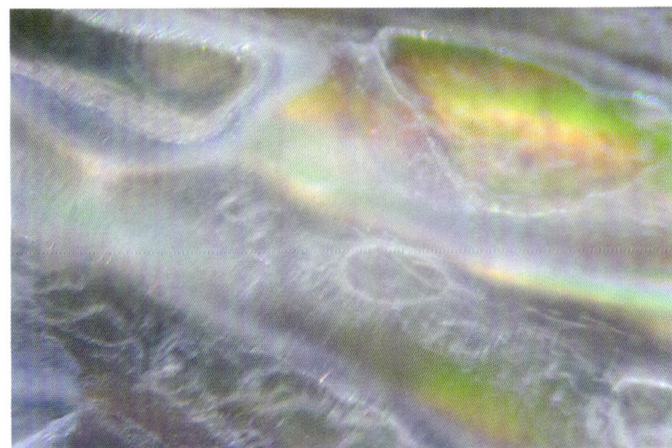

Since 2014, the SCCS has conducted four reviews on this topic, the most recent being in 2024, in which they reviewed data from tests evaluating potential aluminum exposure and its health impacts. These reviews took into account the aluminum content in cosmetic products, the amount used, frequency of use, and how aluminum might enter the body (through the skin or ingestion). Their conclusion: the current reported use of aluminum in cosmetic products produces exposures that are within the established safety limits, meaning that it is generally safe for use in cosmetics. However, as noted in their 2022 report, when considering all potential sources of aluminum exposure—cosmetics, food, and other products—it is possible that the cumulative exposure could exceed safe limits in certain high-exposure scenarios. Therefore, it's crucial to understand that, while individual products are within safe limits, the total exposure from all sources should be considered.

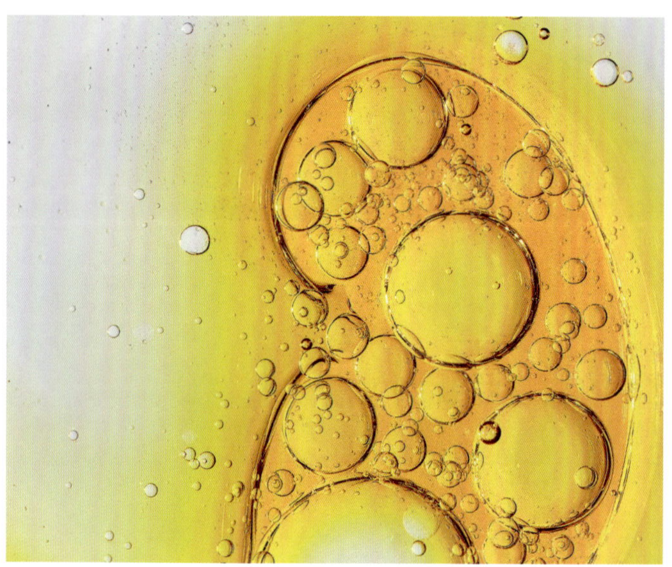

Palm oil

Palm oil is a widely used ingredient in skincare and cosmetics, valued for its versatility in creating smooth textures, enhancing product stability, and acting as a source for many commonly used emollients and surfactants. However, it has also been at the center of environmental and ethical concerns due to deforestation, habitat destruction, and labor issues associated with unsustainable palm oil production. As a result, some consumers perceive palm oil as inherently harmful and seek out "palm-free" products. But the issue is more complex—palm oil is one of the most land-efficient vegetable oils, meaning alternatives like soybean or coconut oil could require even more land and resources, potentially leading to greater environmental impact. The key concern is not palm oil itself but how it is sourced.

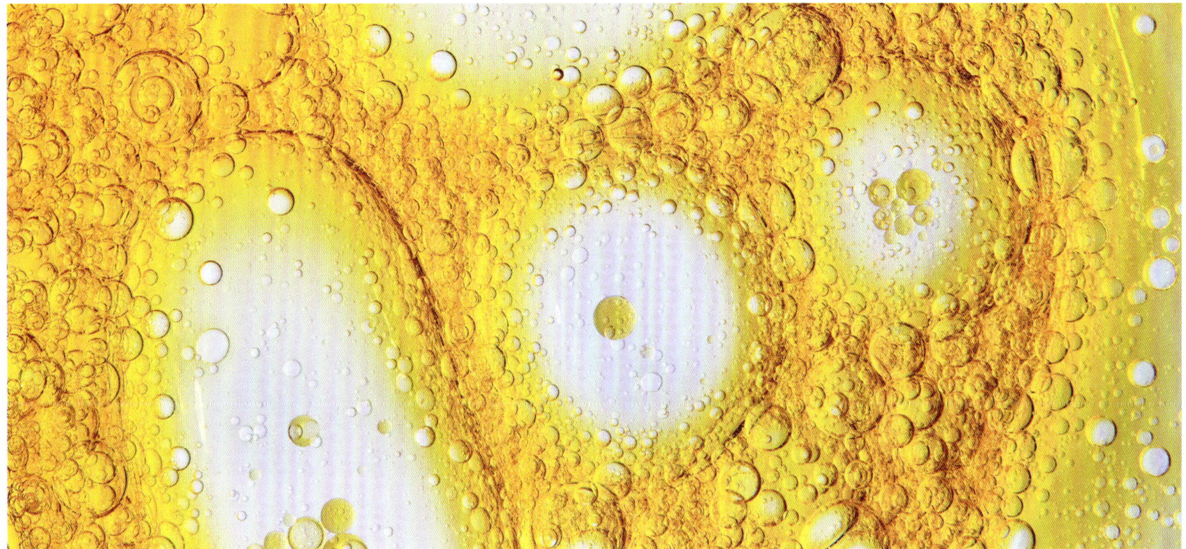

To address these concerns, efforts have been made to improve the sustainability of palm oil production. Organizations like the Roundtable on Sustainable Palm Oil (RSPO) set standards to ensure palm oil is grown and harvested with minimal environmental and social impact. Many cosmetic brands now commit to sourcing certified sustainable palm oil (CSPO) to support responsible practices while maintaining the ingredient's benefits in formulations. While progress continues, the conversation around palm oil highlights the importance of looking beyond a simple "good" or "bad" label and considering the broader context of sustainability, ethics, and supply chain transparency.

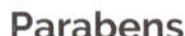

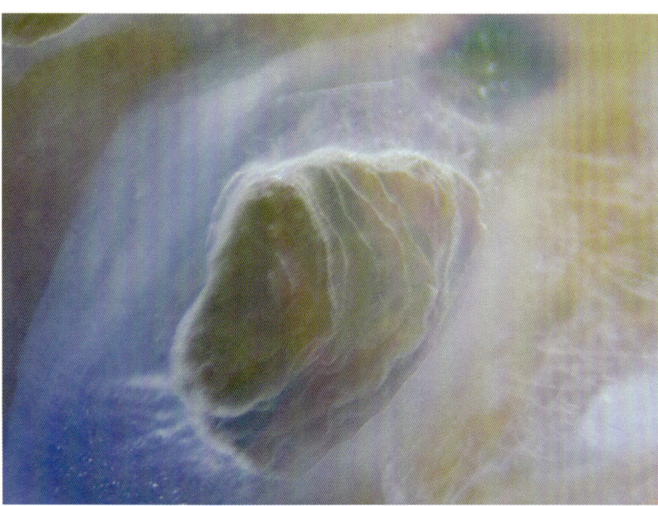

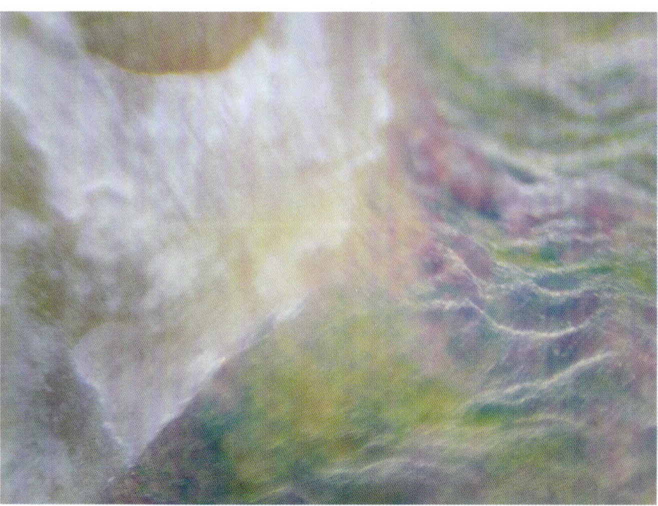

Parabens

Parabens are preservatives that help keep skincare products free from harmful bacteria and mold. The term "parabens" refers to a diverse category of compounds, and not all behave the same way within our bodies or the environment. Parabens occur naturally in some foods and plants, like blueberries, but are also synthetically produced for use in cosmetics. Concerns about parabens stem from their ability to mimic estrogen, leading to speculation about potential hormone disruption. However, global health authorities—including the U.S. Food and Drug Administration (FDA), the Cosmetic Ingredient Review (CIR), and the Scientific Committee on Consumer Safety (SCCS)—have reviewed the evidence multiple times since the 1980s. These reviews have resulted in certain parabens being banned from cosmetics, while more recent assessments confirm that the remaining parabens currently used in cosmetics are safe when used individually at low levels, not exceeding 0.8% of a formulation.

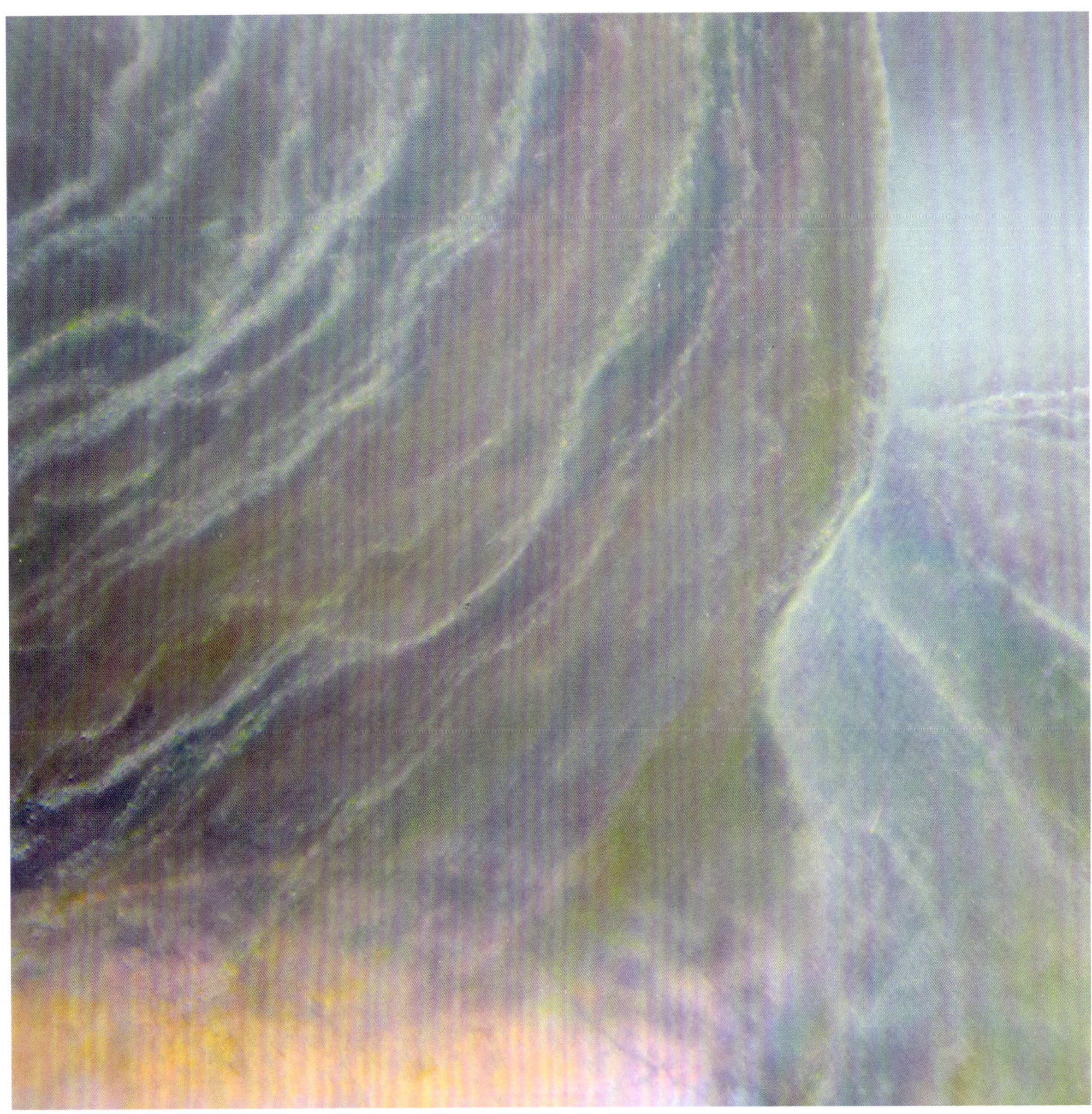

Parabens are also rapidly broken down and eliminated by the body, meaning they do not accumulate over time. Despite this, misinterpretation of data has led to a shift toward alternative preservatives, some of which may be less effective or more prone to microbial contamination. Given their long-standing use and extensive safety evaluations, parabens remain one of the most studied and reliable preservative options in skincare. They also highlight the ongoing work of regulatory and health authorities to ensure ingredient safety based on the most current data, and serve as an example of how, within a given chemical group, individual compounds can behave very differently—underscoring the need to avoid blanket statements about chemical categories.

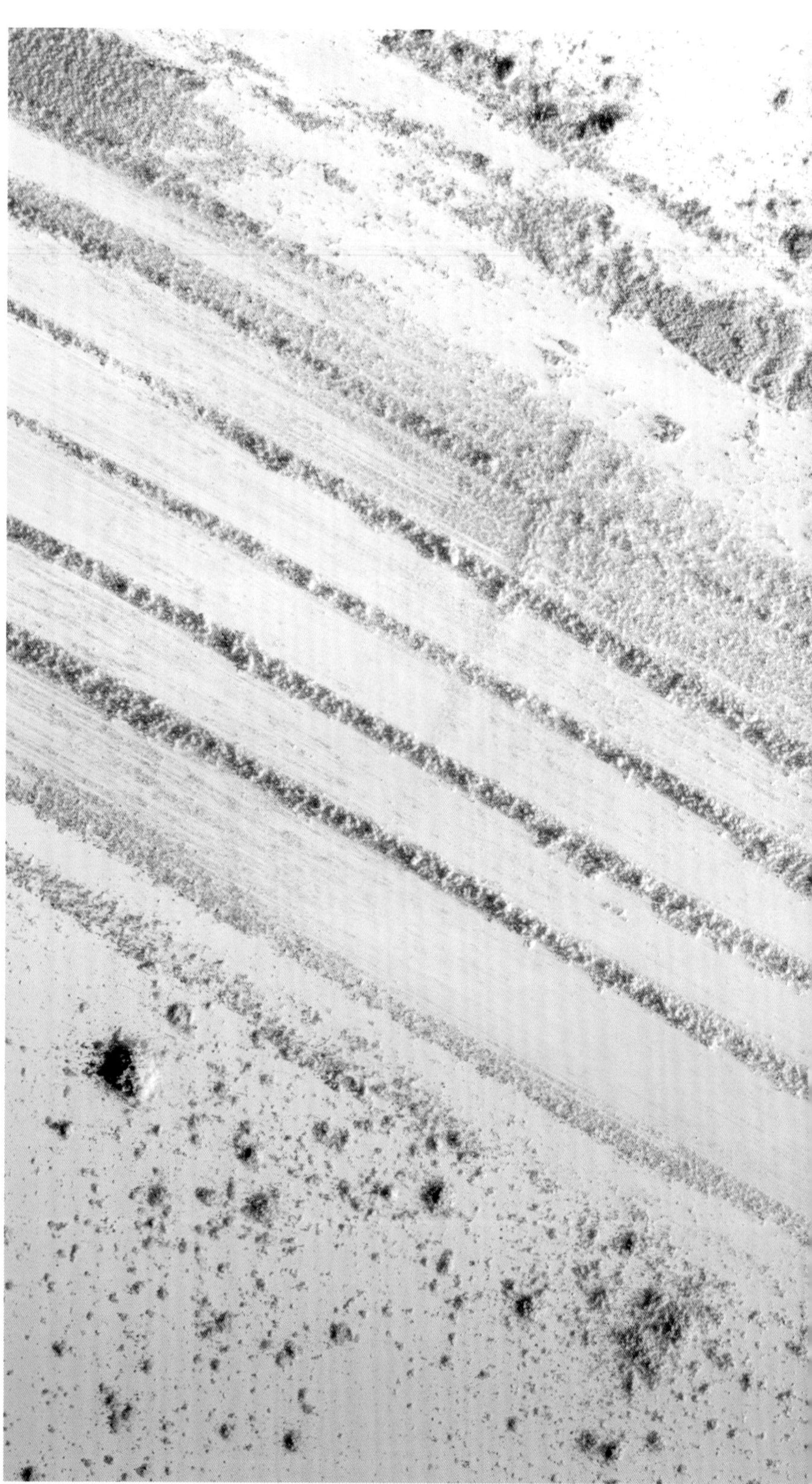

Sulfates

Sulfates are a group of cleansing agents, or surfactants, commonly found in shampoos, body washes, and facial cleansers. They are responsible for creating the rich, foamy lather that helps lift away dirt, oil, and impurities from the skin and hair. The most well-known sulfates, such as sodium lauryl sulfate (SLS) and sodium laureth sulfate (SLES), are highly effective at cleansing, but they have at times been unfairly labeled as harsh or harmful.

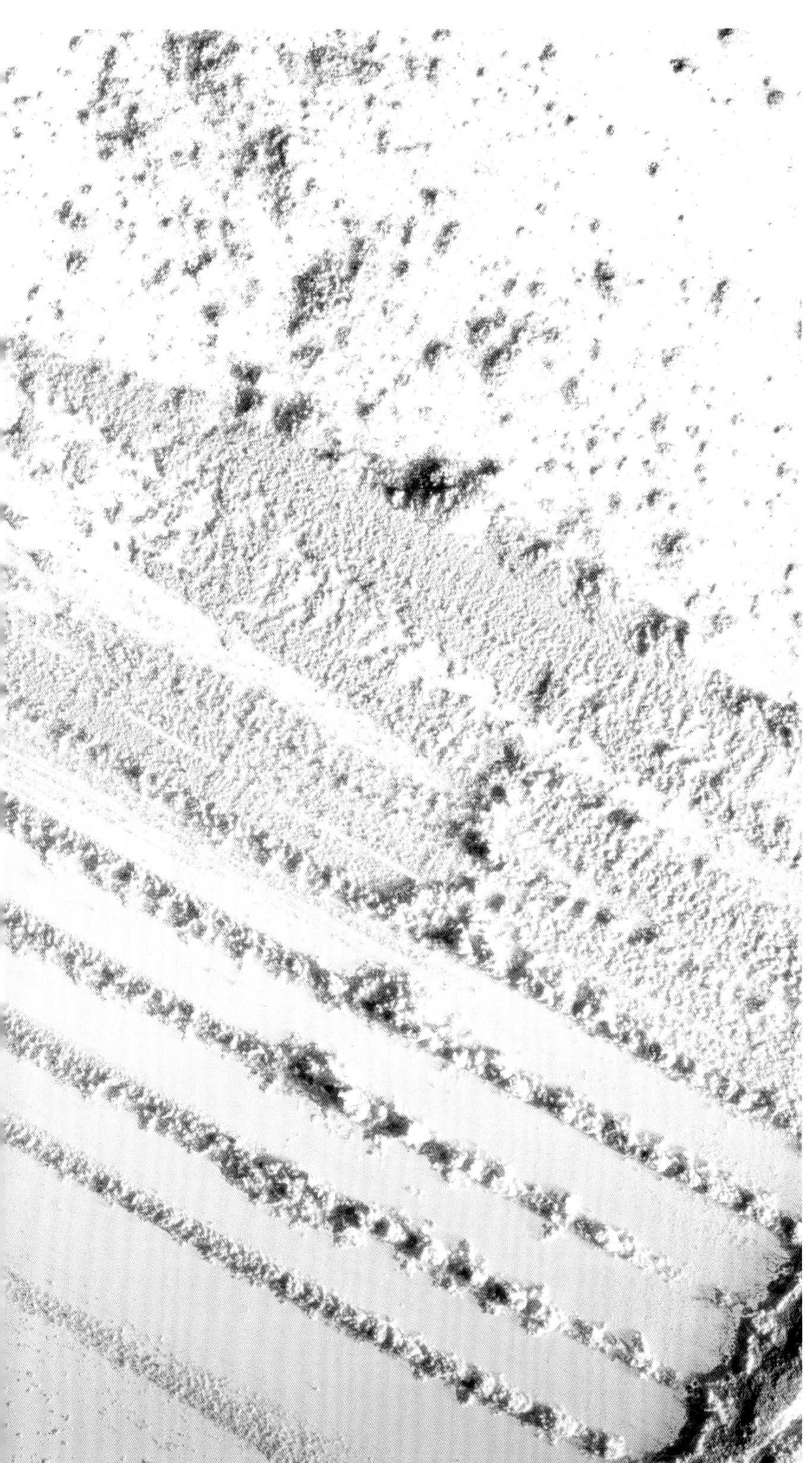

The concern around sulfates largely stems from their potential to strip too much natural oil from the skin or scalp, which can lead to dryness or irritation—particularly for those with a sensitivity to SLS and/or SLES. However, the concentration and formulation of sulfates in a product play a big role in how they interact with the skin. Most cosmetic formulas balance sulfates with gentler surfactants or moisturizing ingredients to minimize irritation. Additionally, most sulfate-containing products are designed to be rinsed off, meaning they have limited contact time with the skin, further reducing the potential for irritation. When used in well-formulated products, sulfates are safe and effective cleansing agents for many skin types.

UV filters

UV filters are the active ingredients in sunscreens that help protect the skin from the harmful effects of ultraviolet (UV) radiation. These filters come in two main types: chemical filters, like avobenzone and oxybenzone, and mineral filters, such as zinc oxide and titanium dioxide.

Mineral sunscreens are often associated with a white cast on the skin. This happens because the particles of these minerals are typically large and visible to the naked eye. To combat this issue, manufacturers have developed micronized or nanoparticle versions of these ingredients, which are smaller and less noticeable on the skin. However, this has led to concerns about the potential for these nanoparticles to penetrate the skin and enter the body. Some studies have suggested that nanoparticles could pass through the outer layer of the skin, but research so far has not shown any significant evidence of zinc oxide or titanium dioxide nanoparticles penetrating the skin and into the living skin cells more than their larger counterparts, deeply enough to reach living skin cells or affect the body. The current consensus from researchers and dermatologists is that mineral sunscreens, even with nanoparticles, are safe to use.

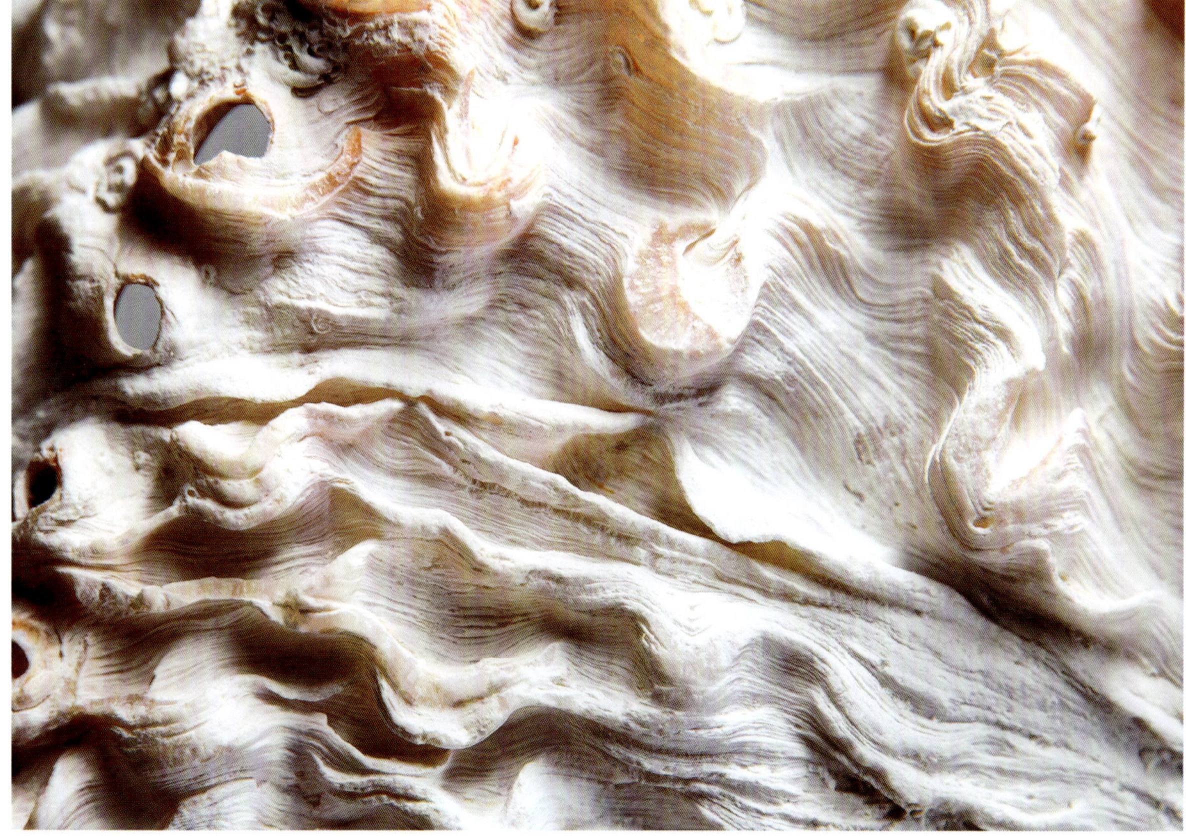

On the other hand, chemical sunscreens have raised concerns about their potential to be absorbed into the bloodstream. Studies have shown that some chemical filters can be detected in the blood after application, but these studies primarily involve higher-than-normal exposure and don't necessarily indicate that these ingredients pose a health risk. While these findings have sparked debate, more research and long-term studies are needed to fully assess the safety of these chemical filters and their absorption. Regardless of whether you choose a mineral or chemical sunscreen, the most important takeaway is that sunscreen remains a crucial part of protecting your skin from the harmful effects of UV radiation, which can lead to premature aging and increase the risk of skin cancer.

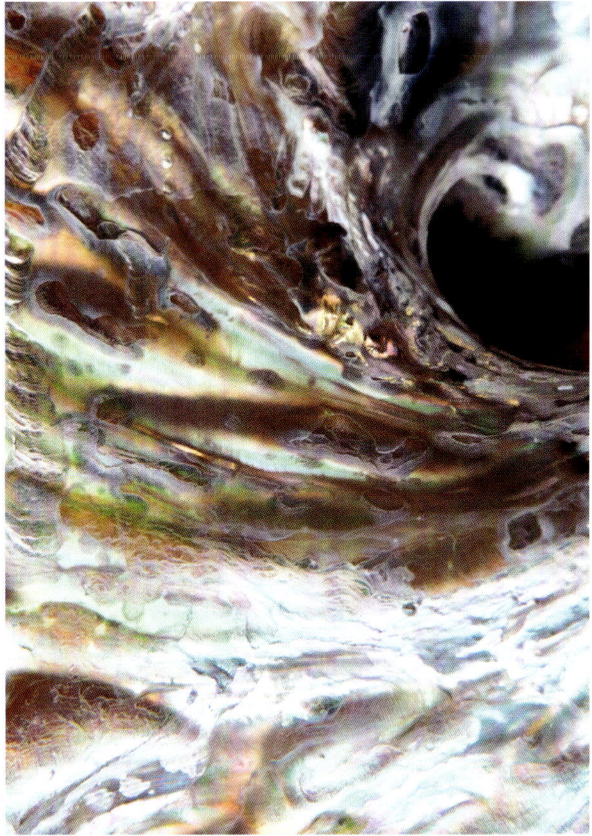

There have also been concerns about the potential impact of UV filters on the environment, particularly regarding the effect of sunscreen washing off and its possible influence on coral reefs. Some policies, like the ban on certain chemical filters in Hawaii, have been implemented based on these findings. While there is ongoing research into this topic, it's important to note that the methods used to assess this impact can vary, and other factors such as water temperature, salinity, and pH levels can also affect coral health. Additionally, the concentration of UV filters in the water is often not measured directly. Although these studies have contributed to the conversation, it's essential to consider other factors as well, such as rising ocean temperatures, which may have a more significant effect on coral reefs than sunscreen. Continued research is crucial to gaining a clearer understanding of the many factors influencing coral health and ensuring that environmental policies are based on comprehensive scientific evidence.

A quick word on what is "sustainable"

We often hear the term "sustainable" when it comes to cosmetics and other consumer product brands, but what does it truly mean? According to the UN, sustainability is "meeting the needs of the present without compromising the ability of future generations to meet their own needs." The reality is, a brand that sells consumer goods—whether skincare products or sneakers—can never claim to be entirely sustainable without fully clarifying what they mean, and without fully understanding what the needs of future generations will be. Ultimately, moving towards greater sustainability is an ongoing process that requires brands to evaluate the entire life cycle of each product.

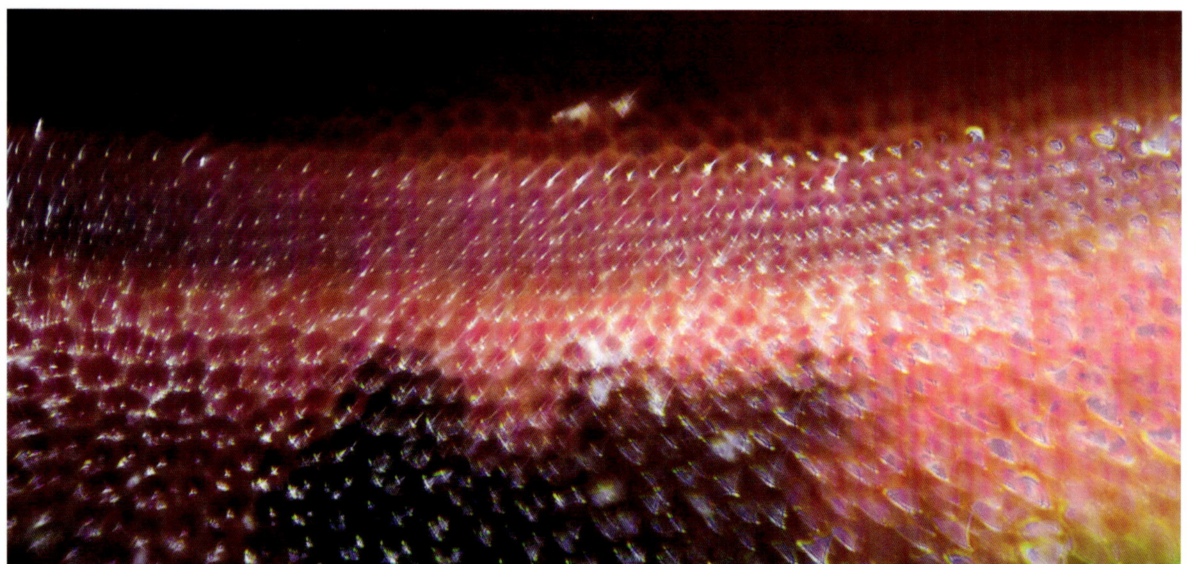

For consumers, the word "sustainable" can be confusing when used on a product. Without specificity from the brand about what exactly is meant by this word—whether it refers to the whole product, just one feature, or what evaluation the brand has conducted to substantiate this claim—it can be difficult to understand its true impact. This lack of transparency has even led advertising regulators to start restricting the word "sustainable" as a standalone claim, urging companies to provide direct evidence and specific detail to substantiate their statements. To truly make a positive impact, it's essential for brands to think strategically and use evidence-backed methods, such as peer-reviewed Life Cycle Assessments or approved testing methodologies and standards, to ensure their sustainability efforts deliver real environmental benefits.

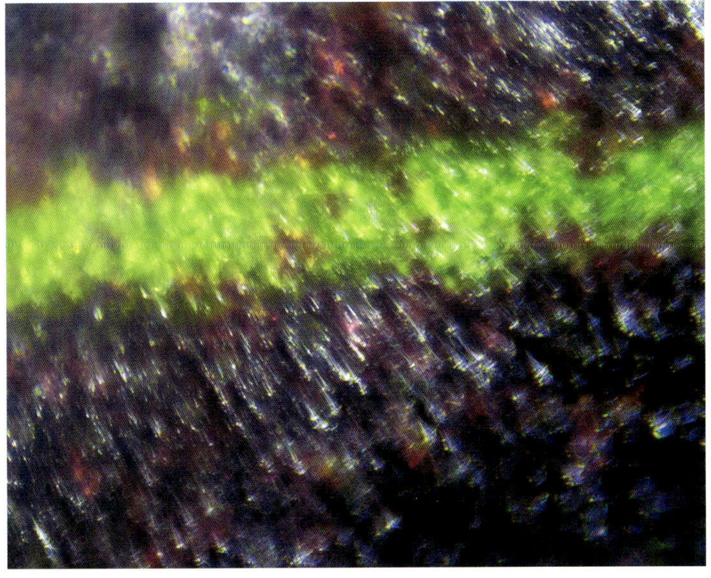

As you've likely seen, the skincare industry—and understanding the controversies within it—can be more complex than it initially appears. However, it's important to remember that skincare is based on science—driven by data and evidence, not personal opinion or hearsay. It's not about one individual's perspective or the findings of a single study, but about the conclusions we draw from multiple, well-conducted studies and continued inquiry. And that shouldn't be controversial.

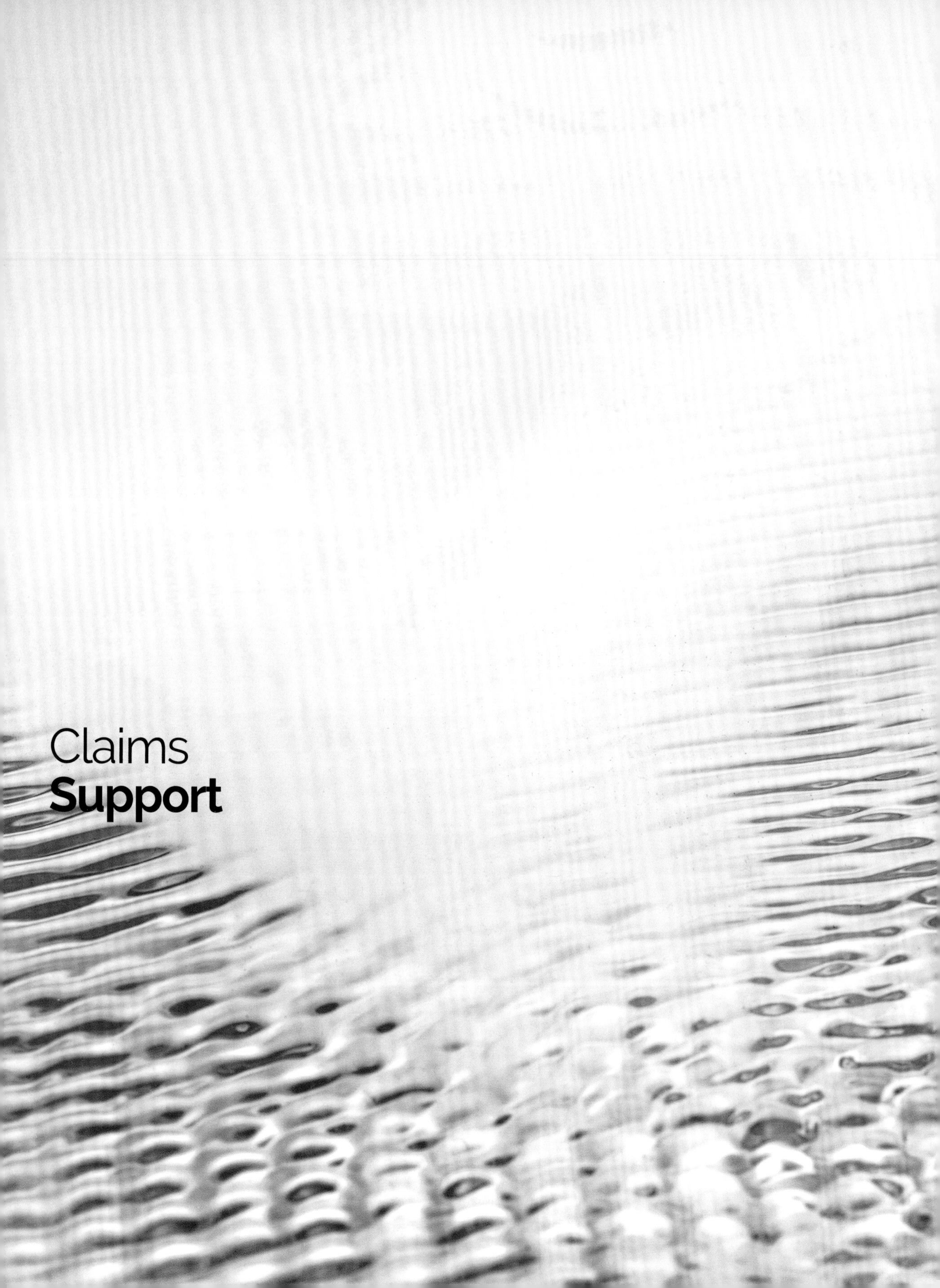

Claims **Support**

Claims Support

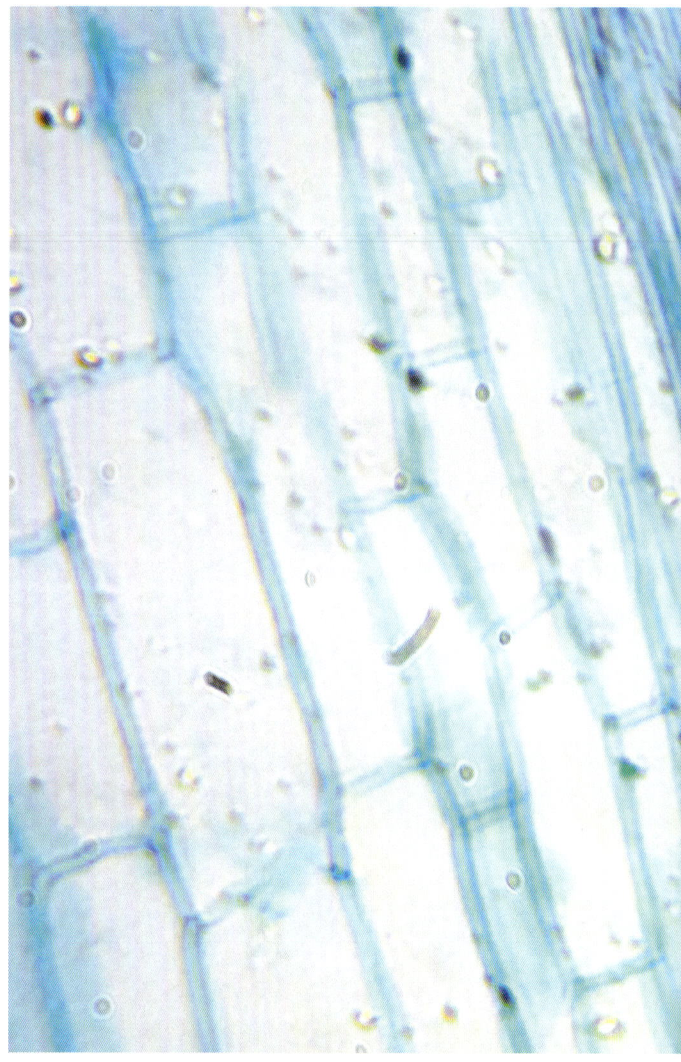

Prove it

When you're looking to buy a new skincare product, there are many factors that might help you make your decision. You might be looking for a specific active ingredient, such as retinol, or a type of product, such as a moisturizer. But you might also be tempted by the benefits touted on the label: that the product won't clog pores—indicated by the term non-comedogenic—that it may reduce the appearance of fine lines, or will make dry skin feel more hydrated. Information like this can help you decide if the product might be suitable for your needs.

All of these statements are known as claims and, as such, must be substantiated by some form of evaluation process for the company to verify that the product performs as advertised.

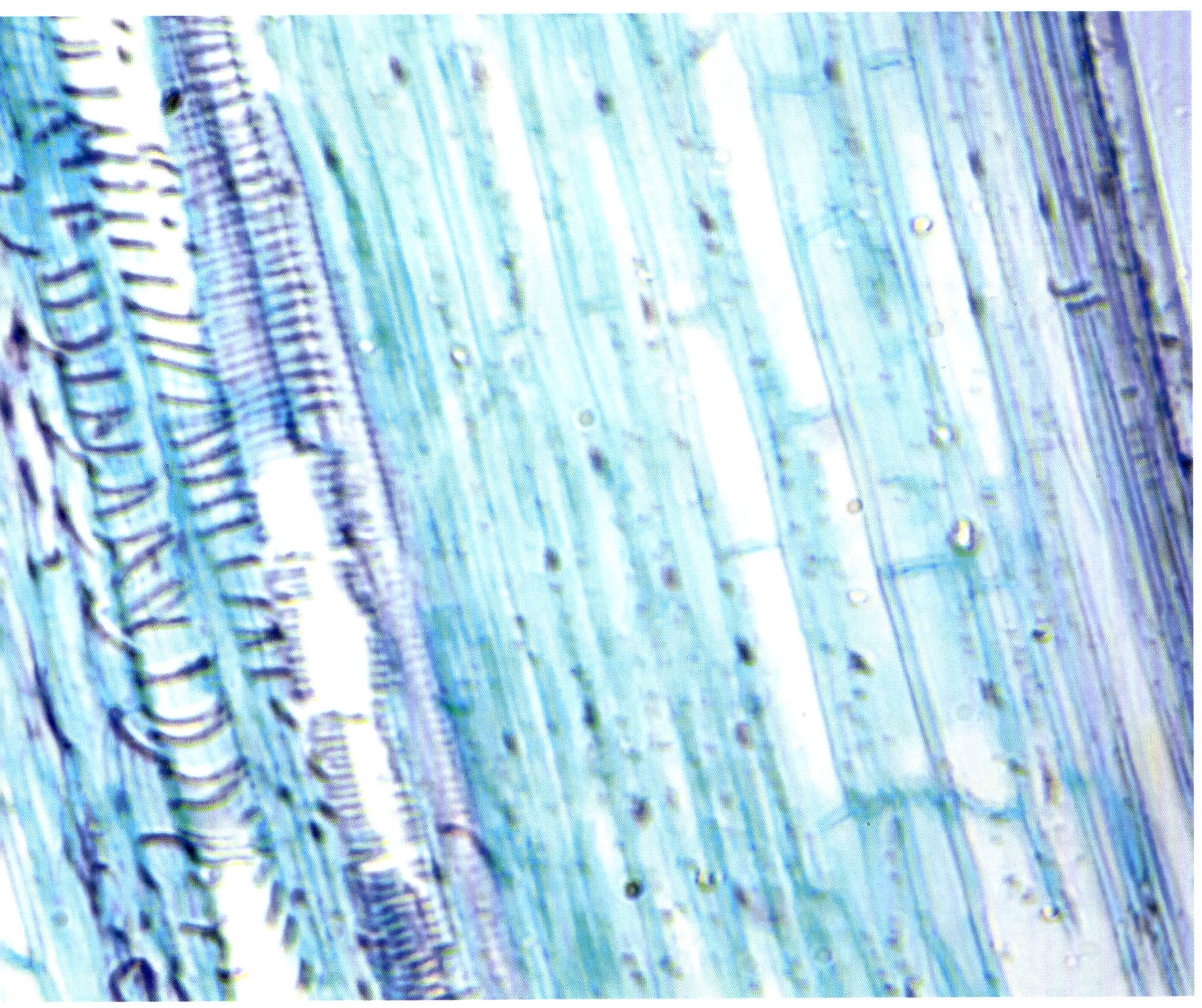

Evaluating: Safety vs suitability

As we've established, when developing a cosmetic product, a series of mandatory evaluations must be performed before it can be sold (see the section "From brainwave to bottle" in Chapter 2). These evaluations ensure that the product complies with global regulatory requirements, is safe for use, and remains stable throughout its expected shelf life. This process may include assessing the safety of the product through regulatory and literature evaluations as well as tests on cell cultures (in vitro), on skin samples (ex vivo), and eventually on human volunteers (in vivo).

Beyond ensuring safety and compliance, these tests can also be used to substantiate claims about the product's performance.

In vitro/ex vivo tests

In vitro and ex vivo tests are conducted on isolated cells or excised skin samples, and can be used to measure a variety of things, including ingredient and formula penetration, antioxidant efficacy, and soothing and hydrating properties.

This type of testing is often done at an ingredient level to evaluate the safety and efficacy of an ingredient at various concentrations. The amount of an ingredient that a formulator ultimately decides to use takes into consideration a number of factors, including safety and efficacy data, assessment of the ingredient supplier's data, published scientific literature, prior formulation samples and products, and the safe limits dictated by regulatory bodies that were mentioned in the previous chapter.

Ingredient tests can result in qualitative claims such as "helps reduce the appearance of pores"—which suppliers will often use to sell an ingredient to a formulator. However, these isolated results should not be used to make claims about the final product. Instead, tests on the complete formula should be carried out to establish both qualitative and quantitative claims, and confirm that the benefits of the individual ingredients—previously demonstrated in isolation—will translate to the consumer when used as directed in the final product.

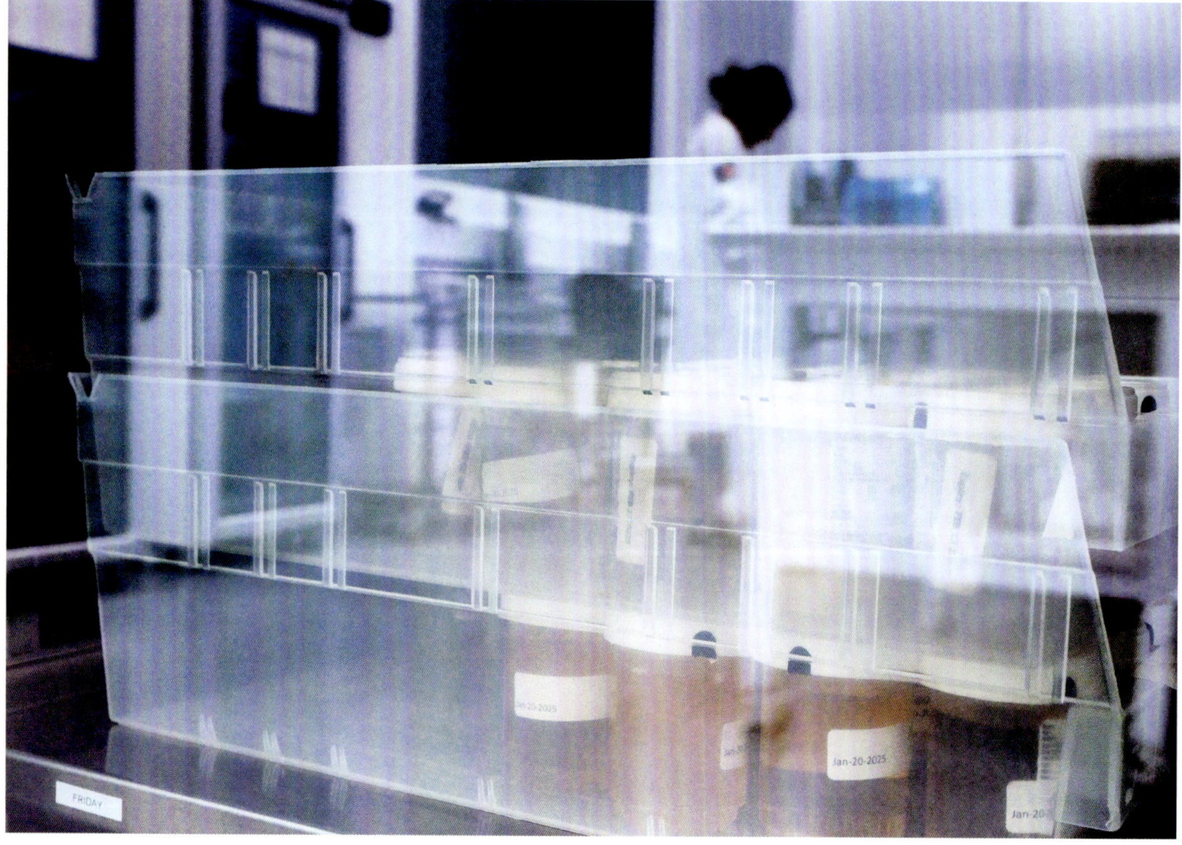

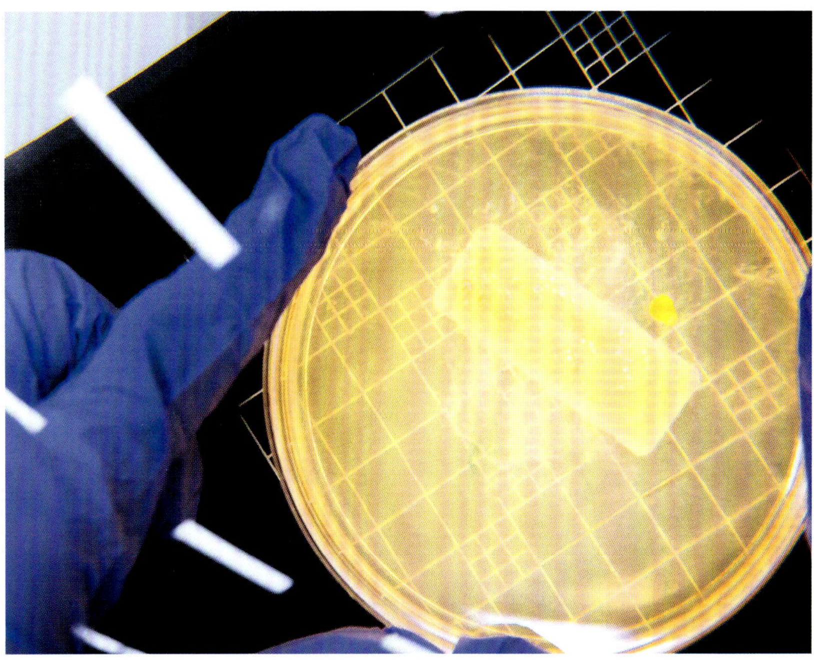

In vivo tests

This is the name given to tests carried out on human volunteers—and ideally on human volunteers with a wide range of skin tones, so that it can be demonstrated that the product is safe and effective for all phototypes.

(As an aside, if you come across claims that a product was "not tested on animals," it's worth taking them with a pinch of salt. In most of the world, animal testing for beauty products is banned, meaning that this is an industry-wide requirement rather than a unique claim that brands can opt to make.)

In vivo tests can be separated into two main types:

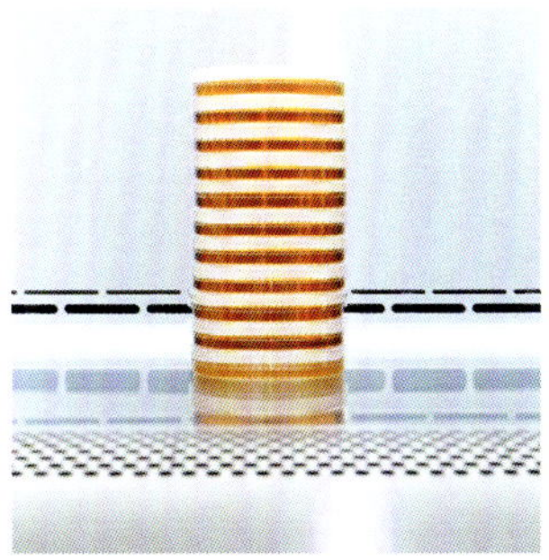

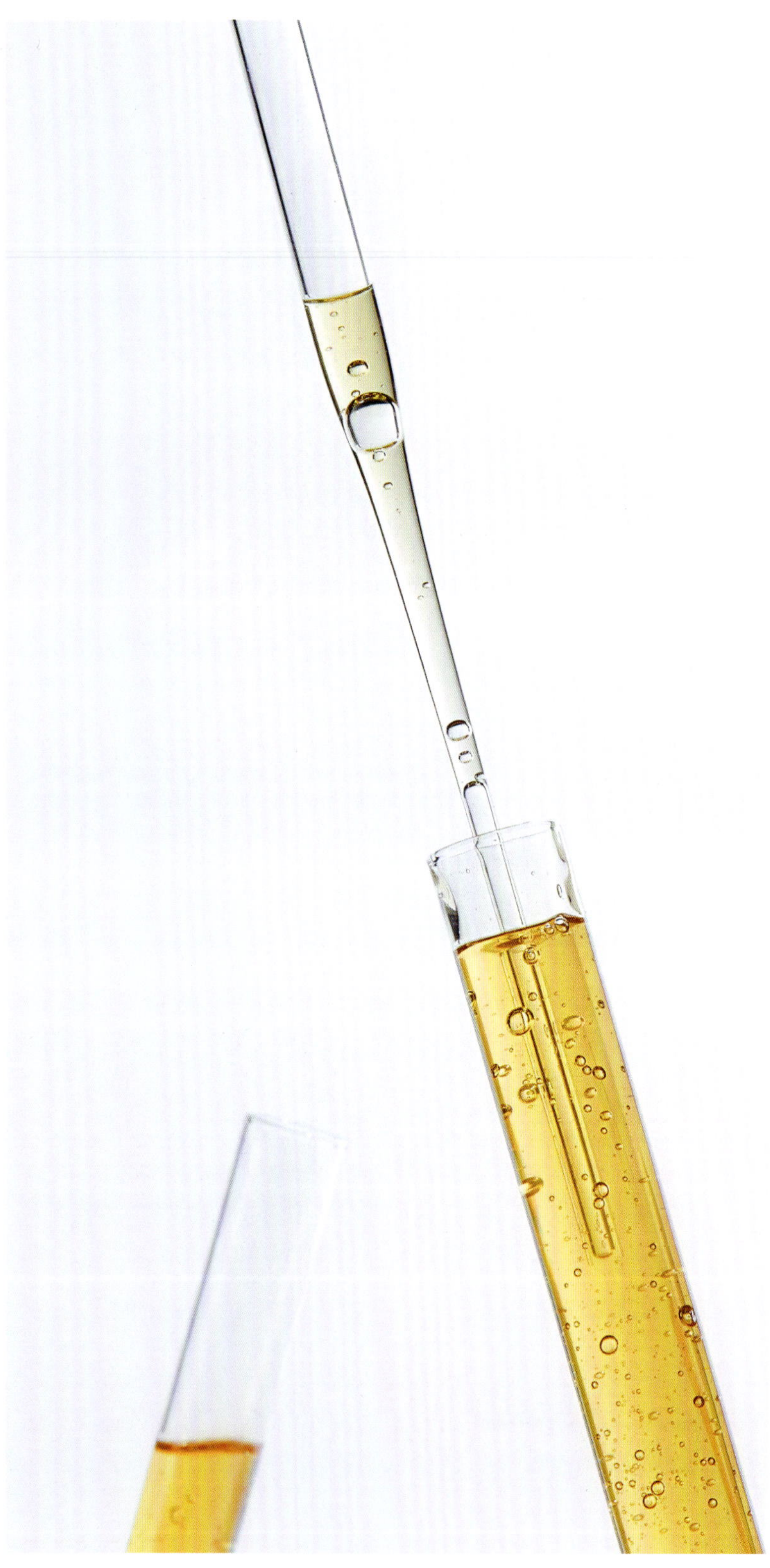

Safety testing

A number of different tests can be conducted to ensure a product is suitable for its intended use. One example is a Safety In Use (SIU) study, where the product is used as intended on a range of different skin types over a period of two to four weeks, with a dermatologist assessing key safety endpoints. Another might be Human Repeat Insult Patch Testing (HRIPT), where the product is repeatedly applied to the skin to check if it causes irritation or sensitivity. Tests that look at whether products irritate the eye, or block pores, can also be carried out.

Some of the claims that can be made based on these tests include: "Suitable for sensitive skin," "Hypoallergenic," "Non-comedogenic," and "Ophthalmologically tested."

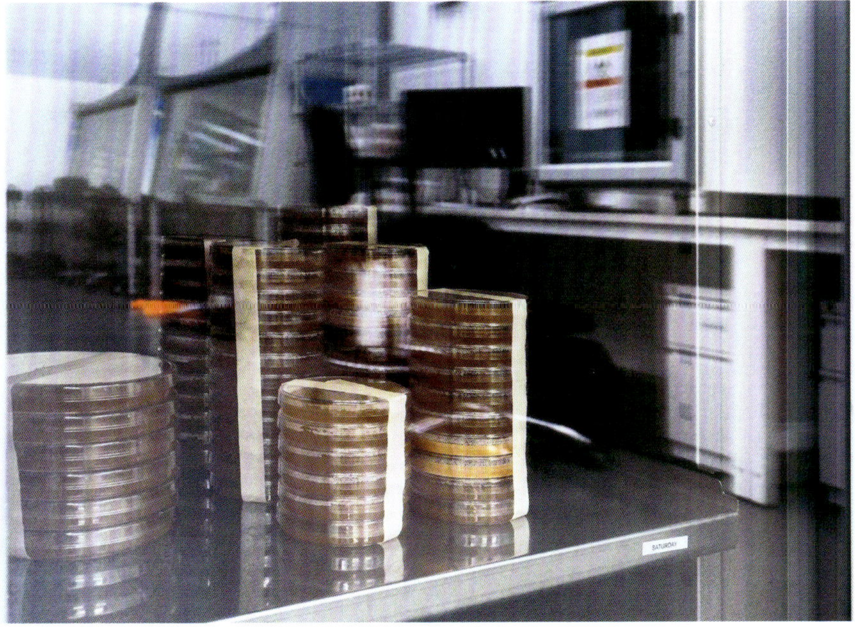

Efficacy testing

A product's efficacy can be assessed in two ways: expert grading or instrumental testing, which objectively measure results, and consumer perception testing (or sensory testing), where users evaluate their own experience of using the product. In both cases, a panel of participants—ideally large enough to generate statistically meaningful conclusions—use a specified amount of the product as part of their routine over a defined period.

Expert grading or instrumental testing studies aim to show clinical relevance and quantify certain changes on the skin surface over time. Devices can be used at intervals to check a variety of properties, such as hydration, the rate at which the skin loses water, skin elasticity, and firmness. Cameras and 3D imaging can also be used to look at changes to the skin topography (or relief) such as fine lines and wrinkles, and changes in the evenness of skin tone over time.

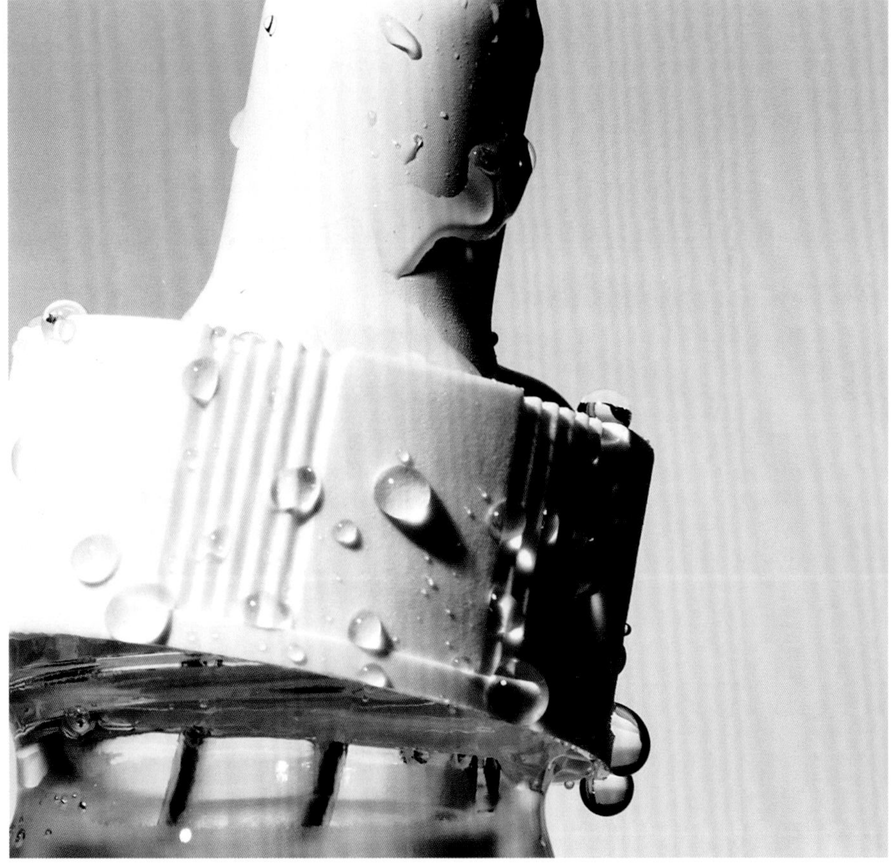

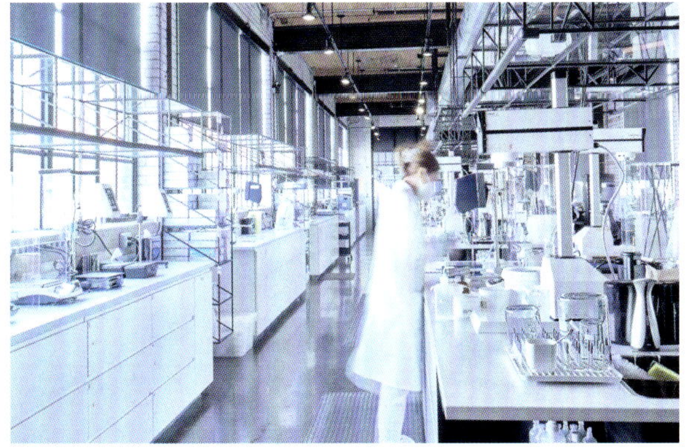

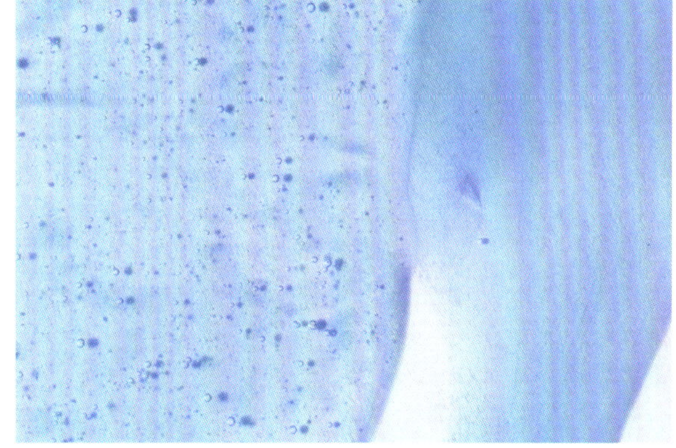

Expert graders, who have been specifically trained in using grading scales to identify changes on the skin, assess clinically relevant changes such as brightness, suppleness, softness, intensity of fine lines and wrinkles, and radiance. Tests like these allow brands to make claims such as "Increases skin hydration by 65% in 1 hour" or "improvement in the appearance of wrinkles after 4 weeks."

While these types of studies demonstrate objectively that a product is effective, sensory and/or consumer studies are also important—after all, there's no point proving something works unless consumers can also see or feel a difference for themselves. In these studies, the results are based on panelists' self-assessment through a questionnaire or interview that participants complete. Claims that might be made as a result of consumer perception studies include statements such as "92% agree their skin felt more hydrated after 1 hour."

Brands might also use before and after images that show participants before starting to use the product and after using it for a specific period of time. Best practice when using images like this is for the pictures to be taken in a controlled setting so that the lighting and the angles are the same, and for any images that are used to be representative of the average result, not a best-case scenario. Similarly, in an ideal world, all efficacy testing should be carried out by a third party to make sure it is objective and independent.

The classification of cosmetics

The claims that companies are allowed to make about their products—and the regulations around those products—vary according to how the product is classified. When the legal category of cosmetics was first developed, it referred to products that would clean, fragrance, maintain, or change the appearance of skin or hair, in contrast to drugs that are intended to diagnose, treat, or prevent a disease or medical condition.

This means cosmetic brands cannot make claims that suggest their products alter the body's structure or function. Doing so would imply that the product falls outside the definition of a cosmetic and should instead be regulated like a drug.

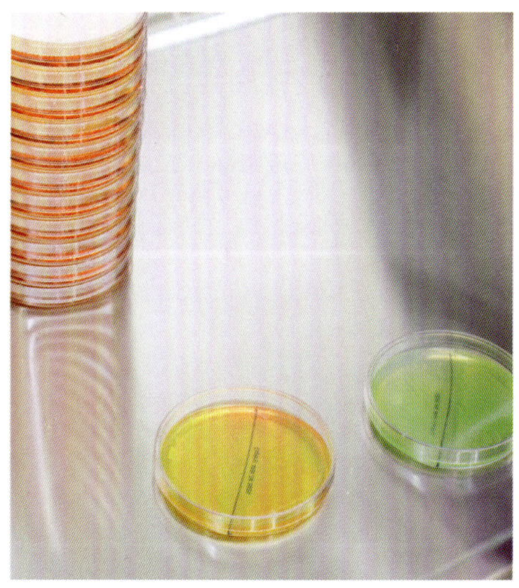

The table below shows the difference between the sort of claims that can be made for cosmetic skincare products, and for drugs that have been licensed for use on the skin.

Cosmetic claims

+	Soothe and calms	Improves the look of uneven skin tone	Suitable for blemish-prone skin

Drug claims

+	Anti-inflammatory	Treats pigmentation	For combating acne

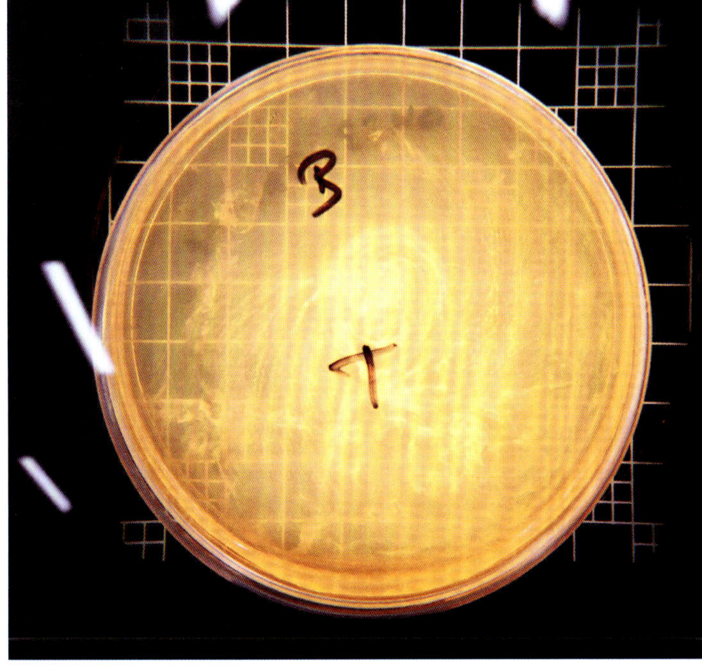

Regulations and terminology regarding drugs differ around the world and so you might find that products that are classified as cosmetics in one territory are classified as Over The Counter (OTC) or prescription drugs somewhere else. For example, in Canada and the United States, products such as sunscreen, dandruff shampoo, and deodorant may be considered drugs, while in the UK and Europe they are regulated as cosmetics.

You may also come across the word "cosmeceutical" used to describe certain products, but this is not a legally recognized term. Instead, it's typically used as an unregulated marketing term to imply that a product is somehow superior, stronger, or more efficacious than other products. However, anything labeled as a "cosmeceutical" is still classified as a "cosmetic" under regulatory standards, and it does not follow any stricter regulations beyond those applied to standard cosmetics.

Testing constraints

There are various limitations that can impact product testing and, in a perfect world, cosmetic companies would be able to work around them, but that's not always possible. Factors that might intervene include:

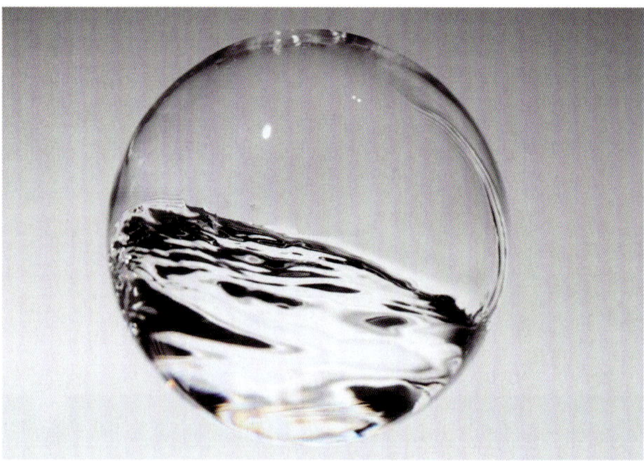

Cost

Conducting the required tests for cosmetics is expensive, and costs are only going up. This is due to changing regulatory rules, the need for a variety of test groups, and advancements in testing tech that make trials longer and pricier. All of this adds up, especially when you consider the product's price and target market size.

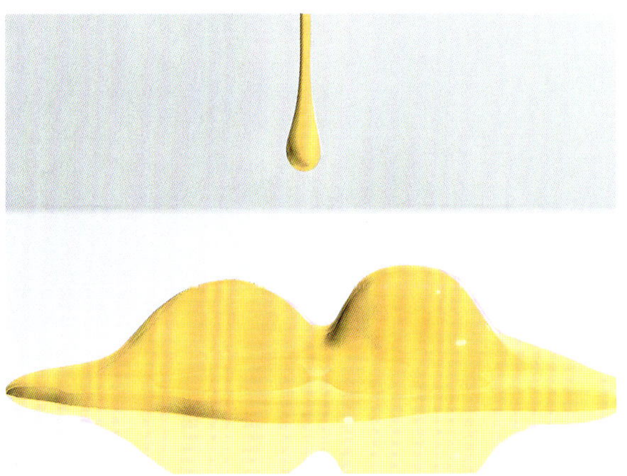

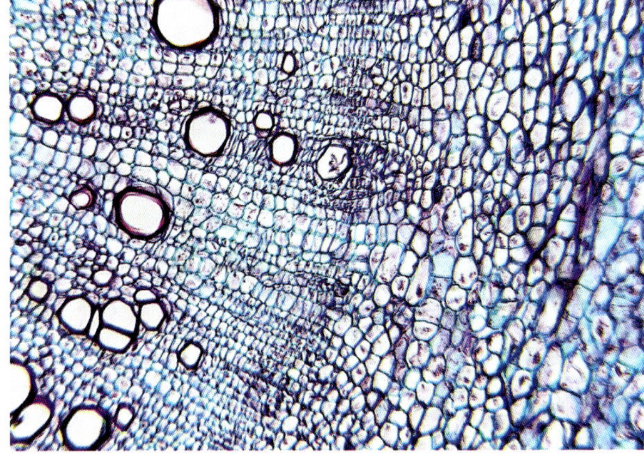

Time

Testing products takes time, and, if commercial launch dates for a product have been pre-defined, this might cut down the amount of time available for testing. This, in turn, can have an impact on the types of testing that a product can be subjected to, and the study length.

Time of year and geographical location

Volunteers who participate in cosmetic testing don't live in a science lab—they're out in the real world, which means weather and geographical location can significantly impact test results, or even determine when and where testing can take place. For example, if you want to show that a moisturizer helps improve hydration, testing in the humid summer heat may not provide accurate results since the air is already filled with moisture. With the effects of global warming, extreme weather patterns are becoming more unpredictable, and this can further complicate testing conditions and locations, and thus increase the competition for testing slots. Rising temperatures, intense heatwaves, or unexpected cold snaps may limit when and where certain tests can be carried out, affecting both the logistics and the reliability of the results.

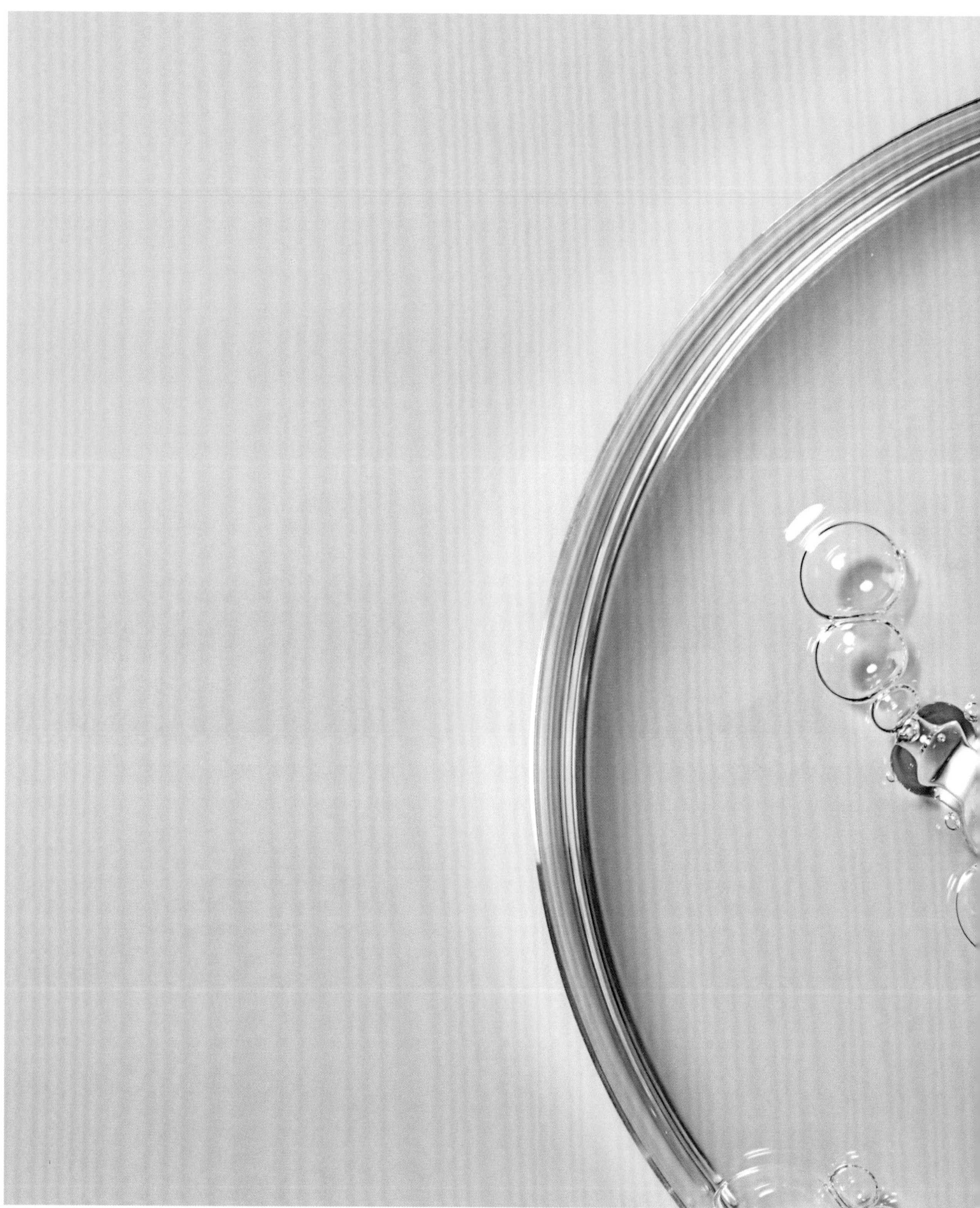

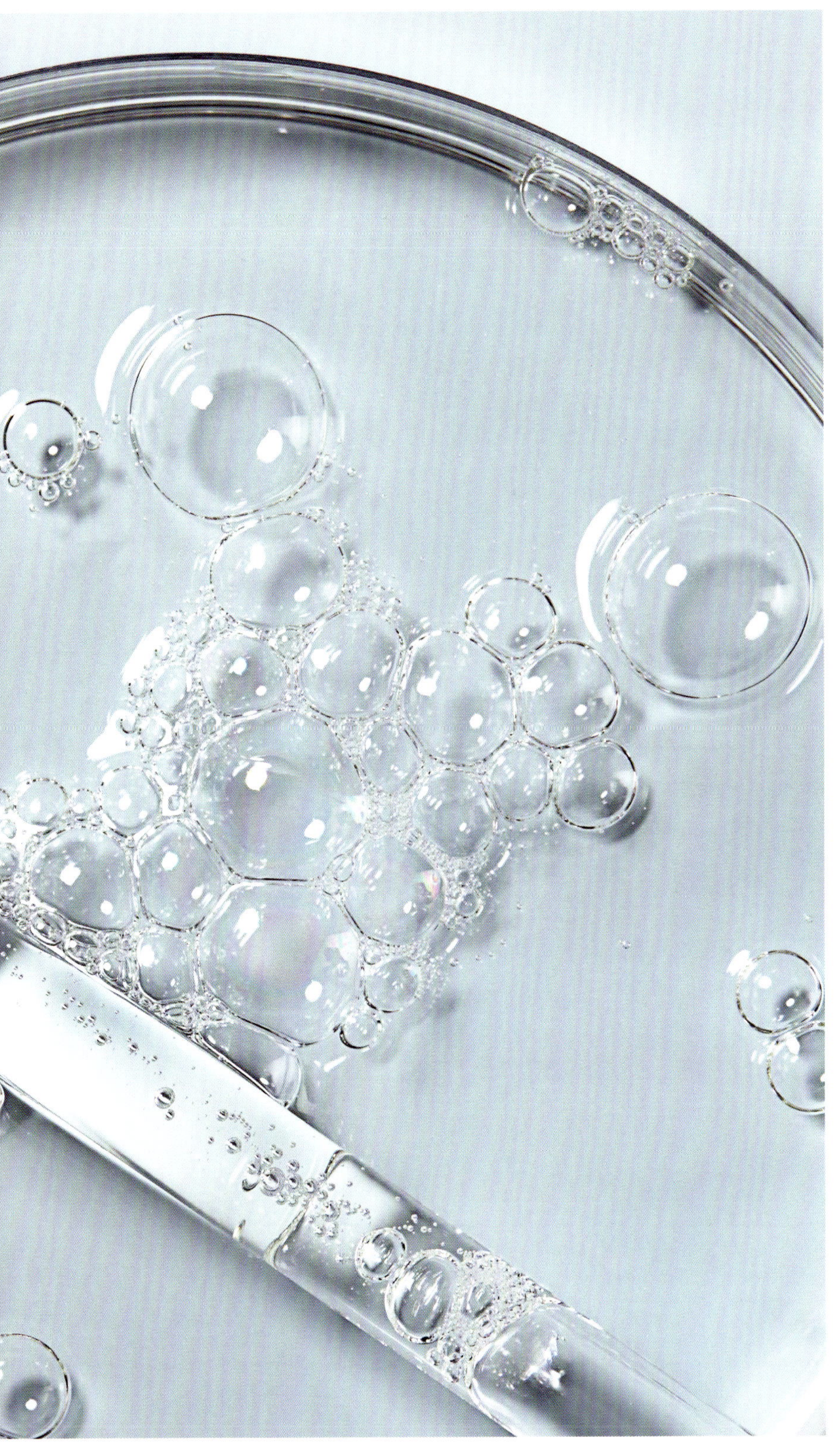

Availability of volunteers

Recruiting a diverse group of participants with the right skin type and ensuring diversity across the panels for one study isn't always easy. As skincare products become more complex, it can be challenging to find subjects who have multiple skin concerns, such as a certain degree of wrinkles, dark spots, and blemishes. This need for a broader range of participants can increase the size of testing panels and, consequently, the overall cost of the study.

So, the next time you see an advert for a new skincare product or are drawn to claims on a label, hopefully you'll have a deeper understanding of the research and considerations that go into validating those claims behind the scenes.

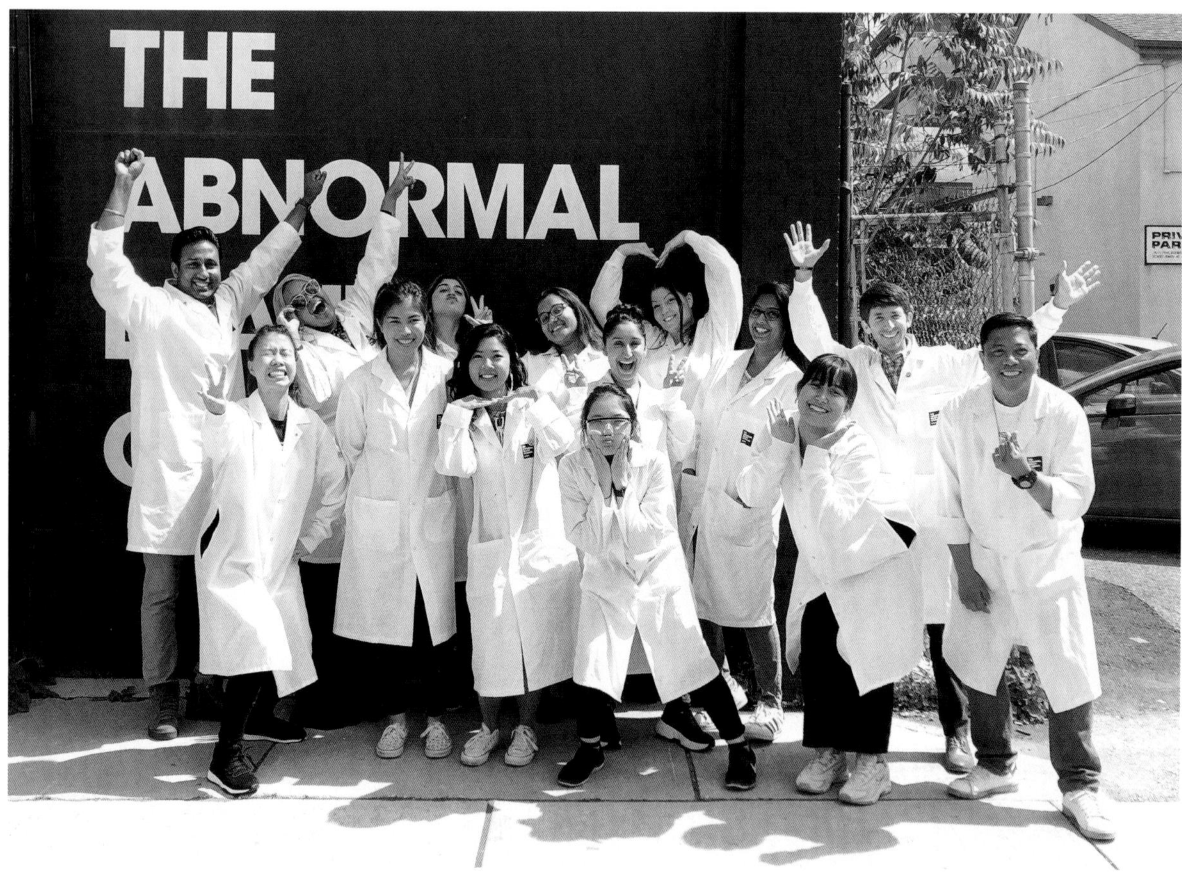

Acknowledgements

DECIEM is home to over 1,400 humans across a vertically integrated structure. Thank you to our incredible teams who have brought this book to life.

To the DECIEM Scientific team who have authored this piece of work—you inspire us daily. To Dina Nicola, Deborah Creatura, Joe Basham, Rita Silva, Bushra Yusuf, and Nafisah Abdalla, who have shared their passion for science, honesty, and integrity through these pages, thank you.

We are grateful to Silvia Stanica for her tireless commitment and exceptional scientific partnership on this project.

Thank you to Angela Bitonti and Heather Leslie for keeping us out of trouble.

This book would be nothing without the brilliant creativity of Esther Rodas, whose creative direction has brought science to life through these pages.

A thank you to Yuliia Matvieieva, Jerome Clark, Liz Brand, Reza Lor, Lucy Brook, Brandon Titaro, Dani Reynolds and Amy Bi for your enthusiasm in supporting (yet another) wild creative endeavor.

We would like to express our deepest gratitude to Claire Coleman. A friend of DECIEM's since the early days, Claire's partnership in bringing these words to life will always be cherished.

To Dakota Kate Isaacs, DECIEM's cheerleader, whose vision and tenacity ensured this book became reality.

A special thanks to Elizabeth Bond and Fionn Hargreaves at Penguin Random House for believing in this project and championing it tirelessly.

To our fearless leader, Jesper Rasmussen, for trusting us to make a book instead of a bottle.

To Brandon Truaxe, Nicola Kilner, Prudvi Kaka, and Dionne Lois Cullen, you changed an industry and each of our lives.

Finally, thank you to the readers. For it is you, after all, who we will always work for.

Index

First published in the United States of America in 2025 by
Rizzoli International Publications, Inc.
49 West 27th Street
New York, NY 10001
rizzoliusa.com

Originally published in Great Britain in 2025 by
Ebury Press, an imprint of Penguin Random House UK
penguin.co.uk / global.penguinrandomhouse.com

For Rizzoli
Publisher: Charles Miers
Editor: Klaus Kirschbaum
Assistant Editor: Emily Ligniti
Managing Editor: Lynn Scrabis

For Ebury Press
Publishing Director: Elizabeth Bond
Project Editor: Fionn Hargreaves
Production Controller: Percie Bridgwater
Writers: Claire Coleman, Silvia Stanica, Deborah Creatura, Joe Basham, Rita Silva, Bushra Yusuf, Nafisah Abdalla, and Dakota Isaacs.
Art Director: Esther Rodas
Designer: Yuliia Matvieieva
Typesetter: maru studio G.K.
Photography: Jerome Clark, Liz Brand, Reza Lor, Hassan Mohamed, Edward Yang, and Brandon Titaro

ISBN: 978-0-8478-7604-4
Library of Congress Control Number: 2025935187
2025 2026 2027 / 10 9 8 7 6 5 4 3 2 1

Colour Origination: Altaimage Ltd
Printed in China

The authorized representative in the EU for product safety and compliance is Mondadori Libri S.p.A., via Gian Battista Vico 42, Milan, Italy, 20123
mondadori.it

Visit us online
Instagram.com/RizzoliBooks
Facebook.com/RizzoliNewYork
Youtube.com/user/RizzoliNY